So you think you know

What's Good
For You?

Dr NORMAN SWAN

So you think you know
What's Good
For You?

ASTER*

Originally published by Hachette Australia (an imprint of Hachette Australia Pty Limited)
Level 17, 207 Kent Street
Sydney NSW 2000
www.hachette.com.au

First published in Great Britain in 2022 by Aster, an imprint of Octopus Publishing Group Ltd
Carmelite House
50 Victoria Embankment
London EC4Y 0DZ
www.octopusbooks.co.uk

An Hachette UK Company
www.hachette.co.uk

ISBN 978-1-78325-529-0

A CIP catalogue record for this book is available from the British Library.

Printed and bound in the United Kingdom

10 9 8 7 6 5 4 3 2 1

UK edition research: Jemima Dunne
Cover image: Brian Hagiwara/Getty Images
Cover design: Christa Moffit

This FSC® label means that materials used for the product have been responsibly sourced

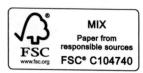

MIX
Paper from
responsible sources
FSC® C104740

FSC
www.fsc.org

For Anna, Jonathan and Georgia

Contents

Introduction

I'm about ten years old. It's Glasgow, where blue sky is a rare event to be rejoiced in. My surname isn't Swan, it's Swirsky, which probably has its origins in the Lithuanian village of Svir. My dad is on the dole looking for a job. Both parents smoke more than 20 a day and all their family and friends do too … inside the house and in their cars with the windows up. On the cooker (despite years in Australia I still don't say stove) is what my mother called the 'chip pan', a pot covered in oil splatter. The chip pan is used once or twice a day to fry chips for lunch and dinner, liberally salted and doused with vinegar. Vegetables are boiled to a mush and it's to be years before I hear there's such a thing as olive oil. Gymnasia are seamy places in side streets where aspiring boxers and wrestlers go to train, and exercise in general is an alien concept although I do have a bike and ride to school.

I'd be at medical school before finding out that at the time Glasgow had the highest rate of heart disease in the world. The life expectancy gap between the richest and poorest suburbs was around 25 years.

I tell you this because it's the driver for this book. What drove this lifestyle was lack of knowledge, lack of money, conformity to the norm, and a swirl of lives where people didn't feel they had much control over their destiny.

I was desperate to escape and gain that control. Medicine wasn't my first choice of career (acting was, which is another story) but a medical training, along with journalism, has allowed me to spend my life offering others the knowledge they deserve so they can make important decisions based on fact rather than opinion or myth, while retaining their right to make whatever choices suit them.

There are two fundamental concepts that sit behind this book.

The first is that there's no such thing as a split between the mind and the body. There's nothing spiritual about the mind. It's a wonderful thing which gives us awareness and identity and creativity but … it's a function of our brains. No brain, no mind. No body, no brain. It's all one. So what goes on in our brains affects every part of our bodies and what goes on in our heart, arteries, gut and even our feet affects our brain and mind. It's why decisions we make about our lives and how to feel good are so important and intertwined.

Which leads directly back to this idea of control.

There are lots of important things in life but when it comes down to the wire, I reckon – and there's evidence to support it – control is the one which matters most. It's not about being a control freak. This is about being able to control your destiny; making decisions which give you independence and an ability to chart your own course, whether that be in your personal life, with kids if or when you have them, and at work. It's also about not feeling oppressed by others who might want to constrain your life or work in some way.

Lack of this sense of control creates chronic stress, which can be damaging to your heart, metabolism, immune system and brain.

This book is about knowledge – that's information plus analysis. It allows you choice and gives strength to some of the key decisions you have to make about how to feel good; sometimes feeling okay about feeling bad; what you put into your body; what you take out of it; what you can add to it; how to ignore ageing as a concept; as well as stuff about sex, drugs, kids and recognising bullshit.

I'm not going to waste your time with unnecessary words. This book is straight, unapologetic and non-judgemental. The world we live in is full of anecdotes dressed up as fact and that creates issues about knowing what to trust. There isn't a single testimonial or human interest story here. There is, however, a lot about emotion, the impact of personal experience and our inner worlds, and just enough so you can apply it to your own circumstances and work out its relevance.

While the book is based on science, I'll tell you when the evidence is wobbly and what's known about the risks versus the benefits of decisions you might make.

Keeping to my promise about not wasting your time, let's get on with it …

The whole wellness thing

Intuitively you know this is bullshit, don't you – 'this' being that somewhere out there there's someone who wakes up every morning feeling refreshed, bounces out of bed, opens the curtains and looks out, skin glowing, abdomen tight and flat, and can't wait to capture the day, knowing they can. Every day. And of course that someone drinks some special green gunk for breakfast, goes to an amazing fitness class, does yoga upside-down at 40 degrees, writes a novel a year, has (or one day will have) three glorious children and a partner who emanates and exudes just like they do.

There's absolutely nothing wrong with aspiration. Just thinking that there is someone like that out there gives us hope that we can be like them and, at its core, a hard-to-tie-down feeling of wellbeing and wellness, which we've all experienced but … just not every day. In fact, we recognise it exactly because it's not an everyday experience. Wellness and wellbeing are intermittent phenomena which are appreciated because they stand out in our lives.

Look, I'll give you an example.

I'm sitting here writing at 5 a.m. I felt totally crap when my alarm went off. I creaked out of bed. Wrangled the curtains. Brushed my teeth, looking in the mirror wondering why I ever thought I could have a six-pack. If I allow myself to think about it, I've pain in my legs and one shoulder from post-exercise soreness.

Made myself a strong coffee to charge up, cut myself off from the world (i.e. turned off my phone and email because they can do my head in). And got down to work. My friends and workmates will tell you that I'm the most focused person they know and yet I sit here and my mind daydreams and drifts to the dramas and joys in my life and I have to keep pulling myself back to the task at hand. If only they truly knew what a fraud I really am.

Maybe I'm as delusional as the person who bounces out of bed, for whom *carpe diem* (seize the day) is their motto. But I actually reckon I'm pretty normal and my point is that it's normal to feel crap in the morning, to have aches and pains no matter what age you are, and it's normal to oscillate between feeling great, anxious, relaxed and energised several times a day. You need that variation to notice light and shade in your life. The always-glowing person I described has a problem. How can they possibly know that what they feel every day is so wonderful when they'd have nothing to compare it with? You and I know what feeling great is like because it stands out above the normal and, at least for me, that's worth cherishing and finding ways to feel like that more often.

There are many ways to weight the scales in our lives towards feeling good and one of them is realising that adversity isn't always what's on the other side of the scale. You need a bit of adversity to rejoice in the 'ups'. Life is like chaos. Not chaos in the sense of clothes lying everywhere and wilfully not having a diary. It's the mathematical idea of chaos; the whirling complexity and diversity of the world. For example, studies of the heart have found that a healthy heart is chaotic and by that I mean the way it beats and its electrical patterns. One way of recognising a heart that's unwell is that there's less chaos – a sameness about how it's working.

We become stronger when we come through tough times or a tough moment or realise that our worst fears didn't happen because we didn't avoid them, or our friends and family rallied to our support when it was needed.

There's no question that adversity can knock us around and there's no shame in that, nor in seeking help to find a way through. Sometimes anxiety overwhelms us; sometimes we need to recognise when we haven't felt great for a long time and aren't enjoying life much and need expert assistance. The thing is that a search for 'always-on' wellbeing will rarely have given you the solution.

So ... be careful what you wish for and ... before we get into the weeds, it does help to understand what you wish for – your aims – since that will affect the decisions you make about exercise, nutrition, kids and living younger longer. If there ever were shifting sands in the course of life, they're our aims.

Personally, I shamble through life with vague aims, which I like being vague because, since I've kept them to myself, they allow me to change my mind without too much embarrassment. Some people are laser-focused. They want to make a shitload of money, or want nothing more than being laidback with friends and family. Of course, when you have kids, you've got to be really careful what you wish for.

Anyway, the point I want to make is that in the real world, like our mood and wellbeing, our aims change through time and life circumstances such as relationships falling apart, losing a job, struggling in a new career or getting a mortgage, kids and the whole deal. Having that insight – which really isn't so profound – makes a difference to the choices we make.

Through the Australian health channel that I co-founded – Tonic Media Network – I do sessions with the same title as this book, for people usually in their 20s and 30s. The sessions were the idea of the talented and highly energetic Jack Mortlock, who worked for us then and who's in that demographic. I don't give a talk, I take questions without notice, anonymously in writing, directly and 'on behalf of a friend'. What I quickly had to contextualise for the audience was that there were no right or wrong answers for each person. How they used the knowledge depended on their aims and this is no different if you're 27, 57 or 77.

For instance, a big mistake is to assume that people go to the gym for their health. It's true for some, I suppose. But most are there for body sculpting, even me who forlornly wishes for that six-pack rather than my hard-to-shift pinot noir abdomen. The handy side effects of the gym are muscle building, better sugar metabolism with a lower risk of diabetes, nerve cell growth in the brain, improved mood, lower cancer rates, cardiovascular fitness and maybe a bit of weight control. But the reason you went there was to look good.

Let's sit for a moment with looking good as an aim. It's perfectly valid but you need to understand the evidence around certain choices so you have your eyes open.

For instance, you might be unhappy with the size of your gut, the plumpness of your lips, the laugh lines on your face, the shape and size of your breasts, or whatever, and are saving up for botox, fillers or plastic surgery. However, you need to be aware that most procedures only last a while then need to be repeated with poorer and poorer results. So there's an argument to be patient and wait so that the number of re-do's you're going to need is fewer.

But maybe underlying that aim of looking good is that at its heart you simply want to *feel* better. If so, that colours a lot of decisions you might make and the knowledge you need to have because – to state the bleeding obvious – it goes deeper than how you look. Some people feel great on a good diet, some feel it with supplements, or the gym, or get it from friends. Others feel good from altruism. Giving back. Giving to others. Others get it from having gone through a spell of feeling bad or a rough time and having come through stronger. We're all different and there's usually no right or wrong answer. Unless of course it's relying on crystal meth.

If, however, your aim is to live longer in good shape, there's less wriggle room for what you need to know and the choices you ought to make. For instance, you don't live longer by inhaling burnt plant material into your lungs. It might make you feel better, which is perfectly fine, but it won't add years at the pointy end when the brick wall is in sight. In fact, it could take many years off your life, as could other habits or behaviours.

If happiness is your aim, then understanding what that really means, and what factors determine being happy is important. You might feel happy on a Friday night after a few drinks, a line if you can afford it or some MDMA, but you know you'll pay for it later.

If kids are your aim, then there's stuff you should know.

If this book is good for you, then you'll have made it so, not me.

PART 1

What you put into yourself

Rise above nutrients

The world is obsessed with nutrients, when we should be thinking big.

How much carb should I eat? Which kinds? What fats are okay – I've heard the whole saturated fat thing is bullshit? Is a low-fat diet really the best thing for me? Coconut milk is really good for you, isn't it? Is there any limit to the amount of protein I can eat? Which protein is best for muscle building? And is it better before or after the gym? Is low fat dairy best? Should I stir butter into my coffee? Which micronutrients do I need to add to my diet? I'm confused by what's meant by a paleo diet but it does make sense to eat like a hunter–gatherer, doesn't it, after all, that's what we were designed to be? I'm convinced I'm short on antioxidants, how would I know?

It really doesn't help to divide up what you eat into nutrients. There are more important things to focus on because if your aims are to feel good, not put on weight and live younger longer, then what counts is your eating pattern, how you cook what you eat, where you eat it, who with and what you add to your food, oh … and yes … what you eat. I know I'm stating the obvious but we didn't evolve to eat protein balls, swallow supplements every morning, or indeed go to the gym at 6 a.m. every day.

Hold on, you might cry. Go to the gym every day? Isn't it fair to say that my throwaway sentence there ignores reality? Surely I'm not arguing that we shouldn't be going to the gym just because there were no Fitness Firsts 10,000 years ago in the African savannah? No, I'm not arguing against gyms. However, we go to the gym or jog every day exactly because our lifestyle isn't what our bodies evolved to deal with and we're making up for sitting all day rather than walking and foraging. So why doesn't that apply to food? Most of us find it hard to escape nutrient-deficient, processed foods and therefore, as with exercise in the gym or jogging, feel the need to make up for the deficiencies, hence the protein balls and supplements.

There's no question that I go to the gym or jog/walk every day for exactly those reasons but exercise is very different from food. It's pretty simple and can fairly easily mimic the physical activity we were designed for, with the purposes of maintaining and strengthening our muscles, keeping our bones strong through impact on the ground, and maintaining and expanding our cardiorespiratory reserve (see If Only You Could Bottle Exercise). What I'm saying is that exercise is a straightforward supplement whereas what we eat is immensely complex and the logic of deficiency doesn't easily apply. As I said, you've got to think big. And while I'm here, it's worth saying that with exercise there is still a bit of a mountain to climb to replace what we were designed to do, which is walk a lot, labour with our hands and plough the fields.

Our bodies are designed to consume fats, carbohydrates (carbs) and protein because when you reduce our bodies to their basics, we need raw materials to build our bodies and energy to power everything. Our energy currency is glucose, the simplest sugar molecule, which is a building block for most carbohydrates. We need fat to store energy and to help protect nerves and even the shrink wrap around our cells. And we need protein to maintain and manufacture muscles, nerves, bones, blood, organs and hormones. Carbs, fats and proteins are the macronutrients.

Micronutrients are the helpers which oil the body's machinery and assist with keeping it bolted together. We know quite a lot about micronutrients like vitamins and minerals from test-tube and animal research and from what happens when we're deficient, say, in vitamin C (scurvy), vitamin D (rickets), vitamin B1 (beri-beri) and so on. But almost all that research is into a single chemical.

And before I go any further, while it may take away the romance of candle-lit dinners, food and cuisine are basically all about chemistry. An experienced chef knows exactly what will happen when you add an egg, oil or heat to a mixture, and such chefs are the first to admit that what they do every day is the world's most complex chemistry. You see, we don't eat single chemicals. Food is a package.

Take an orange. You might eat it for its vitamin C but that's short-selling it and other fruits. The aroma alone of an orange is made up of more than 70 compounds. That's just the smell of an orange. And you eat that smell. Then there are alcohols, amino acids and sugars and, even with all that knowledge, scientists aren't sure what makes a navel orange taste differently from a Jaffa.

That's one orange and it's likely that its natural complex chemistry makes the vitamin C it contains more effective than in a synthetic pill or fizzy, dissolvable tablet.

Just think about what you've eaten in the past 24 hours. Yesterday I consumed:

- Sourdough bread with avocado
  (Sourdough is a dominant carb in parts of the Mediterranean and avocado is filled with good fats.)
- Multiple shots of coffee made espresso style
  (The chemistry of coffee changes according to the method and the roast – with more or fewer antioxidants depending on temperature; heat is better.)
- With hot milk
  (Different chemically from fresh, cold milk.)
- Dark leaf tea with milk
  (Milk affects tea chemistry and maybe reduces antioxidant availability. Too bad. I hate black tea.)
- Natural yoghurt
  (Hopefully teeming with friendly bacteria for my microbiome, see the Microbiome section.)

- An unedifying chicken sandwich for lunch
  (Don't want to think about what was in it.)
- Salad with olive oil and vinegar dressing
  (Vinegar may be at least as important for health as
  olive oil because the acetic acid may affect what are
  called 'short-chain fatty acids' in your bowel and shift
  your microbiome to a healthier profile.)
- Pasta with vegetables and meatballs cooked in olive
  oil and various spices
  (Spices are an underestimated part of our diet. There's
  evidence that, when cooked with vegetables such as
  tomatoes, onions and garlic they have antioxidant
  and anti-inflammatory activity, may subdue cancer
  growth, enhance a healthy microbiome, help with
  keeping your blood pressure down and slow down
  cholesterol damage to your arteries.)
- A glass of red wine
  (There's only a little high-quality evidence that red
  wine is any better than other forms of alcohol and
  in any event may interact with your food and have
  more benefit when taken with a healthy diet such
  as the Mediterranean. And in the end, red wine
  drinkers may have a lifestyle that's healthier, so
  red wine may just be a passenger rather than the
  cause of living healthier longer. You may have heard
  about resveratrol in red wine as an anti-ageing
  supplement ... yet to be proven, at least in amounts
  that are practical to take.)
- Sparkling water
  (Not a fan of still water unless dying of thirst.)

- With a friend
  (Social connectedness is well-documented to have health benefits.)
- With telly off
  (TV on makes you fatter.)
- At the dining table
  (Makes eating an occasion and enhances its importance.)
- Talking
  (Social connectedness is vital for good health.)

You'd go absolutely nuts if you obsessed on all that each day and dissected each meal before you ate it. A global view means that you don't burrow down to individual nutrients. You rise above them to whole foods (preferably cooked) whose beneficial and sometimes harmful effects come from everything in them working together.

#Justsaying

Is it fat or *Game of Thrones*?
There's always a trade-off

Quick trade: If you change your diet – to low calorie, low fat, low carb, high protein, whatever – you'll trade off one nutrient for another, probably unknowingly, and the result may not necessarily be good for you or achieve your goal. You should try to understand what can happen and make up your mind to take charge. Be especially wary of trading fats for refined carbs.

*

I'm just stating the bleeding obvious but you've got to eat something. Your body is designed to survive and has a mind of its own to enable that. For instance, research at the University of Melbourne, Australia, has found that the chemical messengers – the hormones – in your brain which control appetite have their settings set by the end of adolescence. That's why childhood obesity is such an issue because you don't want kids' appetites to be set to feed a body mass index (BMI) of over 30. This shouldn't make you feel hopeless, it just shows how conscious you need to be to make changes.

Here's an example of how things can get tangled and where *Game of Thrones* comes in.

There's been a debate for years now about fat in the diet. There's no question that studies following large numbers of people for many years have shown that people whose diets are high in saturated fats (mostly from farmed land mammals) have a higher risk of dying of heart attacks and strokes. These are called observational studies and can only conclude there's a link between saturated fat and heart disease. They can't prove cause and effect. There could be all kinds of factors which go along with eating saturated fat. Maybe people who like saturated fat are also more likely to watch *Game of Thrones* and what's really killed them was the anxiety between Series 1 and 2 of not knowing whether becoming the Mother of Dragons will save Daenerys, assuming they cared.

To find out cause and effect, you have to test the idea by exposing people to the problematic substance in a randomised trial. For that you need to give half the people the alleged culprit (in this case saturated fat) and the other half a dummy fat. Well, that's not going to happen. No ethics committee is going to approve that experiment.

An alternative is to give a medication which reduces low density lipoprotein (LDL), the bad form of cholesterol in your blood, which is raised by saturated fat. When that's been done using statins, the risk of heart attacks has fallen convincingly. But all that tells you is there's likely to be a cause and effect relationship between LDL and heart disease. It doesn't pin down saturated fat as the enemy. That didn't stop experts for years promoting low fat diets in the hope that saturated fat intake would also fall. The trouble is that large trials of lowering the saturated fat in the diet have been disappointing, which has actually led some nutritionists to flip and advocate increasing your saturated fat consumption, for instance by putting butter in your coffee. They might call it 'bulletproof coffee' but the theory behind it is far from bulletproof.

It turns out that the reason the evidence is weak for lowering the saturated fat in your diet is that it depends on what you trade it for. People who went on a low fat diet and compensated by eating refined pasta and mountains of white rice got little or no benefit, but if they traded saturated fat for a monounsaturated fat like olive oil or, even better, a polyunsaturated fat which actively lowers cholesterol, they saw a reduced heart risk. Highly refined carbohydrates – especially sugar – can behave just like a toxic fat.

I tell you this story simply to warn you that you need to be careful what you wish for. Watch out for unexpected consequences.

Cuisine counts – but not by itself

I grew up in a traditional Jewish family in Glasgow – a city that had one of the highest rates of coronary heart disease (heart attacks, angina and strokes) in the world. The traditional Jewish diet is so unhealthy you might well wonder how Jews have survived as long as they have. Chicken soup with globules of fat floating on top, vegetables cooked to an inch of their lives, matzo balls made with eggs and chicken fat, gribenes – pronounced in a Scottish accent as 'greebinnies' – which are pieces of chicken skin fried on high heat to reduce the chicken fat to schmaltz (cooking fat) and then tossed in salt to be gobbled by children hovering around the cooker, 24-hour slow-cooked pots of potato pudding (laced with salt and schmaltz), beans and lamb shanks (cholent), chopped cooked calf's liver topped with egg, chopped salted herring, latkes (fried potato pancakes) … you get the message. Just writing about it makes my mouth water and induces central chest pain going down my left arm. And that's before we stepped out the door to be tempted by Glasgow specialities like deep-fried black or white pudding and chips (no deep-fried Mars Bars in my day).

Medieval cuisine, which largely describes the Eastern European/Ashkenazi Jewish diet, is full of fat, carbs and calories, and while the people of modern nations are overweight and obese, counterintuitively, we consume fewer calories and fat than our ancestors.

Studies of a similarly unhealthy cuisine – in the Amish – help to explain how we survived. The Amish are a conservative Christian sect living in North America who date back to 17th century Europe. They had a life expectancy in their 70s at a time when most of us died in our 40s. Their diet is high in saturated fat, carbs and calories, yet they're still less likely to develop diabetes than the diet would lead you to imagine. Part of this may be genetics in a culturally isolated population, but a lot almost certainly has to do with physical activity. The Amish shun modern technology and cling to a traditional farming lifestyle. They work hard and burn a large number of calories every day – and their children do too. I tell you this to show again that no aspects of our lives exist in solitude. They interact.

Anyway, back to cuisine.

When it comes to cuisine, it won't shock you to hear that there have been no randomised trials of Jamie Oliver versus Yotam Ottolenghi. The evidence comes from research looking at the health and wellbeing of whole populations and trying to work out what factors are meaningful when you separate them out statistically. It's all very well to say that the Western diet is rubbish but what in fact is the Western diet anymore? Because if it's hamburgers and chips and oodles of sugar eaten sitting in front of the television, then that's no longer confined to what used to be known as Western countries.

I'll expand on the evidence but if you want the quick takeaway here, the elements of a healthy cuisine and dietary pattern include:

- Knowing what's in the food you're eating and how it was cooked – which means only sparingly eating out or using Uber Eats or Deliveroo
- The best way of knowing what you're eating is sticking to fresh, whole foods as much as possible
- Substituting saturated fat for monounsaturated fats

such as olive oil

- Fermented foods like vinegar or soya
- Cooking slowly with lots of moisture (not much high temp grilling and BBQ-ing)
- Fresh herbs of all kinds, including leafy garnishes
- Garlic and onions in most recipes
- Green leafy vegetables
- Using fish, beans, lentils and other legumes instead of red meat
- Chopping tomatoes and red capsicum finely and using olive oil and vinegar in dressings
- Cooking red vegetables in olive oil
- Desserts other than fresh fruit are a treat rather than a daily experience
- Lunch being a more important meal than dinner or breakfast
- Small amounts of alcohol
- Possibly having frugal eating days (see Vegan Fasting)

These days, we're pretty eclectic in what we eat and cook, and when we travel we rejoice in local cuisines. When you visit Greece, Italy or France, for example, it takes you a while to realise that Greeks, Italians and French largely only like their own food and cooking styles. It's reflected in their grocery and local food markets unless you find yourself in a migrant area. The UK doesn't have a specific national cuisine but it has a fascination with foods from all over the world. Throughout the country you'll find almost every national cuisine you could imagine, from Japanese, Indian and Indonesian to European, African and South American. This is even more true in areas where there are diverse communities of different ethnicities.

Even smaller country towns often have a Chinese or Indian restaurant and often a Greek, Italian or French cafe too, which reflects the diversity of the communities within the UK ... and their cultures.

Maybe culture counts more

One of Australia's most respected cancer and nutritional epidemiologists, Professor Dallas English, based at the University of Melbourne, told me, 'We spent years looking at individual nutrients and the results were really disappointing. There were no magic bullets in nutrition. It's a much bigger picture and certainly culture comes into it.'

The excellent research by a group of Australian nutritional researchers informs much of what follows in these sections, particularly the work of Professor Catherine Itsiopoulos and Drs Antigone Kouris-Blazos and Tania Thodis, but many others as well.

Greeks and Italians who cling to their traditional diets are clearly doing themselves a favour.

There's a similar story with Japanese migrants to the United States. Between the 1880s and 1910, around 150,000 Japanese moved to Hawaii and about 30,000 to the West Coast of the United States, mostly seeking economic opportunity. There have been many studies looking at what's happened to these Japanese Americans and comparing them to the Japanese population in Japan and other Americans. Japanese Americans have a lower risk of heart disease than the American average, and this is thought to be due to Japanese cuisine, which contains a lot of fish and soya as well as being less calorie dense. Japanese Americans also have a lower risk of strokes than people in Japan and other Americans. As each generation has put distance between Japanese Americans and their ancestral culture, Americans of Japanese origin have become heavier, and developed a higher risk of heart attacks and a very much higher risk of type 2 diabetes associated with a higher fat and animal protein diet. This probably indicates that thousands of years in Japan has programmed their genes to living with lots of fish and soya and a low fat diet, especially in saturated fat, as well as taking in fewer calories. This genetic susceptibility is so powerful that their risk of diabetes is higher than that of both native Japanese and other Americans. With cancer, rates of bowel cancer have risen with each generation, which is not a surprise since it's related to being overweight or obese and consumption of red meat. Rates of stomach cancer have fallen compared to Japan but remained higher than average – that's because the Japanese diet is high in cured and salty foods – but breast cancer and prostate cancer rates are lower. Swings and roundabouts, as they say. But with all that, the Japanese are the longest-lived people on the planet. So something is going well and, like Greeks and Italians, Japanese mostly prefer their own food.

I can spend a lot of time unpicking genes, culture, diet and physical activity but let's put genes to one side for the moment, because even with genetic variations between populations, we are far more similar to each other than different. For example, type 2 diabetes is a major public health priority in the UK and some have a genetic susceptibility to it especially when faced with a poor diet, too many calories and too little exercise. Among minority ethnic communities, the prevalence is approximately three to five times higher than in the white British population. People of South Asian ethnicity are up to six times more likely to develop diabetes for various reasons but primarily because people of Asian and South Asian background are more sensitive to a poor lifestyle. It's a genetic thing. Whereas the BMI which classifies the white British population as obese is 30, Asian and South Asian ethnicity cruelly lumps you with the risks of obesity at a lower BMI.

Back to culture.

And by that I mean how we live with each other, who we identify with, what values we have and share, what if any religion we follow and how we have fun and recreate.

Research in Melbourne, Australia, many years ago by the late Professor John Powles investigated the health and wellbeing of Greek migrants who came there from the island of Lefkada and compared them to their brothers and sisters who stayed behind. What he found was that Greek migrants lived longer than their Australian-born neighbours – about six years longer, in fact. And the more their children clung to their Greek identity, the more preserved were their lower chances of developing the chronic diseases which would have made them die younger than they should. The researchers also found what they initially thought was a contradiction but wasn't. When they compared the Australian migrants to their close relatives who stayed back on Lefkada, the 'new' Melburnians lived longer than the brothers and sisters they left behind.

Forget the French … the paradox is Greek

There are two migrant groups which have just about the highest average life expectancy in the world and they can tell us a lot if our aim is living longer. They're Greek migrants to Australia and Japanese who moved to live in Hawaii.

Greek Australians have been well researched for many years and what's become known as the 'Greek Paradox' is this.

For decades, elderly Greek Australians have had high levels of risk factors for heart disease. They've been two or three times more likely to be obese and have diabetes, high cholesterol and high blood pressure than Anglo Australians. Yet they are 35 per cent less likely to die prematurely of heart disease and their age-adjusted risk of cancer is lower too. It's mindbending and counterintuitive. I'm not saying that those well-known risk factors aren't important, more that there's something else that's powerful going on. The data come from a few sources including: the Melbourne Collaborative Cohort Study, which is following the health and habits of more than 40,000 people; the Food Habits in Later Life Study of nearly 1000 people; and the European Prospective Investigation into Cancer and Nutrition (EPIC), which included more than 23,000 Greeks. Put together, these studies show that the paradox is even more paradoxical. When these migrants arrived from Greece, they took up the high calorie, high saturated fat Australian diet including lots of red meat, sugar and white bread instead of sourdough. That's what gave them their high risk profile.

But what seems to have saved them was their Greek-ness.

Controlled for other factors, what rescued them was keeping enough of the Greek traditional diet, which is high in plant-based foods and fresh herbs and low in meat, among other things. Then something really interesting happened. When these Greek Australians retired, they returned to what they remembered from their youth and became more traditional. They reduced their meat consumption, increased their plant intake, had a vegetable and herb garden at the back of the house or on an allotment, and became more religious. In the Greek Orthodox church, there are many festivals and holy days which require a degree of abstinence, usually in the form of days when all you eat are plant-based foods. Studies suggest that about one in three elderly Greek Australians have around 100 plant-only days a year. So they aren't fit Adonises with flat abdomens and thin thighs but some things in their cultural and dietary mix work for them.

One clue came from comparing them to Greeks in Greece because they did not live as long as Greek Australians. Ironically, only 57 per cent of older people living in Greece were adhering to a Mediterranean diet pattern, compared to 81 per cent of Greek Australians. Sure, there would have been other lifestyle differences that went along with what and how people were eating but when they were allowed for statistically, the association with the Mediterranean diet pattern remained. In fact, it explained the 30 per cent reduction in the chances of dying at a given age. Put another way, a Greek migrant aged 70 living in Melbourne had two-thirds the chances of dying before his or her next birthday compared to a Greek living in Greece.

There is a caveat to this, though. In the first years of migration, according to John Powles' Lefkada study, the siblings left behind on the island were still adhering to their version of a Mediterranean diet, down to drinking neat olive oil every day and consuming far less red meat than their siblings in Australia. Even so, there were still health differences favouring Melbourne. Part of the reason in the early days was what's known as the 'Healthy Migrant Effect'. People who migrate are generally healthier and better off financially than those who don't. (By the way, the same goes for work. People who are in employment live longer than those who don't work, and again that's partly because you're more likely to have a job if you're healthier to start with.) But after 50 or 60 years, that effect is likely to have washed out and, as often seems to be the case, migrant communities can cling more strongly to traditions than those living in the country of origin.

The bottom line is that older Greek Australians have a cultural affinity with their traditional dietary pattern, which includes growing their own fresh herbs and vegetables, not trusting processed foods (they'll soak vegetables in water to remove chemicals from the surface) and being frugal maybe one day in three or four. It also has to be said that they live in a country which provides a high standard of primary health care and affordable medications to prevent heart disease. But so do non-Greek Australians who don't live as long.

A word of caution, though, before we get carried away with the romance of culture being an unalloyed good. It depends on the culture. You could argue that cultures which value individual endeavour at the expense of communities will also reward enterprise while not taking full account of the costs to others, highly value convenience (e.g. home-delivered meals) making life too easy and kitchens redundant, allow the spread of cities at the expense of good horticultural land, and don't have enough open spaces for exercise or allotments to grow your own vegetables. It wouldn't be surprising that such cultures don't necessarily make you live longer.

Certainly, while the culture which gave me my values was strong, the diet which went with it did me no favours, nor did its disdain for physical exercise.

Rate your diet

Quick snack: I've banged on long enough. Let's cut to the chase. What's the recipe for healthy eating, because a Greek diet looks very different from an Italian one and certainly from sushi and sashimi with soya sauce and wasabi? Well, let's assume that feeling good, not putting on too much weight and living younger longer are your aims. In tune with the theme of staying above the weeds, the Alternative Healthy Eating Index (AHEI) helps to explain how cuisines which don't look the same can have similar health benefits and allows you to rate your diet.

*

In the early 2000s the US National Cancer Institute started a project looking at dietary patterns and how you might measure diets and compare them to each other in their ability to prevent big life-shortening conditions like cancer, heart disease and diabetes. The AHEI has performed well against the others. There is a measure of how Mediterranean your diet is, which performs a little better on predicting cancer prevention, but we're probably quibbling over minor differences.

The AHEI is the result of extensive reviews of the available evidence on the benefits and harms of nutrients and dietary patterns. It was validated by comparing the AHEI to data from long-term Harvard University studies following the health and wellbeing of 110,000 female and male nurses and doctors.

Here's a summary of the evidence. The reasons you'll see me using the words 'linked' and 'associated' is that cause and effect aren't known for sure. It's possible that some dietary patterns work because fruit and veg, for instance, displace unhealthy foods. Anyway, here's the dietary pattern they concluded was healthy:

Vegetables are associated with reduced heart disease, diabetes and cancer. Five servings of vegetables a day are recommended – where each serving is around half a cup unless it's green leafy vegetables where it's a full cup. Green leafy vegetables are thought to be better for diabetes prevention. This excludes potatoes, which are not protective, especially for diabetes.

Fruit consumption is linked to reduced heart disease and cancer. Four servings of whole fruit a day are recommended, where a serving is a piece of fruit or half a cup of, say, berries. This excludes fruit juice, which increases the risk of weight gain and diabetes without the benefits for heart disease and cancer.

Whole grains are associated with reduced risks of bowel cancer, heart disease and diabetes, while refined grains are linked to the opposite effects. Half a cup of oatmeal or brown rice is around 20 g and 75–90 g per day are recommended.

You're probably feeling pretty full by now, but we're not finished.

Nuts, legumes and vegetable protein such as soya or tofu are linked to reduced heart disease and diabetes risks, with one serving of just under 30 g per day being recommended.

Whole fish or fillets (as opposed to fish oil) appear to be good for your heart, with two fish meals of around 120 g each a week being recommended.

Swapping out saturated fats for polyunsaturated ones is good for heart disease prevention. This is independent of a low fat diet, which in its own right has pretty much no benefits although some tout it in a calorie-controlled diet.

So here's what you subtract from the healthy diet:

Sugar-sweetened beverages (including fruit juice) increase the risk of obesity and diabetes. There's even a hint of an increased risk of pancreatic cancer.

Red meat and particularly processed meats are associated with heart disease, stroke, bowel cancer and diabetes. With red meat, the effect may be more due to the healthier protein sources you're not eating but processed meats are risky in their own right because of salt and nitrites.

Transfats are to be avoided, because of their strong link to heart disease.

Excessive salt intake is linked to higher rates of early death, high blood pressure and even stomach cancer.

The health effects of alcohol, if you can keep it to two standard drinks a day, are reasonably neutral although moderate drinking might reduce heart disease events like heart attacks in people who are already at high risk. The more you drink beyond that, the more harm you're potentially doing, but you know that already: heart disease, cancer, injuries, becoming a victim of violence, dementia risk and so on. And no ... you can't store up your two drinks a day and binge on 14 Negronis on a Friday night.

But here's what's not in the Alternative Healthy Eating Index which some researchers believe is important, and it's mainly about what you cook and the actual ingredients.

For instance, bean soups, olives and olive oil, nuts, slow moist cooking (e.g. casseroles and stews with lots of vegetables and a tomato base using garlic, onions and herbs) and of course growing your own vegetables, but for us apartment dwellers that could be substituted for buying at farmers' markets where you get to know the suppliers.

Which brings us to the Mediterranean dietary pattern.

What is the Mediterranean dietary pattern anyway?

I can't remember when I first heard of the Mediterranean diet. It was years ago but what I do recall is that it didn't make sense to me. A glance at a map of the Mediterranean region quickly reveals that there can't possibly be any such thing as one Mediterranean diet, much less a dietary pattern. How could there be, with so much variation in the countries and cultures on its shores? There are North African Islamic countries, a Jewish state, Lebanon with its mix of Christians and Muslims and other groups, Turkey and Syria with their own ancient Islamic and Christian civilisations, the Greek Islands and mainland Greece, and then predominantly Catholic countries such as Italy, France and Spain. Sure, you can eat pita bread and hummus from Greece round to Morocco but there's a lot more to a dietary pattern than your favourite dips.

And before someone tells you that the Mediterranean diet must be terrific because it's thousands of years old, let me disabuse you of that. It's not that old, actually. I bet you the first food that comes to mind when you visualise your idea of a Mediterranean diet is the tomato. Next might be the capsicum or eggplant. All are actually native to the Americas and didn't arrive in Europe until the 16th century. So ancient Romans or Greeks didn't sit around the table mopping up leftover Napoletana sauce with their sourdough bread. The traditional Mediterranean diet is not that old. It just pre-dates the globalisation of food production and easy access to meat and processed foods.

Nutrition and Med diet researcher Professor Catherine Itsiopoulos talks about the basics of the Mediterranean diet being wheat, wine and olive oil with wild leafy greens and legumes thrown in – never forget the huge amount of incidental exercise. Catherine has a great story from her family's island in Greece which she heard from a 90+-year-old who escaped to the hills during World War II. He credits his survival to his mother, who gave him a container of extra virgin olive oil and advice to forage for wild greens and then eat them with the oil.

Of course the romance of the Mediterranean diet is part of its attraction. Sitting in a white and blue courtyard gazing over the Aegean nibbling olives and quaffing red wine is a fantasy that's hardwired into many of us and probably many researchers too. But that doesn't detract from the evidence, which shows that the dietary pattern is closely linked to lower than average rates of heart disease – our biggest killer.

Researchers doing early comparative studies of the risk factors for coronary heart disease were impressed by the diet eaten by men on Crete. In fact, the Cretan dietary pattern is really what most people refer to – probably unknowingly – when they talk about the Mediterranean diet. Lots of olive oil, some wine, sourdough bread, lots of plant-based foods, not much meat, protein from legumes, etc. But there's much more to it than that. Cretans are still among the highest consumers of olive oil in the world. Vegetables are cooked in it and wild leafy greens are doused in olive oil and vinegar, with liberal use of garlic, onions, fennel, spices and herbs, and so on.

For the micronutrient-obsessed among you, the chemistry of the Med diet is fascinating. Extra virgin olive oil (EVOO) used in cooking vegetables, particularly red ones, releases powerful antioxidants and anti-inflammatory compounds like polyphenols which include flavonoids and many others. EVOO also helps with the absorption of fat-soluble carotenoids and increases the bioavailability of green leafy vegetables. Fresh herbs enhance this, especially oregano, but it's also been shown that cooking beans with onions and parsley greatly increases the flavonoid content. Even adding capers to some dishes can release beneficial flavonoids. Crete – being nearer to ancient sea routes – seems to have a cuisine that uses a wider than usual range of spices and herbs, including cumin and coriander.

So rather than take up too much of your time, here's the low mortality, Cretan/Mediterranean package. It doesn't lend itself to easy scoring but the evidence suggests that the closer you can stick to this, the better. And for those of you who prefer Asian cuisine, you'll see there are many common elements; it's just that the flavours and some cooking styles are different.

Eat what you cook, where you cook and if possible with other people

The traditional Mediterranean dietary pattern is anchored in home cooking using fresh ingredients served at a dining table with no television. It's obvious, isn't it? When you cook, you know what you're eating. When the telly is off, you know how much you're eating and savour it more. Restaurants are only interested in exciting your palate and if that needs butter, salt, sugar or refined flour to get them over the line, then so be it. Takeaways are the same. They mostly couldn't care less about your heart, brain or waist and hip circumferences. They want to create an enjoyable experience for you almost at any cost. Great for a treat but not often.

The other thing about meals is that they're a time to pause and connect face to face and here's where dietary patterns overlap with psychological and social wellbeing. Social connectedness is the foundation of wellbeing. The number of people you can call upon for support when times are tough is an important measure of how well you'll be able to deal with adversity.

Cook slowly with lots of flavours

I'll expand on this later (see Brown Isn't Such a Good Colour) but Mediterranean cuisine generally involves cooking more slowly with moisture and often with extra virgin olive oil, garlic, onions, herbs and spices. This allows the best flavours and nutrients to be created and retained and gives your body a hand in reducing inflammation and perhaps long-term cancer risk.

What I've learned: The one purchase I've made which has transformed my ability to cook in this way is one of those heavy iron French cooking pots. They heat up evenly, demand only a medium to low heat on the stove and, most importantly of all, make your kitchen look as though there's a great cook nearby. These pots are expensive but will last a lifetime and I reckoned were the price of a couple of weeks of delivered takeaways and meals out. Call me shallow but this pot has helped make cooking a pleasure. Declaration of interest: did the manufacturer give me a freebie to write this? Sadly, no.

Chop your veg and don't be shy with olive oil and vinegar

Tomatoes and capsicum and probably most other salad vegetables benefit from being chopped up finely and doused with olive oil and vinegar. This releases more polyphenols. You'll notice that most Mediterranean recipes use finely diced tomatoes. That's a good thing. You don't always have to chop, though. I often gently roast halved Roma tomatoes, deeply scored and drizzled with vinegar and olive oil before going into the oven at 150 degrees Celsius.

Garlic, onions, shallots and chives – use lots

They belong to the allium plant family and contain sulphur compounds which look as though they have cancer prevention activity.

Have some fermented dairy regularly

I eat a 500-g tub of natural yoghurt a week. Superb on sourdough and not a clue whether that's a reasonable amount.

Follow recipes

I've changed. Like most men, the Y chromosome has condemned me to:

1. Single tasking
2. Thinking I know where I'm going without a map
3. Thinking that following a recipe shows weakness and lack of creativity

Tick to 1 and 2 (there's only so much biology you can fight) but I've recognised that recipes can be magical things which harness years of chefs' expertise and knowledge. I wouldn't invent my own recipe for a general anaesthetic or an appendicectomy so why do it for a complex piece of chemistry in the kitchen? Professor Catherine Itsiopoulos has great Mediterranean cookbooks and I also heavily use the *New York Times* cooking app.

Dark leafy Viagra?

(#Writingthisforafriend you understand)

Green leafy vegetable consumption is associated with a lower risk of high blood pressure and heart disease. It's thought the reason is that they are high in nitrates. Vegetables which are high in nitrates include rocket, silverbeet, spinach, kale, lettuce and celery. Nitrates get absorbed in the mouth and stomach and can be converted to nitrites then nitric oxide. In addition to their high salt content, products like processed meat have a lot of nitrite (as opposed to nitrate) which might be carcinogenic, but there's no evidence of that risk from the natural consumption of nitrates.

Anyway, nitric oxide relaxes blood vessels and, in fact, there have been trials of organic leafy vegetable consumption (there is evidence that nitrate content varies by season and producer) showing a reduction in blood pressure, and it's thought that this effect is one of the reasons for the benefits of a plant-based diet.

My catchy title (well, it got you in this far, didn't it?) rises from how Viagra-type drugs work. They increase nitric oxide which then dilates the arteries below the belt, so to speak. It won't shock you to be told the evidence that a plant-based diet helps men in the sack is pretty poor, but that doesn't mean there's no effect. The evidence is much stronger that men who have good heart health, aren't too overweight or obese, and take exercise have a lower incidence of erectile dysfunction (ED), at least in part due to the lower incidence of type 2 diabetes, which is strongly linked to ED. So it makes sense that a plant-based dietary pattern will help.

Snoozing and gardening

These are probably the parts of the Mediterranean dietary pattern which are hardest to achieve. The package includes an afternoon snooze after lunch and growing some of your own vegetables. Siestas have been linked to lower blood pressure and heart disease but most of us don't have time for a nap. Mind you, for many years I've had a reputation at the Australian Broadcasting Corporation (ABC) as an Olympic napper. I've trained myself to fall asleep upright at my desk with headphones on, pretending to be editing a story. Fifteen minutes is all I need. Using mindfulness techniques, I force myself to focus on the sounds in my ear. There is an obvious caveat to this for broadcasters, though. Would you air a story that sent you off to sleep? I'll leave that as rhetorical.

With gardening, there's more to it than just the fresh veg. A vegetable garden is labour intensive and involves exercise which is quite vigorous at times. It also gets you out in the sun. As an apartment dweller, my attempt to get around this is to buy vegetables as I need them and if possible at a farmers' market, without a shred of evidence their produce is any fresher than my local supermarket's. But it does get my money directly into the grower's hands.

Is the secret sauce olive oil or vinegar?

Quick splash: There is a school of thought that the normally silent partner in an olive oil discussion – the accompanying vinegar – is actually the food with direct health benefits.

*

Let's start with olive oil. The evidence suggests that the core value of olive oil is that it reduces heart risk by replacing saturated fat. It's worth saying here that if you're aiming to save calories in a low fat diet, there's little health benefit if what you do is replace saturated fat with refined carbs because they too can be toxic for your arteries. Extra virgin olive oil has the extra advantages of containing complex polyphenols in its own right as well as assisting other foods like tomatoes and capsicum to release their natural antioxidants during cooking or food preparation.

There's growing interest in vinegar, which used to be thought of as the tarty passenger in dressings. But there's much more to vinegar than that. It's probably been around for 10,000 years and sold commercially for 5000 years for pickling/ preservation, taste, therapeutics and hygiene. The traditional method involves a double fermentation process using fruit juices, first to produce alcohol and then acetic acid using acetic acid bacteria. These days there are industrial processes for making pure acetic acid but probably with fewer organics or bioactive substances in the mix. There is evidence that vinegar can have anti-tumour and anti-diabetic effects and for those of you quaffing on cider vinegar, it doesn't seem to have too different a bioactive profile from, say, wine vinegars, which may in fact have more. Professor Itsiopoulos argues that vinegar's effects are at least in part on the microbiome and bowel-bugs' by-products such as short-chain fatty acids.

So where does that leave us? Both extra virgin olive oil and vinegar are good for you. They probably work together like so many other foods and just because a little is good, it doesn't mean that more is better (no doubt to the quiet relief of all those nauseous cider vinegar drinkers out there). Remember that when you start to consume nutrients in large amounts, they start to behave like drugs rather than foods, and by that I mean they might not work as intended and have side effects.

The secret sauce is actually complexity and diversity.

Vegan fasting – just what you've been waiting for

#donttellmichaelmosley

Here's the quick takeaway on this. Deny yourself meat, fish and dairy every Monday and Thursday.

Now for the longer version, which requires a bit of mythbusting.

*

Research has found that as Greek Australians age, they become more religious and one of the dominant features of

Greek Orthodoxy is the huge number of fast days there are in the calendar. We Jews only have one major fast day (Yom Kippur) and a handful of minor ones but as I've implied, if you want to live long and healthily, you won't find the recipe in the Jewish diet – at least not the Russian version of it. But the Greeks, that's another matter. If you're devout, you could be fasting for about 100 days a year. Not a Yom Kippur thing where you don't eat or drink for 25 hours; no, most Greek Orthodox fasts are effectively vegan fasts, where, especially on the islands, for a day they don't eat meat, fish or dairy, just plant-based foods, usually grown in their backyards. When researchers look at the plant content of the Greek traditional diet – especially the Cretan one – it's strongly coloured by these plant-only religious fast days, and when scientists try to rate your diet with questionnaires about the way you eat, they almost never take into account the cultural pattern and its potentially profound influence.

And the tantalising possibility is that vegan fasting dates back to the Stone Age.

#donttellPeteEvans

The paleo myth

Quick mythbust: There is no Palaeolithic diet. The Stone Age pattern of living varied according to the physical environment and the fasting associated with it may not be what you think.

*

The usual narrative about fasting starts at the Stone Age – the Palaeolithic era of early humankind. You know the story.

It's feast and famine. Days of eating very little followed by gorging on a hunted animal. This meant that humans who had genes which allowed them to adapt to this cycle of plenty and deprivation would have had a survival advantage. These genes almost certainly facilitated the storage of excess calories easily to get them through the tough times, but that's left us all with an Achilles' heel in times of plenty. Most of us are too good at storing excess calories, especially in our abdomens or on our bums and thighs, and some of us – for example those of South Asian ethnicity – do it even better, which is why they suffer the effects of obesity at a lower BMI than Caucasians.

It may not all be genetic, by the way. Research on the bugs in our bowel has found that obese people have a different, much less diverse microbiome than leaner people. No-one's sure whether obesity does that to the bowel bugs or if people destined to be obese have a microbiome that's very good at harvesting calories and sending them back into the body. That's led to the hypothesis that there's such a thing as a 'thin' microbiome. How you'd acquire that from a thin person is potentially disgusting (#eatshit).

The Palaeolithic diet is misunderstood and romanticised. Just remember, before you jump into the latest paleo fad, that people in the Stone Age lived to their late 20s or early 30s and there weren't many older people around at all. Life expectancy has improved by at least 240 per cent since and while most of that has been gained fairly steadily over the last 150 years, it looks as though it's stalling. So we can't be complacent and there is room for improvement. The question is whether the answer lies 20,000 years ago?

Well, maybe part of it.

Palaeolithic humans were no different from us today in that they too had a dietary pattern moulded by culture, climate and the physical environment. Someone living on the lush, subtropical African savannah was in a very different pattern from someone living in a cave near the Arctic Circle, where it was too cold to go outside several months of the year and when they did go out, there were few plants to be found and they were probably chronically vitamin D deficient. That's without talking about the constant risk of violent death and the debilitating stress of having to conform to complex social rules. So it's ludicrous to talk about a Palaeolithic diet and how wonderful it is.

For most of human history, fasting hasn't been a luxury promoted by diet books. It's been better known as going hungry. Some researchers believe a key to survival was our body clock which helped us adapt to long periods of darkness where hunting, gathering and eating were difficult. On top of that, there are molecular mechanisms in our cells which either speed or slow ageing processes and fasting seems to tilt the scales towards ageing prevention.

Given the proximity to Africa and the gradual movement of humans to the Middle East and around the Mediterranean, it wouldn't be surprising if remnants of the Stone Age pattern survived, embedded in the foundations of Greek culture.

Vegan fasting could well date back to before we learned to tame animals and grasses and grow them for our tables. Prior to agriculture, when we foraged for plants and stalked animals to kill, we generally wouldn't have starved between meat meals. We'd have had the foraged grains, root vegetables and occasionally leafy greens to keep us going. Vegan by necessity, not by choice, and you can imagine a cultural heritage which aims to remind us that we are not entitled to plenty and we need to remember what we came from.

You won't find randomised trials of vegan fasting – at least not yet – and when people have been put on trials of the Mediterranean diet, fast days and veggie gardens understandably haven't been included.

Doesn't mean they're not worth a go.

16/8 and 5:2 … when hunger is a luxury

Fast fasting takeaway: It depends on why you're doing it. For weight loss, intermittent fasting or restricted eating times are about the same as a regular calorie/portion-controlled diet and likely no better at keeping the weight off long term. If you're doing it for health, then from animal studies and some human research, the metabolic stress of fasting is probably good for your body. It improves the action of insulin in keeping your blood sugar down, may reduce heart risk factors and also suppresses the chemical messengers which can make cancers grow. It might also help nerve growth in the brain. Not much harm unless you're on diabetic drugs which could increase the risk of hypoglycaemia (low blood sugar). Interestingly, one of the features of fasting which could help your blood pressure and coronary risk is called 'fasting-induced natiuresis' (sodium excretion). For reasons which aren't clear, fasting can make your kidneys remove salt (sodium) from the blood and excrete it in the urine. It also produces a ketosis (see Keto … Or Low Carb … Or Is It that You Want to Be Ripped?).

*

Declaration of interest: I've always battled with my appetite. If I'm at a drinks party I can only devote 50 per cent of my brain to the chat because the other half of my brain has to be fully deployed to stop me gorging myself on the nibbles and if there's a buffet, I'm a goner. For a while I went to a dietician, renowned for her straight talking and brutal honesty. At the first visit she weighed me then tut-tutted, measured my waist circumference then sighed in an exasperated way and took a long dietary history then shook her head. At the end of this I sat waiting for what I assumed would be a nuanced weight loss regime. What I got instead was (you have to imagine a South African accent): 'Norman, you eat a lot. You're going to be very hungry.' Too true and it worked, at least for a few years.

Hunger is a rare experience for most of us. We tend to eat out of habit; it's 12.30 p.m. so it must be time for lunch, etc. Yet when we do allow ourselves a bit of hunger, it actually feels okay, and many people can tell when they're in a burn (catabolic state) versus laying down fat (anabolic). Going without food for a while isn't a new idea and, as I said earlier, it's been part of life since humans evolved and has become part of many religions. In recent years it's been popularised as intermittent fasting (e.g. the 5:2 day diet) or restricted eating times (e.g. the 16/8 hour diet). In case you're the only person in the known universe who hasn't bought a Michael Mosley book, the 5:2 diet in its latest form involves two days a week of very low calorie intake at around 800 calories. The 16/8 involves 16 hours of fasting with eating restricted to the following eight hours. Both create what many lab scientists believe is beneficial metabolic stress. For weight loss, the research suggests there's not a lot to choose between them. Both tend to make you a bit ketotic, which means you're burning fat for energy (as well as protein from your muscles). The advantage of the vegan fasting concept is that you're consuming highly nutrient dense foods, with a lot of roughage (fibre) and not too many calories.

One area of debate is whether you really can eat anything you like during your eating times in either the 5:2 or 16/8 pattern and it's likely that's not the case, but the evidence is weak since when you're ketotic, you tend to lose your appetite anyway.

For some people, the 16/8 may be easier to maintain, especially if breakfast is a meal you find easy to miss, although a recent randomised trial showed no benefit compared to three structured meals.

How important is breakfast, really?

Declaration of interest – it's my favourite meal of the day: double-shot latte, reading the papers, meeting people, another double-shot latte, trying not to order poached eggs for the third day in a row, ordering the fancy porridge (why do I do that when it spoils the morning?), sourdough toast when I'm not on low carbs. My vegan fasting day breakfast is roasted tomatoes, hummus and avocado with several espressos. (Yep, I know ... doesn't sound like much of a fast, does it?)

Breakfast takeaway: Primary and high-school age children and adolescents should always have breakfast. Kids who skip breakfast tend to be fatter, overeat later in the day and have lower academic performance (see caveats below, particularly on breakfast content). That's definitely true of kids who are nutritionally compromised. For the rest of us, it depends on what you're aiming for. If your drivers are social contact, need for caffeine overdosing and having to feed a poached egg and current affairs addiction, then fine. If it's weight loss, then the balance of evidence tips in favour of skipping breakfast as that tends to reduce your total calorie consumption.

Let's start with kids

When I trained in paediatrics, the absolute necessity of breakfast for children was dogma and, like many things in medicine, there's a lot of anecdotal dogma backed up by rock-solid belief. But when you look for the evidence, it's a bit more like blancmange than rocks. There are heaps of studies, very few of which are high quality and many of which don't properly allow for other features of kids who don't eat breakfast. For instance, how financially stressed the family is, whether there's a functioning kitchen at home, family disruption and culture, and availability of high nutrient, low energy dense foods all play a role in whether a child does well in life independent of breakfast. However, when researchers combine the results of various studies, it does seem that breakfast makes a child or adolescent more alert during the morning; that complex carbs are better than refined ones, perhaps because a slow rise in blood sugar prevents a mid-morning dip; and that if a breakfast is not filled with empty calories, there is a link with lower levels of obesity. Some US school-based breakfast feeding programmes have been accused of making obesity worse because they feed the kids rubbish.

Now for you and me

At the time of writing, probably the best review of the evidence on the impact of breakfast on weight gain or loss is from Monash University in Melbourne, Australia. They found that the quality of studies was not very good but when they sifted out the best, the balance of evidence was that skipping breakfast resulted in an average reduction of 200 calories per day. Everything else being constant, that's a kilo weight loss over five weeks. People did tend to eat more at other meals but not enough to abolish the benefit. As to cognitive performance, there is some evidence in adults that we're less on the ball after skipping breakfast but maybe that effect disappears if you exercise before work. There's also a little evidence that a breakfast without cereals has longer-lasting effects.

So if 16/8 is your thing, looks like the door is open.

Keto ... or low carb ... or is it that you want to be ripped?

#badbreath

Small bite: Keto diets, like paleos, vary a bit according to whose book you buy. Again it depends on what your aim is. A well-designed, properly supervised ketogenic diet can help children with severe epilepsy. It may improve diabetes control and there are tantalising suggestions of dementia prevention. If you're after weight loss, then a very low-calorie diet will induce ketosis – the aim of a ketogenic diet – but you risk nutrient deficiency unless you're very careful or use a reliable meal substitute. Low carb diets can be ketogenic but the long-term benefit depends on what you exchange your carbs for. If fat is the replacement, you may eventually die to regret it. Plant-based foods should be the replacement food. If you want to be ripped, ask yourself why? In men (or women) it can be muscle dysmorphia (see A Warning About Getting Ripped) – a body image issue – sometimes leading to a version of anorexia nervosa. Anyone with diabetes needs to talk to their doctor about a ketogenic diet because you may need to have your treatment adjusted regularly to avoid low blood sugars.

*

Declaration of interest: I gave up on the dream of a six-pack years ago and I don't want to be ripped but I reckon like a lot of men, I don't like my body too much and have struggled with weight since childhood. As such I have tried a very low calorie diet carefully controlled for nutrients, with added leafy greens and protein, and therefore have firsthand experience of ketosis. You feel crap for the first three days, then what the books say is true, there's an energy bounce which is either relative, because you feel good again after the days of crap-ness or it's a real increase. You do lose weight fast, especially if you keep weight and aerobic training going, but it's not sustainable and may make weight loss harder next time around. Anyway, enough of the anecdote.

Here's a biology primer which you probably don't need unless you're the one person in a million who hasn't bought a keto diet book or Googled 'ketogenic diet'. If you think you know it all, skip the next two pars; and if you're a biochemist and do know it all, feel free to send me your critique.

The basic unit of energy in our bodies is carbon, biological coal, which means, by the by, that each of us is a greenhouse gas generator. In a healthy, well-nourished body the carbon comes from glucose. Carbohydrates, which are molecules combining carbon, hydrogen and oxygen – hence the name carbo-hydr-ate – are knitted webs of glucose and other sugars. Table sugar (sucrose), for example, is a fusion of glucose and fructose. The more refined a carbohydrate is, the easier it can be turned into the pure energy of glucose. If we have glucose to spare, it's stored as a carbohydrate called glycogen in the liver and muscles. Once the glycogen stores are full, excess glucose is turned into fat. The main job of the hormone insulin is to move glucose from the blood into cells to be used as fuel. Since the body is designed for survival, it has back-ups on back-ups. If we stop eating for a while or exercise without eating, then our glycogen stores are used up. At that point there are only two stores of energy left: amino acids from the proteins in muscle and fatty acids … well, from fat. But breaking down protein and fat for energy is a less efficient process than generating glucose from glycogen. Proteins are made up of amino acids and when muscle is broken down to amino acids for energy, some of the amino acids are used for glucose production while other amino acids tend to be ketogenic … they're used to make ketone bodies, an alternate source of energy. Hold that thought while I get on to fats. If you're bored, not a fan of delayed gratification and need the punchline right now, skip the next paragraph.

While the building blocks of proteins are amino acids, the basic components of fats are fatty acids. Fatty acids have around 16 times the amount of carbon than glucose, which is the reason fat has a much higher calorie content than carbs. An anabolic state is when amino acids and fatty acids are being turned into muscle and fat. A catabolic state is when proteins and fat are being broken down to amino acids and fatty acids, usually for energy. Like amino acids, fatty acids can be turned into glucose or ketone bodies or both. Calorie restriction produces a catabolic state. The aim with weight reduction is to minimise muscle loss and focus on getting your fat stores into a catabolic state. Ketogenesis is the catabolic process which leads to the production of ketone bodies – substances which can be used by your body for carbon when there isn't much glucose around. Excess ketone bodies are removed from the body in the urine, which is one reason why dehydration is a risk on a ketogenic diet and why a lot of the initial dramatic weight loss is water. Ketone bodies also can make you nauseous and your breath smell (one of the three main ketone bodies is acetone – think nail polish remover). So to preserve muscle you need plenty of protein and you need to keep carbs very low to force fat use (5–10 per cent of total calories).

One of the ways the body compensates for a low-calorie diet is to increase hunger and appetite and one of the sells for a keto diet is that it suppresses appetite. Don't get your hopes up too much, though. Research at the University of Sydney, Australia, has found that ketosis doesn't actually reduce appetite, rather it blunts the increase in appetite which comes with weight loss. Frustratingly, appetite returns in full force when you 're-feed' and sometimes even with a single glass of wine. The good news from the Sydney researchers is that you may not need full ketosis to get the appetite-blunting effect, which suggests that the carb reduction could possibly be less vicious.

Animal research has shown that, within reason, metabolic stress is good for the body and ketosis is certainly a state of metabolic stress (at its most extreme in the highly dangerous ketosis of someone with type 1 diabetes who's lost control of their disease). This metabolic stress appears to renovate your mitochondria, which are the power stations in our cells and whose deterioration appears to drive ageing processes. Metabolic stress also seems to be good for DNA methylation, which influences the shape and function of our genes and changes the way they work. It's called an epigenetic effect because there's no mutation (change to the DNA sequence) involved. Epigenetics is a hot field in biology and partly explains how the environment and the ways we live can change us profoundly.

There's been a lot of interest in the effects of a ketogenic diet on the brain given that it can dampen severe epilepsy in children. There is preliminary and tantalising evidence that people with mild cognitive impairment could be helped by a ketogenic diet, perhaps because it bypasses the mechanism in brain cells which uses glucose as energy and which may be faulty in Alzheimer's disease. There's a long way to go in this but anecdotally people on a keto diet feel energised and alert when it kicks in.

Long-term low carb intake may be problematic. One of the best studies on this came out of Harvard and the University of Minnesota in the US. They followed the health of a group of 15,000 adults for about 25 years and added data from seven other studies involving more than 400,000 participants. They excluded people who were on very low or very high calorie diets, and compared the carbohydrate intake of the remaining participants with their chances of dying prematurely. In addition, the researchers looked at what people swapped their carbs for if they were on a low carb diet. Controlling for variables which could have affected the results, they found that there was a Goldilocks situation with carbs. Low and high carb intake were both associated with higher chances of dying prematurely. The Goldilocks intake over a 25-year span was around 50 per cent of total calories but the risks with a low carb diet depended on what else they were eating. What they concluded was this:

> Low carbohydrate dietary patterns favouring animal-derived protein and fat sources, from sources such as lamb, beef, pork, and chicken, were associated with higher mortality, whereas those that favoured plant-derived protein and fat intake, from sources such as vegetables, nuts, peanut butter, and whole-grain breads, were associated with lower mortality (*Lancet Public Health.* 2018 Sep; 3(9): e419–e428).

Green is a good colour

Quick take: Colours matter in your food and green is good. What can I say that you don't know already? The more plants you eat as a proportion of your diet, the better. According to how plant based your dietary pattern is, you can lower your risks of diabetes, heart disease, some cancers and weight gain, and increase your chances of living longer in good shape. Much as you might identify yourself as vegetarian, vegan, lacto-vegetarian, lacto-ovo vegetarian, pescatarian, etc., unless you're doing it for moral, environmental and ethical reasons, which are perfectly legitimate, the labels don't matter. Think of it as a continuum where you want to aim for the greener end!

*

I'm often asked if there are risks from being a vegan. A few years ago I'd have said yes, because there weren't many food options for people who were strictly vegan and it was easy to end up eating a crap diet full of fat. After all, French fries and tomato ketchup are vegan but it's not a great way to live. In the last few years, though, chefs and food producers have responded amazingly to the growing number of people following a vegan dietary pattern. The diversity of vegan foods in the shops is impressive and diversity is at the core of a healthy diet. There are even upmarket vegan restaurants serving great, accessible dishes – as long as you can afford the bill. The main thing about a vegan diet is not to be any more restrictive than veganism requires. You need to be more attentive to what you consume than omnivores or vegetarians and make sure you're getting a daily dose of sun for vitamin D, lots of protein and iron, plenty of calcium-rich foods, and look out for your vitamin B12 intake. Vegans who are planning to fall pregnant might benefit ahead of time from some expert dietary advice before you conceive. In general, vegan diets are safe in pregnancy but there is a risk of micronutrient deficiency in the foetus unless you're careful.

The evidence is stronger for the benefits of vegetarianism because there have been more studies. The trouble with the data is that they're dominated by studies of Seventh-day Adventists, who have several lifestyle differences compared to the general population beyond their vegetarian diet. There's little doubt that Seventh-day Adventists live longer but when vegetarian diets alone (i.e. in non-Adventists) are looked at, the relationship with a longer life is weaker. It reaffirms the recurring theme that life is a package and diet is just one piece.

Is there a gene for garlic?

A taster: Taste and food preferences are strongly determined by the genes you've inherited from your parents, particularly when it comes to strong flavours like garlic. There are environmental influences as well, so it is possible to modify your and even kids' tastes despite the genes you've been born with. It's worth doing because the consumption of garlic and its cousins from the allium family – onions, leeks, shallots and chives – has been associated with lower rates of cancer, but you may need to grow your own to be sure you're getting the necessary goodies. Cooking with allium vegetables and extra virgin olive oil releases natural antioxidants and other healthy micronutrients.

*

Garlic and coffee are linked to healthy metabolic profiles – at least in women. A study of female twins in the UK matched the metabolic profiles in their urine of seven different dietary patterns, including high fruit and vegetable intake, and low calorie, garlic and coffee intake. Garlic and coffee were linked to a healthier metabolic profile which relates particularly to reduced type 2 diabetes and coronary risk. The relationship of weekly coffee and garlic intake to this healthy metabolic profile was between 44 per cent and 62 per cent genetic.

The same research group in London that did this study has also found that a taste for garlic is significantly genetic. They found a genetic effect for food and distinctive taste preferences of around 50 per cent. Their conclusion was that we naturally drift to what we prefer, but the fact that the genetic contribution is only around 50 per cent leaves a lot of room for the environment in which we grow up being able to influence what we like and dislike by learned eating habits and patterns.

Some studies have linked the allium family to lower rates of cancer, including tumours of head and neck, oesophagus, stomach, bowel and breast. They may also enhance the effects of treatments. No-one is too sure which compounds might be involved but they're thought to be natural antioxidants like flavonoids and sulphur-containing compounds. But if you think this is simple, one study of garlic has found that whether these compounds are in the garlic you buy in your supermarket depends on the kind of garlic, whether there has been water stress, the adequacy of fertiliser and the colour of the skin. White-skinned bulbs, for example, according to the study, have higher levels of natural antioxidants. Purple bulbs were higher in vitamin C. Sulphur levels tend to depend on where the garlic has been grown and how much sulphur was used in the fertiliser. And if that isn't complicated enough, late harvesting also helps with the sulphur content, which of course affects taste and odour. Storage time is important, with the bioactive substances starting to disappear after 6–8 weeks. In terms of cooking, it seems that stir-frying garlic is best for retaining the active compounds, which is another reason to cook your garlic and onions in olive oil first before adding the other ingredients.

Speaking of cooking, there is also evidence that cooking other vegetables with the allium family helps to release micronutrients that might otherwise be locked up. The added element which makes a difference is extra virgin olive oil.

That's a bit of a warning to people who are dedicated raw food eaters. You may be missing out on some important nutrients associated with cooking. Remember, Palaeolithic men and women only lived to their late 20s or early 30s.

Allium vegetables are associated with various benefits in addition to cancer prevention. There is evidence of protection against heart disease and kidney damage.

Red is a very good colour

Quick take: Red and reddish vegetables are potent sources of natural antioxidants like beta carotene and lycopene, which have a particularly strong antioxidant effect. Chopping the vegetables and cooking them in extra virgin olive oil releases these antioxidants and makes them more available for absorption into the body. Cooking vegetables together heightens the effect (for example, sofrito – the cooked mixture of extra virgin olive oil, onions, garlic, tomatoes – sometimes carrots – and herbs).

*

The vegetables and fruits we're talking here include tomatoes, watermelon, capsicum, carrots and beetroot, and the antioxidants include lycopene (especially in tomatoes and watermelon), beta carotene and flavonoids. Beetroot contains betalain pigments, which also have antioxidant activity.

Why does it matter? Well, repeated studies have shown that low levels of carotenoids and lycopene are associated with heart disease, premature death and poor cognitive function. That doesn't mean it's cause and effect but changing your dietary pattern to boost their levels isn't linked to harm, so why not do it? (See Be Bioactive: On Antioxidants and Tubas for caveats about antioxidants from supplements rather than food.)

While studies have shown that red, orange and purple vegetables in their raw state have a variety of antioxidants, how you cook them counts, at least when it comes to lycopenes and other carotenoids.

Experiments done in Melbourne, Australia, compared chopped tomatoes cooked with and without extra virgin olive oil and found that the people in the study absorbed more lycopene when olive oil was used. The same group did this with grilled red capsicum after drizzling with extra virgin olive oil. Other studies have suggested that this is specific to olive oil and does not seem to happen with sunflower oil.

It's also been shown that when carrots are chopped and cooked, their beta carotene is more bio-available, and when you cook carrots and tomatoes together, lycopene becomes more available.

This culinary chemistry-set all comes together in sofrito, the basic sauce in Mediterranean cooking, using diced tomatoes, onions and garlic lightly fried in extra virgin olive oil. Some cuisines include carrot. In one experiment with sofrito, a group of antioxidants from tomato was increased and made more bioavailable compared to raw tomato, and the onion helped to preserve the effect.

The other benefit of many of these vegetables is that they make the platelets in your blood, which set off blood clots, less sticky. That's likely to be one reason vegetables are good for heart health.

Be bioactive: on antioxidants and tubas

#saveyourmoney

The message: We do a deal with the devil to stay alive. Without oxygen we can't survive much longer than four minutes. Yet oxygen is also a poison. It 'rusts' our tissues, drives ageing and is part of the process which causes blocked arteries, dementia and possibly even affects cancer. This 'rusting' is called oxidation. So, in theory, substances which slow or block oxidation – antioxidants – should be good for us. Indeed they are good for us in food, especially when cooked in certain ways, but there's no evidence of benefit from antioxidant *supplements*. You see, diversity matters. Our food contains hundreds of different antioxidants which do a lot more than stop rusting. Supplements will never be able to mimic that at the right dose with the right chemistry. Save your money on them and spend it on extra virgin olive oil and red, purple and orange vegetables, watermelon for dessert and a Mediterranean cookbook.

*

Here's another biology primer. If you can't be bothered reading it, no sweat, skip the next two paragraphs although, in my defence, it will help you understand the rationale for how you might increase your effective antioxidant consumption and reduce your intake of pro-oxidants, the substances which speed up rusting and ageing.

When we eat, the food gets broken down in our intestines and absorbed into the bloodstream. When we breathe, the oxygen from the air is transferred to the blood passing through our lungs. The blood then transports the nutrients and oxygen to cells throughout our bodies. Cells are the biological bricks, if you like, of our blood, muscles, brain and other organs, and are surrounded by a kind of shrink wrap called a membrane. So as blood passes by our cells, the nutrients and oxygen are transported across the membrane into the cell 'soup'. In this 'soup' are tiny machines called mitochondria which make the energy that fuels the cell to do its work. As part of that process, the mitochondria eject waste in the form of what are called 'reactive oxygen species' – toxic forms of oxygen – which, if not mopped up, can damage the tissues of the body. Another way these species can be produced is by white blood cells if the immune system is activated by infection or disease. By the way, these mitochondria do other important stuff. They help cells to talk to each other and can tell them when it's time to die. That's called 'apoptosis' and while it sounds awful, it's actually part of maintaining healthy tissue and preventing cancer (which can be a failure of apoptosis – in other words cells don't die when they should).

Another name for these reactive oxygen species is 'oxidants' and they create what's called 'oxidative stress'. To counter that, the body has an army of antioxidants which help to slow down or stop oxidative stress, but in fact it's a bit unfair to call them antioxidants because that's only part of what they do. They help signals to be sent within cells and between them, and have other important functions which are quite specific to each antioxidant and little to do with mopping up oxidants. For that reason, some researchers prefer to call them 'bioactives' rather than antioxidants.

You can start to see what an unreasonable expectation it is for vitamin C or E or beta carotene or selenium supplements to make a difference. It's like throwing a very large tuba into an orchestra thinking it'll make for sweeter music. You need the whole band in concert. It can't be achieved by a single instrument. That's why food and cuisine and even factors like exercise are so important. Coming back to the tuba, its sound – the dose of the tuba in the orchestra – may be too big, too powerful, and knock out the balance between the instruments. More is not better. Dose and balance matter with bioactives and there's even a little (and controversial) evidence with some supplements like vitamin C, that in high doses they can turn from an antioxidant into a pro-oxidant. In the next section, you'll find out how certain kinds of cooking also produce pro-oxidants. Tobacco and saturated fat are pro-oxidants, as is too much sunlight.

Excessive oxidative stress is behind ageing, dementia and heart disease and gets caught up in cancer. For instance, with heart disease, the way the bad form of cholesterol – low density lipoprotein (LDL) cholesterol – causes atherosclerosis (which by the way starts in childhood and progresses through life) is that the LDL experiences oxidative stress and becomes oxidised. It's actually the oxidised form of LDL in the artery wall which triggers inflammation, scarring and thickening, leading to narrowed, vulnerable arteries in the heart and brain, and increasing the risk of heart attacks and strokes when you grow up. And if that wasn't enough, tobacco smoke – either yours or breathing in someone else's – is a pro-oxidant which makes it easier for the LDL to become oxidised.

Yep. The bastards work together.

There are several families of bioactives including carotenoids (e.g. beta carotene and lycopene), flavonoids and biophenols, and they are sometimes co-dependent. By now it should be no surprise to you that when you look at populations, low levels of lycopene and other carotenoids are associated with lower cognitive function and premature death from all causes. It should also be no surprise that you need to have a dietary pattern which includes as many bioactives as possible in the most absorbable way. Hence the value of cooking in extra virgin olive oil which itself has lots of biophenols and usually replaces saturated fat. Even the microbiome gets in on the act by producing butyrate which, along with other bioactives, drives a biochemical pathway called Nfr2/ARE which reduces oxidative stress and inflammation, slows tissue ageing, protects the brain and helps with a healthy level of cell death (apoptosis).

Finally, if I haven't convinced you about antioxidant supplements, there have been large-scale and repeated analyses of clinical trials which show no benefits. One suggested a slightly higher risk of dying but that probably wasn't a valid conclusion. Even so, you've better things to do with your money.

Now to the colour brown.

Brown isn't such a good colour

Quick take: Cut back a bit on roasting, BBQ-ing and grilling – high-heat cooking – and move to slower, lower temperature, moist cooking. High heat browns food. Browning and high-temperature cooking causes something called the Maillard reaction, which is tasty and results from a chemical reaction between proteins, fats and sugars. Caramelisation from heating sugars by themselves is similar. There is debate about this among researchers, but the concern is the production of substances called advanced glycation end products (AGEs) which induce oxidative stress (see Be Bioactive: On Antioxidants and Tubas) and are linked to diabetes and other chronic diseases. AGEs can occur in high fat foods even before cooking.

*

This is yet another issue where cause and effect is hard to prove. In looking at groups of people, those with high AGEs have higher rates of heart disease, type 2 diabetes and dementia. In animal studies, you can increase the risk of heart disease by giving AGEs and block the effect by blocking the AGEs. There is also evidence that some AGEs can hang around in your body and accumulate.

The best way to produce AGEs is by using high temperature, dry cooking. Conversely, you can reduce your exposure by slow cooking with moisture, and possibly by marinating your food in lemon juice or vinegar before cooking since an acidic environment also inhibits AGE production. Dietary patterns like the Med diet are lower in AGEs.

One study compared cooking scrambled eggs over a medium or high heat. Medium heat produced half the amount of AGEs. Likewise roasted or grilled chicken has around four times the level of AGEs compared to poached or steamed chicken. Interestingly, microwaving was reasonably neutral and letting beef sit in an acidic marinade for an hour halved the level of AGEs after cooking. Foods which are low in protein, such as vegetables, whole grains and fruit, have low AGE levels even after cooking.

People who already have type 2 diabetes seem to be even more vulnerable to AGEs in their diet, as are people whose kidneys aren't working well – often in fact because of diabetes (AGEs are excreted from the body in urine).

Immune boosters, *Pulp Fiction* and *The Sopranos*

Quick lift: Although a lot of people will take your money saying their product will enhance your immune system, it's not complete bullshit. Here are the things for which there's some evidence for boosting your immune system: immunisation, including the BCG vaccine for tuberculosis; an anti-inflammatory, micronutrient-rich diet like the Mediterranean dietary pattern; moderate to vigorous exercise; short-term stress; and probiotics (maybe).

*

I got a surprise with this one. I thought it was mythology until I really got into the evidence.

A biology primer here would take the rest of the book. The main things you need to know are that there are only a few categories of moving parts in your immune system but there's a lot going on in each category: the 'snitch' (or dendritic) cells which recognise invaders and dob them in; the first responder white blood cells (B cells) which produce antibodies; 'Harvey Keitel' white blood cells (didn't you ever see *Pulp Fiction*?) which clean up the mess (macrophages); 'Tony Soprano' white blood cells (T cells) which bear a grudge and have a long memory for past invaders; and 'Godfather' white blood cells which attack invaders themselves (Killer T cells). Then there are the consiglieri – chemical messengers who meet regularly and advise the immune system on how to respond. The messengers go by various names including interleukins and chemokines. Sometimes the immune system can be turned on when there's no infection, for example: when a rogue cancer cell appears and needs to be mopped up, a lousy diet loaded with saturated fat inflames the immune system, or with an autoimmune disease like rheumatoid arthritis. These latter two produce chronic inflammation which accelerates ageing, makes it easier for cholesterol to damage your arteries and probably increases the risk of cancer.

So … be careful what you wish for. Just blindly boosting the immune system isn't always a good thing. For instance, you don't want more chronic inflammation.

Here are a few things which are known or strongly suspected of boosting the immune system in a good way.

Immunisation in itself is an immune booster and one in particular, against tuberculosis (the BCG), appears to have a generally enhancing effect on how well your immune system works. That's why it was trialled in health care workers to see if it protected them against the COVID-19 virus, and a suspected reason why people in low-income countries with high rates of TB seemed to have low rates of COVID.

Nutrition profoundly affects the immune system in a variety of ways. A poor diet, low in protein and micronutrients, especially as you age, reduces the effectiveness of the immune system in fighting off infections.

The dietary pattern I talked about earlier in the Rate Your Diet section is strongly associated with an immune system which is not wasting its energy on chronic inflammation and all the havoc that can cause in your arteries and other parts of your body, including your brain. The ageing effects of this inflammation are also linked to a decline in immune function, so by inference, a low inflammatory diet is actually an immune booster. The problem starts in childhood and what appears to happen is that an unhealthy meal alerts the immune system as it's absorbed in the intestine. Researchers have compared the inflammatory effects of an egg and bacon kind of breakfast to one which includes food containing natural antioxidants such as polyphenols and found that the gut's immune system didn't react as much. Children who eat junk food have unhealthy levels of immune messengers which switch on inflammation compared to kids on a Mediterranean diet.

Obesity certainly switches on this damaging immune activity. If you have cancer, these immune effects can tone down the natural attack on cancer cells. Part of the effect of a micronutrient- and plant-rich diet is that it changes the bacteria in your gut which help to tune up and train your immune system.

Exercise also has a profound effect on your immune system. It was believed for a long time that elite athletes were immune deficient; in other words, that extreme exercise inhibited immune function. Part of the reason is that after sports events, athletes seemed more prone to upper respiratory infections. This is now thought to be a myth. Studies have not reliably found evidence of viral infections associated with the symptoms, nor indeed a true increase in symptoms at all, which appear to be more like irritation than infection. And, in any event, competitive athletes are often abnormally exposed to large numbers of people who might be carrying viruses themselves.

There's also been misinterpretation of a finding which suggested that the immune system was suppressed in the hours following extreme exertion. Instead, what happens is that in the first hour or so after intense exercise, the immune system goes into hyperdrive with lots of T cells flushed out into the bloodstream. Then the levels drop for a few hours and rather than an immune deficiency, this seems to be the army being told to deploy itself at points of entry such as the respiratory system and intestinal tract. It's thought that this helps clean up stray cancer cells and induce apoptosis, which is natural cell death and part of the heathy cycle of cell renewal throughout the body. This has been called 'exercise immunotherapy'.

Looking at responses to immunisation, people who exercise regularly develop a deeper level of immunity. Older people in structured exercise programmes have been shown to have significantly more competent immune systems and regular exercise seems to reduce what's becoming known as 'inflammageing'.

Short-lived episodes of stress are linked to a tuned-up immune system possibly through the effects of adrenaline, which may also be the reason intense exercise, such as high intensity interval training (HIIT), benefits the immune system. Chronic stress is a different matter. This is where you feel out of control of your life and work and find it hard to make your own decisions. Chronic stress is linked to immune suppression and perhaps even an increased risk of inflammation and cancer (see The Control Factor).

Probiotic supplements (as opposed to the prebiotic effects of a whole dietary pattern) have a little evidence to support an immune-enhancing effect, but the studies have been small and fragmented and not consistent when it comes to the actual content of the supplements. Different bacteria have specific effects and maybe not all are the ones you want.

Epigenetics rule: The good news is that a healthy dietary pattern, including exercise, is likely to change the way your genes work (epigenetic effects) in a way which can lock in longer term benefits.

Is butter that bad? The dairy paradox

Quick spread: Butter fits into the mould of this book, so to speak. Don't get confused by single nutrients. You've got to think about the whole food. Saturated fat intake is linked to an increased risk of coronary heart disease: angina, heart attacks and strokes. The logic should then follow that butter, which is 80 per cent fat and most of that saturated, is bad for your heart and arteries, along with other full-fat dairy products. Do as I do, if you like. I have full-fat milk in my coffee (life's too short to pollute coffee with soya or almond unless you're lactose intolerant or allergic) and happily consume Greek yoghurt. I rarely put anything on bread other than avocado but if a recipe requires some butter, I'll use it. The saturated fat story is nuanced.

*

I need to take you through this slowly because if you take it the wrong way, you'll be devouring high fat meats, grilled on the barbie, thinking it's okay. Well, it's not. But that doesn't mean that butter is off the menu.

Here's the story on saturated fat. What's happened is a revolution in thinking based on relatively recent research and that's caused confusion, especially if doctors and nutritionists haven't kept up to date.

Fat basics

#chooseyouroil

Measuring your fat intake by the amount of cholesterol in your food is pretty meaningless because it's not absorbed as cholesterol. It's broken down to building blocks for fat called fatty acids. What matters more are the kinds of fats you're eating. Trans fats from food processing are very unhealthy, and saturated fats moderately unhealthy but that depends on the food which the saturated fat comes from and what else is in your diet.

The cholesterol in your body is mostly manufactured by your liver. You need cholesterol because it keeps the membranes – the shrink wrap around our cells – in good shape and is also the raw material for some hormones and other essential substances. Cholesterol is not a single fat. It's a balance of good and bad which are themselves mixtures. The good mix is called HDL (high density lipoprotein) and is said to be 'good' because it can hoover up cholesterol from the arteries. Having said that, trials of drugs to raise HDL have been mostly unsuccessful. LDL (low density lipoprotein) cholesterol is the bad one and just to make it more complicated, it is a mixture of LDL particles of different sizes where the smallest are the most toxic when it comes to atherosclerosis, the disease which blocks arteries and makes them more fragile. Trials of medications to reduce LDL have shown a significantly reduced risk of heart attacks. There's a third mix of fats which reflect the fat content of your diet and are routinely measured in blood tests: triglycerides. High triglycerides can make your LDL particles smaller and therefore increase the risk of atherosclerosis. Weight loss reduces triglycerides and increases HDL. Smoking, saturated fat and trans fats all make things worse.

Why doctors can be confused is that they may have missed the results of research over the years. Originally the equation was simple. All cholesterol was bad and caused heart disease. Then they discovered the good and bad parts of the story. Tobacco cessation and the introduction of indoor smoking bans in Scotland in 2006, and in 2007 in England, Wales and Northern Ireland alone reduced non-smokers' exposure to other people's smoke, and made a huge difference to heart disease death rates. Public Health England's Local Tobacco Control Profiles network show that by 2015 heart disease death rates had fallen by more than 20 per cent. Public health authorities also tried to eliminate trans fats from food production and they made saturated fats the evil players which had to be reduced at all costs. The trouble was that trials of reducing saturated fats in the diet were disappointing and it took a while to find out why. Critics said the lack of results meant that saturated fats being a problem was wrong. But when researchers examined the trials in more detail, an interesting pattern emerged. If people went on a low saturated fat diet and replaced the calories from fat in their diet with carbohydrates, there was no benefit. However, if they replaced saturated fats with olive oil or polyunsaturated fat, there was a reduction in heart disease risk.

Refined carbohydrates are not good for the heart, nor are animal-origin saturated fats, whereas polyunsaturated fat lowers cholesterol levels and extra virgin olive oil has lots of goodies which help to prevent atherosclerosis, particularly if it's used in cooking.

What they also found was that just having a mildly raised cholesterol level did not necessarily condemn you to an early death or always need statins to lower the levels. Most people who die of a heart attack or stroke have blood pressure which is a bit raised, cholesterol which isn't sky high, they might be a bit older, have a family history, and have fat around the belly with a bigger waist circumference than is healthy. This bundle of factors can be brought together and calculated by a health professional, such as your GP, into a QRISK assessment, which looks at a number of health factors that together give a picture of your risk of having a heart attack or stroke in the next five or ten years. In people who have not got diabetes or heart disease already, a QRISK is a better guide to whether you need medications like statins or blood pressure lowering drugs.

Back to butter and the dairy paradox

Full-fat dairy products like butter contain a lot of saturated fat, so they should be bad for you, but the evidence that's true is lacking. The reason is – yet again – that doctors and others have focused on a single nutrient – saturated fat – and ignored the fact that fats come from whole foods and their effects are influenced by cuisine, whether we're eating too many calories overall, the state of our microbiome, and whether we're experiencing a lot of oxidative stress (see Be Bioactive).

Reviews of the evidence on butter consumption from several countries involving more than 600,000 people found a slightly increased risk of dying prematurely from any cause. Followed over many years, people had a one per cent increased risk of dying prematurely from any cause for every added 14-g portion of butter consumed per day. But paradoxically, the studies found no link between butter consumption and heart disease, and maybe a protective effect against type 2 diabetes.

The reasons are not known but it could be that the mix of saturated fats in dairy isn't that bad. In addition, dairy foods have other fats such as mono and polyunsaturates as well as bioactive antioxidants, all of which may counteract the negative effects of saturated fats in dairy products. In addition, fermented dairy products such as yoghurt may influence the microbiome and inflammation in a beneficial way.

So ... the most reasonable spin on this is that butter is fairly neutral when it comes to our health, but it's still the case that if you were to replace butter with extra virgin olive oil, polyunsaturated fats and nuts, and not with potatoes or sugar, the result would probably be better for you. So don't believe those who argue that butter is so good for you, you should slop it into your coffee. You're not that bulletproof.

What about other foods containing saturated fat?

Well, red meat appears not to have the goodies that dairy has which protect against the effects of saturated fats.

Coconut products contain varying amounts of saturated fat depending on whether it's the cream (more) or milk (less). The structure of coconut saturated fats suggests they could be toxic for the arteries and heart, and there appear to be fewer protective compounds than dairy unless you're consuming extra virgin coconut products, which may behave more like olive oil than butter. Studies have found that coconut consumption increases both good and bad cholesterol levels but there isn't a lot of reliable evidence one way or the other on actual heart disease.

Finally, remember that any fat is high in calories so if your aim is controlling your weight, you don't want to go over the top with any of them.

Which milk? (This is the farting bit)

Quick sip: You'd have to pin me down and tube-feed me to get me to drink a soya or almond latte. I'll take the risk and have full-fat milk in my coffee, but as you now know from the dairy paradox, that may not be as much of a risk as you've been led to believe. Anyway, there are so many different types of milk these days that it's hard to keep up but unless you have an allergy to cow's milk, or are lactose intolerant, or are vegan, or – perfectly rationally – want to minimise the carbon footprint of your morning muesli and coffees, nutritionally, cow's milk is pretty good.

*

The milks from cows, goats or sheep have a complex mixture of fats, carbohydrates, vitamins and minerals including calcium, phosphate and vitamin B12, including all the essential amino acids. They're the protein building blocks which can't be made by your body and therefore must be sourced from food.

Full-fat cow's milk has a fat content of about 3.5–3.8 per cent per serving size, compared to semi-skimmed at 1.5–1.8 per cent and skimmed at 0.3 per cent.

Lactose intolerance: The most common symptoms are bloating, farting, tummy pain and maybe loose motions after consuming dairy foods. The reason is that the enzyme which breaks down lactose – lactase – is deficient in your intestine, which means undigested lactose hits your colon where the bacteria hoe into the lactose. But that's inefficient and generates gas. There are many causes of lactase deficiency. The commonest is genetic. Depending on your ethnic heritage, you can be born with low lactase levels – for instance, people from parts of Asia, the southern Mediterranean and Africa. Gastroenteritis may cause it temporarily as can bowel surgery, as well as coeliac and Crohn's disease and cancer treatment. Usually your story gives the clue to the diagnosis, especially if reducing the lactose in your diet relieves symptoms. A breath test can help but can be falsely negative or positive because of medications, smoking and even exercise just beforehand, so sometimes a lactose challenge test is used. Interestingly, lactase levels may decline through life and therefore someone might develop symptoms in later adulthood. People with lactose intolerance often tolerate some dairy but soon learn what their limit is.

Cow's milk allergy: Symptoms such as a rash or difficulty breathing after eating dairy suggest it's a cow's milk allergy and need to be checked out (avoiding dairy until you do). It's pretty unusual for cow's milk allergy to start in adulthood but that doesn't mean it can't.

Could it be irritable bowel syndrome (IBS)? It'd be a

shame to limit your dairy intake if what you have is IBS and sometimes it's hard to differentiate. IBS comes and goes with various foods, not just dairy, and sometimes hits you out of the blue. IBS also usually alternates between constipation and explosive motions, whereas the effects of lactose intolerance on your bowel motions is almost always just diarrhoea.

Dairy alternatives: The main alternatives are soya or almond milk. There's rice and coconut milk, too, but they're not in the same nutritional league as the more common plant-based options.

Researchers from McGill University in Canada published an article in 2017 saying that 'while plant-based milks are popularly advertised as healthy and wholesome, little research has been done in understanding the nutritional implications of consuming these beverages in short and long term'. While soya milk has reportedly been overtaken by almond milk as the most consumed alternative, soya products have been used for centuries in many parts of the world, which you might find reassuring. The Canadian researchers concluded that soya is the best alternative because it's so rich in protein. That might matter for people following a vegan diet. However, some of us are put off by the 'beany' flavour of soya milk, which might explain the take-up of almond milk over the past decade.

You've got to be a bit careful about almond milk. To soften the taste, it can be pumped full of sweeteners. So check the sugar content. If it's high, it could offset beneficial elements including monounsaturated fatty acids.

Milking the environment and cow farts: Some believe that soya milk production is less harmful to the environment than dairy milk because it requires less water and has a smaller carbon footprint (cows are major emitters of methane). Almond trees require vast amounts of water so aren't necessarily environmentally friendly.

Our salt addiction (well, mine at least)

#doasIsaynotasIdo

Quick shake: Wherever you look in the world, salt intake is higher than it should be. Of all the deaths from heart disease, excess salt intake is a significant cause in more than 1.5 million of them. Salt raises blood pressure and makes the natural increase of blood pressure with age worse and as a consequence the risks of stroke and heart attacks go up. But that's just part of the story. There are growing suspicions that salt increases oxidative stress and inflammation and may increase the risk of Alzheimer's disease and autoimmune diseases like rheumatoid arthritis. Salt is, of course, 'addictive' and makes food taste good. Most salt comes from processed foods rather than the salt you add and even that can be reduced by making flavoursome, herb-dense meals. Reducing how much you eat through portion control will effortlessly lower your salt intake simply because you're eating less.

*

Okay, this is a tough one. I am a hardcore salt addict. I find it very difficult to pass the latest brand of pink salt flakes on the supermarket shelves and it takes a huge act of will to ignore the salt instructions in a recipe or stop myself from adding salt to my local cafe's scrambled eggs before I've tasted them. However, after researching this section, I've realised I've been denying reality and started reforming. Promise.

Let's start with the confusion that reigns over knowing how much salt you're eating. There are two measures: sodium and salt. Sodium is what does the damage but it comes in salt, which is sodium chloride, and salt weighs 2.5 times more than its sodium content. The aim should be to keep your *sodium* intake to 2 g a day. That's 5 g of *salt*, which is about a teaspoonful. So if the pack says there's 500 mg of salt in a serving, that's 200 mg of sodium which is 10 per cent of your target intake. Current NHS guidelines recommend that adults should eat no more than 6 g salt a day, and children far less. On average though, a British adult's intake is 8 g, so 25 per cent too much. That's a lot of extra sodium a day and 75 to 80 per cent of it is coming from processed foods such as ready meals, soups and sauces as well as bread, breakfast cereals, cheese and cured meat.

Salt increases your blood pressure and your risk of heart attacks and strokes in various ways. Too much sodium in the blood makes your kidneys retain more water and that raises blood pressure. It's also pretty clear that excess sodium can damage arteries in its own right and is linked to stiffer, less elastic arteries that in turn can make high blood pressure worse as well as the kidney damage it can cause. High blood pressure and diabetes are the commonest reasons for kidney damage as people age, and to complete this deadly cycle, kidney damage in its own right increases the risk of premature death from heart disease.

The damage that salt can do to arteries – particularly the lining (endothelium) could explain the observation that salt intake is related to the risk of Alzheimer's disease. Experiments in mice have shown that dietary salt can induce the production of the tau protein which gums up the brains of people with Alzheimer's. A recent review of the scientific literature by researchers at the University of New South Wales, Australia, found that the link with salt – at least in mice – occurred even without an increase in blood pressure. One possibility is that salt increases oxidative stress in the memory part of the brain called the hippocampus. This oxidative stress may also increase the chances of LDL cholesterol damaging the arteries and causing atherosclerosis.

Excessive salt intake is moderately associated with the risk of stomach (gastric) cancer. Salt may make the effects of the ulcer germ *Helicobacter pylori* worse and probably damages the stomach lining directly.

There's growing evidence of a link between salt intake and autoimmune diseases such as rheumatoid arthritis and perhaps multiple sclerosis (MS). It's early days in this research but the suggestion is that excessive sodium takes the foot off the brake which holds back the abnormal immune responses which activate the immune system to attack various parts of the body such as the linings of the joints (rheumatoid) and nerves (MS).

Before getting to tips about reducing salt intake, there are other non-drug ways of lowering your blood pressure. Reducing alcohol intake, moderate exercise on most days of the week, perhaps mindfulness meditation and possibly yoga can help, but if your QRISK score is high (your risk of a heart attack or stroke in the next five to ten years) or you've already had a heart attack or stroke, then you might need medications to get it under control more urgently.

Reducing your salt intake requires a bit of effort. A weight loss or weight maintenance diet with portion control will lower sodium intake just because you're eating less. Cooking your own food rather than buying processed foods will help because you will be in control of the added salt. There is also evidence that you can fool your tastebuds with aromas from herbs, adding lemon juice to salads or cooked vegetables, using coarse pepper and even tiny amounts of ham. (Jews and Muslims can console ourselves that adding ham still adds salt but indirectly.)

Unlike cholesterol where you really can't go too low, with salt there's probably a sweet spot at around the recommended levels of 2 g of sodium/5 g salt per day. While some people are more salt sensitive than others, there's little doubt that if we can shift the average salt intake by the population downwards, it would have an enormous impact on a lot of people.

Our sugar addiction (yours and mine)

Short and sweet: There's nothing good about sugar other than its taste. I like desserts probably more than the average person (I wish you could try my tiramisu) but don't delude myself that they're doing me any good. They're purely for the pleasure … but I try to minimise sugar intake otherwise. A calorie from sugar is an empty calorie with no nutritional benefit and it's easy to consume vast amounts of calories very quickly in sugar-sweetened foods, especially beverages. Sugar rots your teeth because it feeds the bacteria in your mouth which cause dental caries but the well-publicised (and researched) effects on obesity and type 2 diabetes are more nuanced. It's likely that the really harmful effects of sugar occur when your calorie intake is high and therefore your body is at higher risk of being in a state of metabolic disorder. If your energy intake is not high (i.e. your weight is normal for your height and stable – fat chance), then sugar in your diet seems to have a neutral health effect apart from rotting your teeth. In other words, according to some experts, sugar is at its worst when you're taking in too many calories overall. So it kind of feeds on itself. Almost all processed foods have some sugar added (as well as salt). And if you shift to sugar substitutes, there is mixed evidence about their benefits versus risks. They appear to alter your microbiome and may increase appetite but, on the other hand, are linked to weight loss when studied as a substitute in sugar-sweetened beverages.

*

Even with the above caveats, there's good evidence that sugar and refined carbohydrates stress your insulin system, behave a bit like fats on your heart and blood vessels, and are strongly linked to obesity and adult onset (type 2) diabetes, and as a result, probably pancreatic cancer, which you don't need me to tell you is best avoided. And did I mention tooth decay? When you trade off saturated fats in your diet for refined carbs, there's no reduction in heart risk, whereas if you trade saturated fats for olive oil or polyunsaturated fats, there is (see Is it Fat or *Game of Thrones*? There's Always a Trade-off).

There is no doubt about the evidence, much as the sugar industry would like to suggest otherwise. What there's also no doubt about is that if we as a population reduce sugar consumption, our average weight reduces as well. Coming back to harm, most of the research has been into sugar-sweetened beverages but enough evidence exists about sugar itself that you can be sure it's harmful. However, when the accumulated evidence is reviewed, it looks as though sugar's harm is exerted when your calories are high. I know that's a bit mindbending since sugar is a powerful cause of high calorie intake, but what it means is that if your weight is stable and your calories controlled at an appropriate level, some sugar in your diet is unlikely to do you any harm apart from your teeth. But the proportion of people whose weight is stable is self-delusionally small.

I know I'm going on about your teeth but dental caries – tooth decay – is often missed as a toxic effect of sugar. I grew up in Glasgow – sugar and fat central – and, as a result of the sugar bit, have a mouth full of fillings. Dental caries, according to the World Health Organization (WHO), is the commonest non-communicable disease globally. Sugar feeds bacteria in the mouth that produce acid which destroys the tooth enamel and tooth itself. The cost worldwide is in the hundreds of billions of dollars and for people who can't afford dental care, it magnifies poor nutrition and is even a cause of unemployment since bad or missing teeth stigmatises people.

An addiction? Some believe it may be, in terms of how sugar can act on the reward centres of the brain. I'm not sure, though, that I've ever met someone who's seen pink spiders crawling up the wall when they've gone sugar-free cold turkey. But there's no doubt about the craving, which can be for fat at the same time, perhaps because fat can give sweet food its aroma.

Artificial sweeteners: The science is a bit confusing and conflicted. There is evidence that artificial sweeteners may increase appetite, change the microbiome, damage glucose metabolism and be linked to weight gain. On the other hand, in trials of encouraging switching from sugar-sweetened beverages to artificially sweetened ones, there has been weight loss.

How do I deal with this conflict? I don't consume anything that's artificially sweetened and confine my sugar-sweetened beverages to the mixer in an occasional cocktail. Sparkling and tap water are good enough for me most of the time.

Enhanced foods – be careful what you wish for

Quick take: There are aisles in your local supermarket chock-full of products advertising what's been added to them for your health and wellness. By and large the additives are there because marketers in the food industry have researched our anxieties and what health gurus we're following. Enhanced foods tread a fine line because they're trying to increase sales through implied benefits which often relate to feeding an idea that our diet is somehow deficient. Why you've got to be careful is that the core products which have been enhanced are often not that healthy because they contain large amounts of salt and sugar to make them palatable. The enhancements can be a distraction. I ignore what vitamin or micronutrient they're using to divert my attention and look at the salt and sugar content, which is usually enough for me to put it back on the shelf.

*

The chilled food section in the supermarket is a quagmire.

I get stuck in the yoghurt section.

Which type of yoghurt is best? One with added protein? More vitamin D? As an experiment, I picked up a tub labelled 'added calcium' and compared it to the same brand's 'original' version. There's 262 mg of calcium per 100 g, compared to 160 mg in the original. Granted, that's a higher volume of calcium, but I reckon I'm getting an adequate dosage from the original.

Every aisle has products with added chemicals or enzymes to make these staple foods more attractive to the consumer. The many buzz-words include 'plant-based' and 'organic'. And while organic methods of production may be more attractive, they don't always make for a higher nutrient content.

If you know you need more calcium in your diet, perhaps the tub of yoghurt I just mentioned is the right choice. But I suspect these enhanced foods tell us more about modern marketing techniques than any breakthroughs in nutrition.

The point of this book is to take a 360-degree look at your health, rather than fixate on the minutiae. There's little in the scientific literature which suggests that injecting food with additives makes any difference to our overall wellbeing.

The dizzying array of product information and choice makes the process harder than it needs to be, particularly if you're shopping with young kids.

It's important to stop here and acknowledge the few exceptions to this rule. A handful of staple foods in the UK (and around the world) are fortified with additives to help protect us against chronic problems and disease.

In the UK wheat flour is fortified with thiamine (vitamin B1) to reduce the incidence of a potentially fatal neurological disorder linked to excessive alcohol use. If you drink too much, your diet is probably suffering as a result and you might even inflame the lining of your stomach, making it harder for your body to absorb vitamins. All brown and white flour in the UK must also be fortified with calcium, iron and niacin (vitamin B3). The UK's Scientific Advisory Committee on Nutrition (SACN) has also recommended that wheat flour is also fortified with folic acid (the synthetic form of folate – vitamin B9), but it is not yet mandatory. It's important that women in their childbearing years have added folic acid so that when they fall pregnant their foetuses are protected from neural tube defects (spina bifida). This is where a baby's lower spine does not develop completely. In severe cases, it leaves the nerves in the spine exposed and easily damaged after birth, causing paralysis and serious disability.

You can also buy salt that is enriched with iodine, a mineral essential for the proper functioning of the thyroid gland, which can prevent deficiency in unborn children. However, iodine-enriched salt is not widely available in the UK.

Margarine and low-fat spreads are routinely fortified with vitamins A and D, but it is no longer mandatory in the UK. It's up to specific milk producers and cheese makers if they add it to their products. Some breakfast cereals and yogurts have added vitamin D.

In the UK, some foods, such as breakfast cereals, are voluntarily fortified with folic acid. In addition, non-wholemeal wheat flour and products (for example biscuits cakes and pastries and some stuffings and gravy) are fortified but it's not yet mandatory.

Many countries do mandate fortification with folic acid.

Professor Carol Bower at the University of Western Australia's Telethon Kids Institute was a driving force behind mandatory fortification with folic acid in Australia. She says that before this public health initiative, neural tube defects were much higher, especially in disadvantaged and remote communities because of lack of access to a healthy diet. In the UK it has also been shown that neural tube defects are more common in disadvantaged areas and in certain ethnic groups whose diet may put them at higher risk.

It's important to remember that a baby's neural tube develops very early in pregnancy. So in order to protect against spina bifida, mothers must consume adequate folate/folic acid before the sixth week of life. The problem is, about 45 per cent pregnancies and one third of births in the UK are unplanned. So, unless you're getting folate in your diet anyway, you might miss the crucial window of time.

Adding folic acid to staple foods like wheat flour was mandated in countries such as the United States and Canada long before Australia, with positive results. Fortification began in Australia in 2009 and Professor Bower says that neural tube defects are much less common now across the country. In the UK it's recommended by the SACN and manufacturers do add it to some foods, but it's not mandatory. This makes it all the more important in the UK that women of childbearing age keep in touch with their GP so they start supplementation before there's a chance they're pregnant.

Okay, I've held off this long ... time for the microbiome

The take: The microbiome is the trillions of living organisms on the surfaces of our bodies. They are integral to our health and wellbeing because they foster a healthy immune system, efficient use of energy, recycle nutrients and help the absorption of by-products which can counter the oxidative stress of ageing. Some of our gut bugs may have effects on the brain, influencing mood. The microbiome can help to make you obese or lean, and imbalances in the microbiome or damaging it with antibiotics can make cancer worse or interfere with cancer treatment. Trouble is that, with some exceptions, interventions with specific probiotics have been disappointing so far, possibly because the range of bacteria used is too narrowly based or there are inconsistencies in manufacture and quality control. At the moment, the best option is to take a prebiotic approach, namely a diet with huge variety, lots of fermented foods and complexity, and allow the microbiome to self-adapt to a healthier profile.

*

Inside out: What you think is 'inside' your body when it comes to the microbiome are actually exterior surfaces. The skin is obviously on the outside but if you think about it, the nose and bronchial tubes in your lungs and the entire gastrointestinal tract from mouth to anus are external surfaces. They're actually tunnels and therefore, like tunnels, are exposed to the outside world and whatever we throw at them. To really get inside the body, whatever is on these surfaces needs to be absorbed across the walls of the gut or respiratory tract into the bloodstream and that includes germs, nutrients, toxins and bioactive compounds.

It's the frontline: These surfaces are therefore our first lines of defence and humans would not have survived as a species without a sophisticated and adaptable immune system ready for warfare at the frontlines. Like any army, constant training is essential to maintain an effective immune system and it gets its training in live action right from the first days of life on the battlefields of the respiratory and gastrointestinal systems. Those battlegrounds are covered in murky soups of bacteria, viruses and fungi, most of which are friendly but some are dangerous and need to be neutralised. The COVID-19 pandemic started in the microbiome of bats who manage to harbour untold numbers of viruses which happily exchange genes with each other and occasionally transform themselves into viruses which can attack humans. The microbiome is a fact of life whether you're a bat or a human. Bats have evolved to cope with a disgusting array of organisms that are unknown to our immune system and are therefore 'invisible' on the battlefield until it's too late. Just as micro-organisms get everywhere, including in unlikely places such as hot vents deep under the sea, so bacteria, viruses and fungi inveigle their way past the hydrochloric acid in the stomach, past the enzymes in the small bowel which break down proteins and fats – far away from any sunlight – into the large bowel – the colon – and once there can mindlessly affect how our bodies work without, for the most part, causing disease. That's as long as there's balance because the pattern of living organisms in our bodies can increase or decrease the risk of chronic diseases over time.

For example, it's known that some organisms affect the level of acidity and even oxygen in the gut, and produce fatty acids including one called butyrate which can boost genes which have an anti-inflammatory effect as well as influencing messaging within cells. Butyrate is largely produced in the bowel from bacteria which ferment fibre and other carbohydrates. It provides energy for the cells lining the bowel and the family of fatty acids to which butyrate belongs also contributes to our total calorie needs, maybe up to 15 per cent.

So why, you might ask, have interventions like specific probiotics often been disappointing? Well, the microbiome is lock-in-step with the recurrent theme of this book. Our bodies, our culture and the world around us are mind-bogglingly complex and all the elements work together. So it's hard to pick out one or two players and bet on them to do a particular job.

Here, though, are some areas where manipulating the microbiome has been a help or a hindrance.

Babies: Unfortunately, at the time of writing, there's no convincing high-quality evidence that infant colic – a controversial label given to the many babies who cry a lot and draw up their knees as if they have tummy pain – is helped by probiotics.

Necrotising enterocolitis (NEC) is a dreadful, life-threatening intestinal inflammation primarily affecting pre-term babies, who enter the world with an unprepared immune system, often need antibiotics and who sometimes miss out on breast milk. Over the years there have been many trials of different probiotics in an attempt to protect these babies' fragile guts. The studies have not been particularly well conducted and are inconsistent, which makes it hard to compare them to each other. Also, what can happen in a neonatal intensive care unit is that babies given a placebo end up getting cross-colonised with the microbiome of the others! Anyway, there is a signal that probiotics can reduce the risk of NEC but exactly which bacteria are best is still unclear.

Irritable bowel syndrome: There is some evidence that probiotics can help but it's uncertain what exactly the right recipe might be.

Bowel cancer: The microbiome has been repeatedly implicated in the cause of colorectal (bowel) cancer. Fatty acids in the butyrate family (short-chain fatty acids) are produced in the bowel from the fermentation of fibre. They're critical to the health of the bowel lining and stimulate immune messengers called interferons which keep the local immune system on its toes. Without these fatty acids, the bowel lining loses its way; it doesn't repair damage as well and becomes more inflamed. This means that when we eat a cancer-causing chemical, the depleted bowel doesn't shrug it off as easily as it might. For decades, a diet high in vegetables has been recommended for the prevention of bowel cancer with fairly strong supportive evidence. In relation to the microbiome, a plant-rich diet with lots of soluble fibre, particularly containing lignin and beta glucan, which have been shown to reduce bowel polyps in animal models, is actually a *pre*biotic approach.

Antibiotics are important if you need them but ... There is evidence from both animal and human studies that antibiotic use increases the risk of cancers in general and bowel cancer in particular. For instance, multiple antibiotic courses throughout life, including childhood exposure, have been linked to colon cancer development, although it's complicated.

It may be that the impact of antibiotics on the microbiome may be different depending on the segment of the bowel. For instance, antibiotics may for some reason only increase the risk of cancer in the first part of the colon on the right side of your abdomen. Another complexity is that people who need antibiotics may have other things going on which predispose them to cancer risk from another source altogether. However, there are disturbing indications that antibiotic exposure can increase resistance to bowel cancer chemotherapy and reduce the effectiveness of some new anti-cancer immunotherapies.

Bioactive rescue: The good news – although so far it's mostly from animal studies – is that the bioactives from a diverse plant-rich cuisine (see Be Bioactive: On Antioxidants and Tubas) look as though they can enhance the effects of cancer treatment and may ameliorate the damage from antibiotics. Probiotics could also be important in the future once researchers can sort out exactly which ones make a difference and manufacturers standardise the quality and content of their products. There is laboratory evidence that some probiotics can induce programmed cell death (apoptosis), the failure of which creates the immortal cells of cancer.

The microbiome and your mood: One way of looking at the microbiome is as an organ in its own right, sending messages around the body and interacting with the gut, which has remarkable similarities to the brain. When the gut talks to different parts of itself or to other parts of the body, it uses chemical signals that are pretty much identical to the ones used by the brain. So it wouldn't be a surprise to find that the gut can influence our mood and the way we react to the world. The evidence for that mostly comes from animal studies. Faecal transplants from people with major depression into rodents seem to induce depressive behaviour, and depressive behaviour in rodents is associated with a less diverse microbiome. Work in Canada – in rats – found suggestions of an antidepressant effect from a bacterium called *Bifidobacteria infantis*. They've similar results using *Lactobacillus rhamnosus* in mice, and evidence that the brain then sends messages back to the gut via a nerve called the vagus. So the brain and the gut are likely having two-directional conversations all the time, perhaps mediated by the microbiome. But in humans, randomised trials of probiotics to treat depression have been disappointing. That doesn't mean the idea is wrong, maybe just too simplistic. In parallel with the research on the microbiome, there's been more awareness that the immune system can have a profound effect on the brain and is linked to mental health issues such as schizophrenia. And if you're not confused enough by now, another factor which may throw a spanner in the works is that while antibiotics can wreck the microbiome, they might have direct effects all of their own on the brain which haven't been fully recognised.

Other brain problems? There's been lots of excitement about whether there's a link between the microbiome and autism, dementia and Parkinson's disease. It could be real but meaningful evidence is so far lacking. It'd be wonderful if it proves true but in the meantime there's no harm in getting going on a bioactive diet.

Exercise: Aerobic exercise is associated with a more diverse and healthy microbiome.

Weight control: Obese people seem to have a less diverse microbiome and there is evidence from animal studies that thin people may have a microbiome that isn't very efficient at recycling calories back into the body. That's led people to suggest that a treatment for obese humans could be faecal transplants (i.e. almost an entire microbiome) from thin people. The jury is a long way from coming back in on that or the use of probiotics in weight loss. Let's hope, because it'd be nice if it worked out.

Allergies: Too early to say at the time of writing.

Immunisation: There is experimental evidence to suggest that antibiotics prior to being immunised can reduce the effect of the vaccine and perhaps increase an inflammatory response. That might become important now that COVID-19 immunisation has been implemented.

Spices as possible prebiotics: An interesting US study of seven spices – black pepper, cayenne, cinnamon, ginger, oregano, rosemary and turmeric – found strong antioxidant activity and that they enhanced the growth of 'good' bacteria such as *Bifidobacteria* and *Lactobacilli* and inhibited 'bad' ones such as *Fusobacteria* and *Clostridium*.

You get thirsty for a reason – and don't bottle it up

Quick mouthful: It's a marketing triumph. We have the world's cleanest, safest water which also protects our teeth and it's free. Yet we pay for water in environment-polluting plastic bottles, which denies us the tooth protection of fluoridation (water contains additional fluoride only in some areas of the UK) and for which the best that can be said is that it's better for us than energy drinks or carbonated sugar water. We've also been conned into believing we need to force ourselves to drink litres of fluids a day – even if we spend most of our time indoors not exercising much. Ask yourself, why did evolution give us thirst? Bottom line, unless you've been advised otherwise or are in unusual conditions, let thirst be your guide, even if you're exercising. Water is best but my fluids of choice when I'm not exercising are coffee, tea and sparkling water. Also, remember that a plant-rich diet has a fair bit of water in the foods themselves, particularly complex carbohydrates. If you're an extreme endurance athlete, take the advice of experts but note that the world's best endurance runners – the Ethiopians – run a little bit dry and rarely drink before or during training. Never drink so much you gain weight because you risk a serious condition called hyponatraemia. Exercise-associated muscle cramps are generally not due to dehydration or electrolyte imbalance. They're probably due to fatigue and in fact may also be associated with overdrinking.

*

Thirst is a highly evolved physiological feedback mechanism designed to keep us alive by controlling the level of fluids in our bodies. As such, it's a perfectly good driver of fluid consumption in most people. The brain is highly tuned to fluid load and has sensors throughout the body which give constant feedback to the thirst centre which tells us to drink to top up. There's little reason to drink ahead of thirst and 'Drink to Thirst' is the current recommendation to athletes to prevent the risk of potentially dangerous low sodium levels (hyponatraemia) from overhydration. One guide to this (again) is never drink so much you gain weight.

If you're anxious about your intake, don't obsess on it,

there's enough to worry about in life, so drink if it makes you feel better. Your urine should not be too strongly coloured or odorous (unless asparagus was on last night's menu). By the way, if you're peeing large volumes frequently and it's not as a result of forcing yourself to drink vast amounts of bottled water in the misguided notion that it's natural and doing you good, then you do need to get checked up by your GP to make sure you don't have diabetes or kidney disease.

Older people with cognitive impairment, people on diuretics or who have kidney damage may not have a reliable thirst drive and need more regular reminders.

People with heart or kidney failure or liver problems need to carefully follow medical advice on fluid intake. There are also medications which can either make you retain water, such as non-steroidal anti-inflammatory drugs (like ibuprofen), or affect your thirst, such as opioids and some antidepressants.

All of the above needs to be tempered with a dose of common sense such as on a hot day when you might have had too much alcohol and need to push water to get ahead of alcohol-induced dehydration. I wouldn't wait for thirst to act on that one.

So … for the task-focused among you who love being given a target, is there a daily volume of fluids you should be drinking every day? Trouble is, it's hard to generalise between winter and summer, days when you're exercising and days when you're not, whether you're pregnant and your blood volume is bigger because of the baby, whether you're breast feeding, whether you're otherwise healthy or have a fever and might need added fluids.

Research suggests that people who drink water are generally

healthier and are more likely to have a better diet. But that's not cause and effect, they go along with each other.

The guide to this from official sources is a bit loose.

Primary aged kids probably need around 1 to 1.5 litres a day but that's an average with none of the specificity about whether they've been at sport on a hot day, for example. Needless to say, a litre is four 250 ml cupfuls. The recommendations for adults vary but surveys suggest that without prompting, we drink around 2–3 litres a day – again an average – more if someone's pregnant. You can see how thirst and having the occasional look at your pee is so much simpler.

Is the sparkle worth it?

The spritz: Indulge me on this one. I consume considerable amounts of mineral water and needed reassurance. There's no effect on your bones and a fair bit of evidence that, as long as there's not too much salt in the water and the sodium is in the form of sodium bicarbonate, blood pressure doesn't go up and may come down. It could have a beneficial effect on gastric fullness (satiety) and blood fats – although f..k knows why that would happen. Bottom line – there will still be mineral water in my fridge for years to come.

*

I'm talking here about unsweetened, unflavoured, carbonated water, which can commonly come in the form of mineral water which, depending on its source, can contain a variety of minerals such as salt, calcium and sodium bicarbonate. There have been all sorts of rumours about mineral/carbonated water, from rotting your bones, to increasing weight gain. For your benefit (mainly mine) I have trawled the scientific literature and here's what I've come up with. Carbonated water stimulates receptors on the tongue which in turn send messages to the brain. What the brain does with these messages is a mystery. In my case it's 'drink more mineral water'.

Generally, there's been little research on the effects of carbonated water compared to sugared fizzy drinks.

Appetite: The most commonly cited research in recent years – at least by the media – came from a study in 2017 from Birzeit University near Ramallah in the Palestinian Territories. It was called 'Carbon dioxide in carbonated beverages induces ghrelin release and increased food consumption in male rats: Implications on the onset of obesity' and was published in the peer-reviewed journal *Obesity Research and Clinical Practice*.

Male rats (yes, rats) were subjected to different sorts of drinks and evaluated for one year. It found the rats consuming the gaseous beverages gained weight at a faster rate than those consuming tap water. The researchers concluded that this is due to elevated levels of the hunger hormone ghrelin, which could explain the greater food intake in rats drinking carbonated drinks compared to control rats. Moreover, they showed an increase in liver fat in fizzy-drinking rats compared to control rats on tap water. In a parallel study, the levels of ghrelin hormone in 20 healthy young men rose upon drinking carbonated beverages compared to controls. It found they also had higher blood ghrelin levels after drinking fizzy drinks than after flat soda or water. They implicated carbon dioxide in this effect on hunger.

Call me a biased, carbon dioxide junky but this was one

study where there could have been all sorts of other causes of the ghrelin production. The balance of evidence from other research suggests more health benefits than risks. In fact, there's some evidence that carbonated water can increase a sense of fullness and presumably help control food intake. Sadly, that's not been my experience.

Blood pressure (and bones): A trial of people on a low salt diet to reduce their blood pressure showed a beneficial effect from a low sodium chloride, high sodium bicarbonate mineral water as well as reduced excretion of calcium. Another trial in healthy people showed inhibition of the blood pressure-raising hormone aldosterone in women consuming a high sodium bicarbonate mineral water, suggesting a protective effect against high blood pressure. In general, sodium enriched mineral water seems to have either no effect or a beneficial one on blood pressure if it's sodium bicarbonate rather than sodium chloride (salt). A review of the available evidence suggested that mineral water may be good for the metabolic syndrome, blood pressure and even blood fat (lipid) levels, although that may say more about the diet of mineral water drinkers than the bubbles.

And here's the clincher on bones. Egg-laying hens are less likely to break their tibial bones when drinking carbonated water. If you don't find that convincing, you could be right. There's no evidence of bone remodelling in postmenopausal women drinking mineral water.

Indigestion and constipation: There are a few studies showing improvement in dyspepsia (indigestion) and constipation. One small trial suggested carbonated water can help gallbladder emptying. This could be a combination of the direct effects of carbon dioxide and gastric fullness from the gas.

Other stuff: Interestingly, there have been studies showing that carbonated water improved swallowing in older people.

And in kids there's no evidence they drink more when there are bubbles in tap water compared to plain tap water.

Weird stuff: Immersing your legs in warm carbonated water in the hope that the carbon dioxide opens up the blood vessels didn't play out. A pity since it could have been good for people with heart or arterial disease.

Caffeine hits

Espresso: Again, a declaration. I'm a hopeless coffee addict but I have tried to be dispassionate about the evidence. Coffee is actually pretty good for you. People who drink up to five cups a day, and – importantly – don't smoke, have a reduced chance of dying prematurely and a lower incidence of heart disease, kidney stones, Parkinson's, diabetes, perhaps some cancers, and mental health issues like depression. And many of these effects are associated with coffee rather than caffeine. (Again a declaration, I drink caffeinated coffee until midday, so like hearing these stories.) Caffeine, on the other hand, can cause anxiety and insomnia. Tea seems to be associated with similar benefits to coffee. Our preferences for these beverages appear to be significantly driven by genetics.

*

My first coffee of the day is a double-shot normal sized latte. My second coffee of the day (usually within minutes of the first) is a double-shot normal sized latte. An espresso shot is about 200 mg of caffeine.

Obviously, I can't speak for you but on the whole, caffeine is a need not a want.

There have long been concerns that coffee and caffeine more generally may increase the risks of cancer and heart disease. A *New England Journal of Medicine* review of the available research refutes that. In fact, it says that if you drink up to five standard cups of coffee daily, there may even be a reduced risk of several chronic diseases. Prospective studies in the US, Europe and Asia have shown a strong inverse association between the risk of Parkinson's disease and caffeine i.e. more caffeine, less Parkinson's.

In one study with 4 million 'people-years' of follow-up, one to five cups of coffee per day was associated with lower chances of dying prematurely from any cause but this was predominantly in people who had never smoked. Five or more cups a day had a neutral effect on premature death. Unlike other studies, they found no influence on deaths from cancer but they did for heart disease, neurological diseases such as Parkinson's disease (but not dementia), depression and suicide, and this was for both caffeinated and decaf. Coffee consumption – in multiple studies – also reduces the risk of type 2 diabetes. Yes, we're back to the whole food argument here rather than crediting or blaming a single substance. The reasons may be components of coffee such as chlorogenic acid, lignans, quinides, trigonelline and magnesium which reduce inflammation and improve the function of insulin.

Coming back to smoking and coffee: Our preferences for

coffee are anywhere between 40 and 70 per cent driven by our genes; the rest is the environment in which we live – in other words, the influence of family, friends, marketing and availability. Older people prefer tea. The more tea we drink, the less coffee, and vice versa. Smoking is more common in coffee drinkers and vice versa. There's no evidence that coffee drives us to cigarettes or nicotine drives us to an espresso habit. What seems to be the case is that some people have genes – a shared genetic trait – which give a preference for smoking and coffee consumption.

You may be a smoker without realising it: As an aside here, you may not identify as a smoker because you might have two or three cigarettes after food or are a weekend smoker when you're out. The evidence is strong that the first ten cigarettes are the most dangerous. No question that smoking 20 a day is worse than ten, but you have to reduce to zero to get the maximum health benefits.

Anyway, back to coffee.

The problem with coffee research is how you consume your caffeine.

Sweet isn't so sweet: Soft drinks, energy drinks or coffee and tea with added sugar might make it more likely that you eventually have to unbutton your jeans before you sit down for a breather.

In your cups: Variation in cup size, brew strength, type of bean and whether you drink black or white coffee are generally not captured by epidemiological studies of coffee consumption. It's easier to consume more caffeine in a cold sugared drink, or in an espresso martini.

The concentration of the cholesterol-raising compound

'cafestol' is high in unfiltered coffee such as French press, Turkish, or Scandinavian boiled coffee; at medium levels in espressos; and almost non-existent in drip-filtered, instant and percolator coffee. But the population-based studies which fairly consistently show a reduction in heart disease suggest that the risk from cafestol is more theoretical.

What I will say here is that you're the one who's best placed to make a call about what constitutes a healthy daily dose of caffeine. If you're anxious, or stressed, or having trouble with sleeping, caffeine can make that worse. You'll know how much is too much even if you don't do anything about it.

Smoking increases the metabolism of caffeine and oral contraceptives slow it down, as does pregnancy. You do need to be careful in pregnancy because caffeine intake has been linked to low birth weight and perhaps pregnancy loss.

You can get a bit addicted to caffeine, if your definition of that includes craving when you haven't had your daily shots and withdrawal effects. The commonest withdrawal symptom is a headache but can include fatigue and flu-like symptoms which peak one or two days after reducing your caffeine intake and hang around for up to a week.

Perhaps the biggest downside is that while I may be in a steady state of balance with four shots in the morning, for some people the more you consume, the more you need to get the same buzz. Also, caffeine won't compensate for extended bouts of sleeplessness. The stimulation is not the same as the refreshment of a night's kip. There's no doubt that if you're prone to anxiety and sleep disorders, caffeine is likely something you should avoid.

Quick cuppa: The benefits of black and green tea look quite similar to coffee but you still get a whack of caffeine.

Tea is more popular than coffee globally and maybe that's a combination of availability and the belief that it's seen as a healthier option. The potential benefits of tea are thought to have been first documented by the Tang Dynasty in China in 700 AD. The rest is history, as they say.

Most teas are made from the processed leaf of *Camellia sinensis*. Black tea is fermented leaf and green is non-fermented, which determines its taste and chemical composition and thus the debate about the medicinal advantages of each. The bottom line is probably that there aren't too many differences in potential benefits.

Green tea: A typical cup of green tea usually contains 250–350 mg of tea solids, of which 30–42 per cent are catechins or antioxidants and 3–6 per cent is caffeine. The most abundant of those catechins is epigallocatechin gallate (EGCG) and is usually credited with the cancer-protective properties of green tea. But if you've come this far in the book, you'll know to be sceptical of single foods and single substances within them. Tea, like every other food, is a package that's hard to dissect into individual elements.

The balance of evidence on green tea is that it has some anti-cancer and heart-protective effects, at least in the lab, although there are some human studies – but again not so protective that it will overwhelm the toxicity of cigarettes if you're a smoker.

Part of the problem seems to be that scientists are yet to find a specific dose of tea components that assist with cancer reduction.

The bottom line is that the antioxidants in green tea are

good for you. It's much better to brew a pot of green tea than consume a highly sugared energy drink which will rot your teeth and make you fat. There is a little evidence that adding green tea to your diet is good for weight control.

Black tea? It has plenty of antioxidants too. A 2010 study from the Netherlands surveyed 37,000 healthy men and women over 13 years. It showed that the age-adjusted risk of death from cardiovascular disease dropped with daily consumption of 3–6 cups of black tea.

A standard black tea bag has about 40–50 mg of caffeine, which is slightly greater than a green tea bag at 30–40 mg of caffeine. But black tea still gives you less caffeine than your average shot of coffee.

Gender may play a role too. Many studies suggest the benefits of tea are greater in women than men. This may be related to men generally drinking more alcohol and smoking more than women (at least in the past). There's only so much you can reasonably expect from a cuppa.

Just on that issue of men's versus women's alcohol habits: a study by Professor Maree Teesson and her colleagues in Sydney and New York, showed that at the beginning of the 20th century, men had a 360 per cent greater chance than women of experiencing alcohol-related harms. By the end of the century, that gap was down to 30 per cent. Pretty dramatic, and the reason is not that men have quit booze. It's that women's use has increased significantly, for complex reasons in part due to changing gender roles, greater independent financial resources, access, attitude and less hidden consumption.

Negronis and other alcoholic drinks

The slug: Most of us drink, some far too much. There is no sweet spot for alcohol consumption. The more you drink, the more harm you're risking from accidents, violence, cancer, brain and liver problems. Two standard drinks a day can't be traded for a ten-drink binge at the weekend. Alcohol is bad for unborn babies, not good for teenagers and a risk in the elderly, not to mention increasing the risk of breast cancer in women. The kind of alcohol probably doesn't matter and the only benefit may be for people with heart disease who drink modestly. It's a myth that it's good for parents to allow children and adolescents access to alcohol, for instance at the dinner table. It does not teach good habits and risks distorted brain development.

*

What's a binge? Drinking enough that your mental state changes. You feel tipsy or a bit drunk. To be more precise, it's four or more drinks in women at a sitting, and five or more in men.

In Scotland, where I grew up, drinking is a national sport. We were taught in medical school that any patient who said he or she worked in a bar was alcohol dependent until proven otherwise and anyone in a bar before lunch was also alcohol dependent. I can't tell you how often, as a junior doctor, I was woken up in the middle of the night to get to the bedside of a patient who was seeing pink spiders crawl up the wall. Alcohol withdrawal can be ugly and when you've seen the brain damage from alcoholism, it does make you circumspect about your own drinking. But that's the extreme end where the strong preference for alcohol is inherited in tandem with a drinking culture which tolerates – even respects – bingeing.

Having said that, I make a mean Negroni and have a cupboard full of malt whisky. The fact that it's full is significant because I don't drink much of it. I'm notorious for leaving alcohol in the glass. For some reason (and I so wish it'd happen with food), I seem to know when I've had enough and I was lucky that I never tried cannabis until my late teens and never smoked, so never had to quit.

The recommendations for safe drinking are that the less you drink the better. In England in 2018 around 82 per cent of adults drank alcohol in the previous 12 months, with around 49 per cent drinking at least once a week. The Chief Medical Officer's guidelines are that healthy adults (men and women) should drink no more than 14 units per week. This should be spread over 3 or more days for those who regularly drink 14 units. If you're otherwise well, this reduces your risk of dying of alcohol-related harm. However, around 24 per cent of adults in England and Scotland exceed the recommended rates. If you've been born into a hard-drinking family, it's wisest not to drink at all.

Professor Maree Teesson, a leading researcher into mental health and substance use at the University of Sydney, Australia, argues that since the human brain is still developing and maturing well into the 20s, drinking alcohol during the teenage years can disrupt healthy brain development. For this reason, teenagers are advised to avoid drinking for as long as possible. Starting to drink at an earlier age also places young people at greater risk of developing alcohol-related problems later in life. It's a myth that you can teach a young person to drink by giving them alcohol at an early age.

So the later young people delay their first alcoholic drink, the less likely they are to develop an alcohol use disorder.

The good news is that alcohol use among young people has declined quite quickly in recent years. In the UK almost a quarter of young adults don't drink alcohol. A study at the University of Sheffield concluded that abstinence rates among 16 to 24 year olds rose from 10 per cent to nearly 25 per cent between 2001 and 2016. The trouble is that young people who are drinking are often still doing so at high risk levels.

Women who are pregnant or planning a pregnancy should not drink at all. There is no completely safe level of alcohol consumption during pregnancy and even when planning pregnancy, it's safer to quit drinking. Any alcohol consumption from conception through the entire pregnancy can affect brain development. With breastfeeding, you need to ask yourself, do I want my little baby to have a drink? If I might answer that on your behalf, no you don't. Alcohol goes into your bloodstream and into your milk. Hang tight for a few months more.

A huge study of 10,000 nine-year-olds in the US, including MRI brain scans and their full histories, showed that any alcohol consumption in pregnancy was linked to depression, anxiety, attention deficits, impulsiveness, sensation seeking, memory problems associated with learning, ability to plan ahead and make decisions, and physical symptoms such as a manifestation of psychological issues (somatising) in these children. Those findings were associated with brain structure differences on the scans.

There is also disturbing evidence of an association with

alcohol in pregnancy with young children sipping alcoholic drinks.

So the results are clear.

One group of people who are at particular risk are the over 50s, which is an age group who are increasingly likely to be drinking at unsafe levels. As people age, their body composition changes, not to mention having lower brain reserves. This makes their ability to cope with alcohol much lower. Over 65s risk shrinkage of brain volume at a time when they need all the brains they can get.

People who have heart disease may benefit from two standard drinks a day if they are aged over 50 although alcohol does increase blood pressure and the risk of stroke.

Type of alcohol? It probably doesn't matter that much although my Negronis do have lots of sugar. It's worth remembering that what makes you addicted to a substance is a quick hit followed by a drop in blood levels of the drug. That pattern is a major reason why smoking, cocaine, crystal meth and heroin are so addictive. So when it comes to alcohol, drinking shots of spirits and bingeing in general are not a good idea. Mixers which are carbonated increase rapid alcohol absorption, and beer increases the risk of bladder cancer. There's not a lot of evidence that red wine has much extra to offer apart from its taste.

The main differences between alcohols are congeners, which are by-products of sugar fermentation and help to give alcohols their taste. Drinks that contain high quantities of congeners may increase hangover symptoms. Clear beverages like vodka, gin and white wine contain fewer congeners than darker drinks like brandy, whisky, rum and red wine. Mixing your drinks may be more about mixing your congeners and amplifying side effects like gastritis.

Having food with alcohol does slow down its absorption and reduce the risk of gastritis. Another technique to slow alcohol intake is to start the evening with a soft drink then alternate alcohol with soft drinks like soda water after that. That also helps to prevent the dehydration which accompanies alcohol consumption.

Mixing alcohol with other drugs: Not a good idea. To put it more positively, it's a bad idea. Sedatives, anti-epilepsy medications, heart rhythm drugs, arthritis medications and pain relievers, medications for ADHD and blood thinners all have a reasonable risk of serious consequences when mixed with alcohol.

When you hear about drug deaths, they are often because of drug-mixing including prescription drugs, alcohol and illicit drugs. (See overleaf.) They make each other more potent and can together cause profound suppression of the centre in the brain which drives breathing.

Alcohol and other drugs

Quick-ish shot: It's all too easy to be judgemental about drug use and in so doing emphasise the dangers, when individual experiences might be different. Take methamphetamine (ice, speed or base), for instance. It's an unpleasant drug in terms of addiction, behaviour change and serious heart complications. Luckily the prevalence of methamphetamine use is fairly low in the UK in terms of the proportion of people who've used it in the last year, but that's no cause for complacency. In Australia, for example, ice consumption as measured by lifetime use shows that nearly 6 per cent of Australians aged over 14 have tried it sometime. While not all of those people have come to harm, clearly a proportion have. People try or use legal and illicit drugs for all sorts of reasons. According to Australia's Professor Maree Teesson, the thing is to be aware that there's always a risk of drug use becoming a problem. Common reasons people give for trying or using drugs include: to fit in or feel part of a social group, to reduce inhibitions and increase confidence, curiosity, to escape the reality of life, to relieve boredom, to manage mental health issues like low mood or the effects of trauma, to forget problems like unemployment or financial difficulties, and/or to enhance sexual experiences and intimacy. No drug is without its risks so don't delude yourself, and mixing them increases the potential danger and certainly the chances of feeling crap on Mondays or even Tuesdays.

*

There's not a lot of difference between most legal and illicit drugs. Alcohol and tobacco do the most damage to public health. Heroin, cocaine, meth and tobacco dealers are selling drugs which are exquisitely designed to create addiction and keep you as a customer. Even cannabis can cause dependence. Most people control their use, but there's often one person in a social group who starts off being charming and amusing on their drugs of choice but over time slips out of control. Sometimes the reason is that they're self-medicating for mental health issues such as depression and anxiety, which means they need to be encouraged into more productive ways of helping themselves. Alcohol is okay in moderation but what's moderate to one person can be quite high consumption. Alcohol is also a gateway drug in that, on a Friday night, it can reduce your inhibitions and lead you to using other drugs such as cocaine. A big message is don't start any drug when you're young because it'll change your brain. Knowing where to get support is sometimes hard. There are several organisations where people and families troubled by alcohol or drug-related problems can get help – www.nhs.uk/live-well provides a list of resources.

The age you start on alcohol or other drugs counts: The time most people acquire their drug pattern (or avoid an unhealthy one) is in adolescence. Childhood is a period of huge brain growth and development and we enter adolescence with overgrown brains. Adolescence is a period of development where that overgrowth is pruned and the brain knocked into shape for the rest of your life. Use of drugs – any drug – during adolescence risks disrupting the pruning and directing the pruning shears in a bad direction which can cement drug use into the complex networks of nerves in our brains. It's physical programming which can influence our propensity to crave alcohol, tobacco, cannabis, cocaine or other drugs, not to mention the risk of mental health issues such as anxiety, depression and psychosis.

Our brain is the most important organ for a successful, healthy and long life and we need to pay attention to brain health at all ages. The evidence with alcohol is that there are three very vulnerable periods to neurotoxicity and brain damage: even low level drinking during pregnancy and adolescence (especially binge drinking in 15–19 year olds), and low to moderate drinking in the over 65s.

Mental health issues and drugs: About half of people who have trouble controlling their substance use (legal, illicit or prescription) have a mental health issue, including anxiety, depression or psychotic illness. And it works the other way, too: people with mental health issues often have problems with alcohol, tobacco and other drugs. Sometimes the mental health issues came first, with people trying to self-medicate to make themselves feel better. Sometimes the drug use appears first and seems to have caused the mental health problem. Either way, it's important to be alert to this because you won't fix either problem unless both are dealt with. Smokers have higher rates of distress than non-smokers, and the coexistence of mental health problems in crystal meth (ice) users is high.

Drug use in the UK: The proportion of 16–59 year olds in England and Wales who took drugs in 2019 currently stands at 9.4 per cent. In Scotland around 12 per cent of the same age group took drugs in 2017–18, an increase from 7.6 per cent reported on the 2014–15 survey. Northern Ireland has the lowest prevalence in the UK of drug use – only 5.9 per cent of 15–64 year olds reported it in 2014–15.

Cannabis usually comes from the *Cannabis sativa* plant although there are synthetic forms on the market. There are many cannabinoid substances in the plant which act on receptors in the brain but the main ones are tetrahydrocannabinol (THC) and cannabidiol (CBD). Cannabis is the most commonly used illicit drug in the UK. There are an estimated 22 million people worldwide with cannabis dependence. It can be associated with depression and psychosis, lung damage and heart complications including heart attacks and abnormal heart rhythms. Rates of usage have been relatively stable over the past 20 years (around 11 per cent in the previous 12 months) and the average age of users has risen by about five years, which reflects a general downwards trend of young people in the UK using drugs of most kinds.

Crystal meth/methamphetamine is a stimulant sold in three main forms: ice, base and speed. Ice is the most potent. It comes as small clear or white crystals, and is smoked or injected. The use of speed has declined, replaced by ice, and while, for example, fewer than 2 per cent of Australians have used ice in the last year (a similar proportion to the UK), the harms have risen. People taking it often feel agitated and nervous. Some have anxiety attacks and the comedown after use can include low mood and nervousness. Other harms include hospital admissions, dependence and psychosis (delusions and delusional behaviour). In Scotland in 2018, there was the highest number of deaths on record. In a warning for the UK of what can happen, Australian deaths have risen as well and some emergency departments have become used to seeing young people having heart attacks and other cardiac complications from ice and cocaine. The treatment of ice dependence isn't easy but there's a growing body of evidence on what works.

Cocaine is a stimulant derived from the coca plant and these days mostly used in powder form by snorting through the nose. Its use has increased in the UK and is particularly prevalent in higher socio-economic areas. An estimated 5.3 per cent of people aged between 15 and 34 in the UK took cocaine in 2018. Users report more energy, confidence and sociability and an increased libido. Your temperature, blood pressure and heart rate go up and because the effects last less than an hour, often just 30 minutes, there's a tendency to binge and with that in some people the risk of toxic effects and overdose increase, especially if other drugs are involved. The comedown effects include low energy, demotivation, irritability and sometimes paranoia. Regular use of cocaine can damage the heart, liver, lungs and kidneys, and cause thinking and memory problems, sexual dysfunction and strokes. Cocaine also produces dependence.

Opioids/heroin: While heroin use among the UK general population is low, other opioid use is rising in the UK and around the world. Worldwide, about 0.5 million deaths are attributable to drug use. More than 70 per cent of these deaths are related to opioids, with more than 30 per cent of those deaths caused by overdose.

Synthetics: These are emerging drugs like synthetic cannabinoids, phenethylamines and novel benzodiazepines, and mimic the effects of existing illicit substances. People who use drugs like ecstasy are more likely to use these drugs than the general population. One-third of regular ecstasy and stimulant users reported recent use of these drugs, which are poorly understood in terms of their risks.

Non-medical use of pharmaceuticals: This is a growing health problem, with evidence suggesting increasing prevalence of misuse and associated harms including death. Worldwide, opioid pain-killers (excluding over-the-counter) have been the most commonly misused pharmaceuticals followed by tranquillisers and sleeping pills.

In the UK, a study published in 2014 showed 7.7 per cent of respondents admitted misuse – comparable with US figures. Despite the adverse publicity, there has been a trend worldwide of increased dispensed prescriptions for pharmaceutical opioids.

Supplements for big muscles

Performance- and image-enhancing drugs (PIEDs) and performance- and image-enhancing social media: We've just got to be a wee bit careful about the risk of moral panic over this because idolising the image of a perfect male form which is highly muscular with low body fat and a flat abdomen is nothing new. The ancient Greeks did it. Michelangelo did it. The almost cult status of Angelino Siciliano, the fabled 97-pound weakling who turned himself into the Charles Atlas bodybuilding and money-making machine in the 1920s, did it. And now social media are doing it, particularly Instagram sharing among gay guys. Even anabolic steroids aren't new and have been part of a toxic gym culture for gay and straight men for many years. Like the other cultural and health anxieties in this book, striving for the perfect male body becomes a problem when it's an obsession which interferes with your life and relationships, and involves risk-taking behaviours such as unhealthy dietary restrictions (Charles Atlas developed heart disease) and injecting drug use – all of which could be covering for psychological problems.

*

Are PIEDs a quick route to a six-pack? Maybe, but the desire for muscle sculpting using artificial enhancement could be a sign of mental health issues and has risks including poor sexual performance.

We're talking here mainly about anabolic steroids to bulk up muscle and help with body sculpting in bodybuilders, fitness trainers, amateur athletes, older men, police and security workers. According to UK Home Office figures, anabolic steroid use in 16–24 year olds fell from 0.5 per cent in 2014–15 to 0.1 per cent in 2015–16, but 0.2 per cent of adults aged 16–59 reported using them. These drugs are injected and not always with clean needles so there is a risk of local infection (cellulitis and abscesses) and blood-borne viruses such as hepatitis C and HIV, although it seems at a lower level than intravenous drug users. There is also an issue about coexisting mental health issues in this group because perhaps around 50 per cent are also on psychoactive medications such as antidepressants. So it's likely that the drive to body sculpt in some people is about trying to satisfy a psychological need.

Potential harms from the steroids themselves include liver damage, which is usually reversible when the drug is stopped. One Dutch study found that common side effects were loss of libido, erectile dysfunction, acne and agitation. There is, possibly, an increased risk of heart disease but that is probably in older, longer term consumers of these steroids.

Is testosterone worth taking?

Testosterone in men

Quick take: It depends. If men haven't got what's called hypogonadism, then testosterone supplements don't benefit them much at all in the medium to long term.

*

There is evidence in men that falls in testosterone and other hormone levels are linked to an increased chance of dying prematurely. In women, low levels of testosterone have – controversially – been blamed for lack of libido. This has created a multi-billion-dollar industry for testosterone replacement therapy or supplements with dehydroepiandrosterone (DHEA) which is used by the body to make sex hormones like testosterone. Unfortunately, trials in men have found no benefit in vitality, muscle strength or weight loss. There are small but short-lived improvements in sexual performance. There also may be small and mostly theoretical risks of heart disease and prostate cancer but most trials haven't gone on long enough to really know.

If you're a bloke and want to raise your testosterone levels, lose weight and get some exercise. Studies following large numbers of men have found that older men can have the testosterone levels of younger ones and that's usually associated with good metabolic health and not being overweight or obese. One study of healthy ageing men found no age-related decline in testosterone at all. It was a smoking history, obesity and other medical conditions which were linked to lower testosterone levels.

If you're not suffering serious symptoms suggesting hypogonadism, then it's not worth asking your GP for a testosterone test. Adult-onset hypogonadism is relatively rare and associated with symptoms including psychological changes, erectile dysfunction, loss of libido and male pattern facial and body hair, breast enlargement and fragile bones. This is a situation where testosterone replacement does help.

The disappointment has been from trials in ageing men with the kinds of testosterone levels you'd expect for their age. One reason could be that a decline in testosterone is just a result of other problems and not a cause of them.

Testosterone in women

Quick take: This is a minefield with explosive medical and social arguments based on an inadequate research base. There are some reported benefits from testosterone supplementation in women in terms of physical performance and sex, but that should not divert attention away from the social, psychological and couples' interventions which can help women who experience distress from low sexual desire and arousal.

*

In healthy young physically active women, testosterone cream has been shown to improve aerobic running time and increase lean mass. Not a reason for young women to get into testosterone cream because safety is still an unknown.

In premenopausal women there is no link between a woman's levels of most hormones and sexual function including arousal. There may be a small association with testosterone levels but the researchers weren't sure it was a significant finding.

One of the battlegrounds in women is a condition called hypoactive sexual desire disorder (HSDD). This is defined as a persistent deficiency in sexual fantasies and the desire for sexual activity and more recently in the fifth edition of the *Diagnostic and Statistical Manual of Mental Disorders* (*DSM-5*) was brought under the category of Female Sexual Interest/Arousal Disorder. Making this a medical condition infuriates many women since they see this as trying to explain away issues such as exhaustion from an unfair burden of household and childcare responsibilities, men's failure to give women what they want and need, and perceived societal expectations (not helped by the explosion in internet pornography) that high sexual performance is the norm. The corollary of that is some people, seeing deeper causes, have a resistance to treat this with a medication. Having said that, when researchers have brought together the available evidence, there is a bit of support for using testosterone patches to improve arousal and desire. But be wary. Long-term safety hasn't been proven.

Vitamins and mineral supplements

You know what my take on this is by now (see sections on diet, nutrition and antioxidants): It's a multi-billion-dollar industry based on very little science. Largely a con. Over-the-counter supplements give you large single whacks of vitamins and minerals at doses which potentially turn them into drugs rather than nutritional supplements. Unless you have a deficiency, there's little proven benefit compared to whole foods which have more potent combinations of nutrients, especially when cooked. Don't be beguiled by simple answers to complex questions. Vitamin D supplements in people who don't get outside enough, the elderly or those with dark skin and other high risk groups are exceptions, as may be vitamin B12 in older people who may not be absorbing it well from the stomach. But seek advice from your GP.

*

There's certainly money in supplements. Data from the British Nutrition foundation survey conducted in 2018 showed that 59 per cent of respondents bought vitamin, mineral or other supplements, and an average of 34 per cent took a supplement daily – 38 per cent of women and 29 percent of men. Whether supplements are seen as a replacement for a healthy diet is not known for sure but research has found that most adults and children in the UK don't meet the recommended dietary guidelines for fruit and vegetables.

The trouble is that supplements can't replace that deficit because what's lost is a vast array of micronutrients which have to interact with each other to give you the benefits. No supplement can live up to that challenge.

I'm only going to focus on five supplements which have various levels of evidence and confusion.

Vitamin D: If you're getting out in the sun enough (you can check with your GP or health practitioner about the right amount according to skin colour, latitude and time of year) then vitamin D supplementation isn't needed. Nor, in most circumstances, is vitamin D testing. During the spring and summer months in the UK, most people should be able to get the vitamin D they need through sunlight exposure on the skin and by eating a healthy, balanced diet. During the autumn and winter months, supplementation may be recommended. If your doctor thinks you're at risk of low vitamin D levels, then simply getting going with supplements is low risk.

Vitamin B12: There is a relatively rare form of anaemia called pernicious anaemia, where the stomach lacks a factor that allows vitamin B12 to be absorbed. Anyone with the symptoms of B12 deficiency needs to be investigated because there is a risk of developing stomach cancer if it's pernicious anaemia. The symptoms of B12 deficiency include tingling, muscle weakness, fatigue, a smooth tender tongue, depression and becoming easily irritable. Other causes of B12 deficiency are being on a strict vegan diet, having an autoimmune disease, Crohn's disease, surgery on the stomach and upper intestine, and being elderly.

The risk of starting B12 supplements without a doctor checking you out first is that pernicious anaemia could be covered up until it's too late. There is an argument for routine B12 supplements in people with types 1 and 2 diabetes, particularly if you're taking the medication metformin.

There isn't a lot of evidence for the neurological benefit (or indeed the value of B12 testing) from clinical trials in the elderly.

Some experts believe that if you are elderly and have diabetic kidney damage and need B12, then the formulation counts but it's controversial.

Folic acid: Women of childbearing age should be taking folic acid supplements so that if or when they fall pregnant they've reduced the risk of having a baby with spina bifida.

For the rest of us, as long as we're getting plenty of folate rich green leafy vegetables, then folic acid supplements should be unnecessary. There is a theoretical increased risk in older people of accelerating cancer development from folic acid supplementation but not in younger people.

Fish oil/omega 3 fatty acid supplements: A lot of people are taking fish oil supplements. There is some evidence that they improve mood and protect the heart but as more and more evidence accumulates, these benefits seem to disappear, and recent research has also identified a possible risk of atrial fibrillation. The real heart benefits appear to come from eating actual fish a couple of times a week.

High-dose fish oil is anti-inflammatory and can help relieve the discomfort of arthritis. Sadly, the supplements seem to have no impact on cognitive decline or dementia prevention but further research is needed.

Selenium: This is a mineral which is sometimes deficient in soils and, in trials of antioxidants, selenium hasn't shown harm. While there's been a little evidence that selenium supplements help to prevent cancer, large trials of selenomethionine have not shown benefit.

PART 2

What you take out of yourself – making sure it's not too much

Do as I say but ...

I've put off writing this section ... procrastinated ... gone back and added bits to the diet and nutrition stuff ... major avoidance. Why? Because I'm totally crap at managing the 'balance thing'. Totally. I learned as a lad in Scotland that the early bird catches the worm. Be the first at work and one of the last to leave. Never say no. A training in medicine is partly about learning you have to suck in as much experience as you can, never let a patient down and suck it up. Yes I know that's changed with medical schools trying to adapt medicine to a balanced life and employers bending over backwards to provide warm and friendly workplaces … but in the end you have to see, learn and do and be as good as you can. And when I abandoned medicine for journalism and broadcasting, I never lost that. My medical training seeped into my bones even though I haven't seen a patient for years. To this day, when doing a long interview on radio, I apply the history-taking skills I learned in psychiatry – which was my first choice of specialisation before I went into paediatrics. And coming back to the balance thing, you know something? I don't think anything's changed. When I look around the Australian Broadcasting Corporation and industries like advertising and media and government, in general, the people who prosper are those who finish the job and do it beyond expectations and aren't driven by lunch or a 5 p.m. knock-off. In fact, one of the predictors of good physical and mental health is having a job. Chronic unemployment is a bad risk factor as far too many people found during the Year of Plague. Work is part of life, and the relationships we develop at work are often our most lasting and supportive.

But we need a life; we need people we love and care for physically and emotionally and who will do the same for us and we need to be interested in the world and what it has to offer. Connected and engaged and in control of our choices and decisions as much as possible, and there's lots of evidence that this is at the core of wellbeing. The challenge is to find the time and freedom. One of the benefits of COVID has been an enforced shrinkage into our own worlds to learn what counts.

To bring this home before I get on and write more, here's what I've learned about myself. I'm selfish and have to fight that self-centred urge many times a day. I know in my life who counts and who I love and who I'd give my life for. I also know that I need structure in my life in balance with a sense of control over my destiny and some tangible 'giving back' with no expectation of reward. I'm a pretty anxious person who can drift into low mood but recognise that ups and downs are normal and to be expected. The downs strengthen us more than the good times but it's important to know when things are spinning away and we need to call for help.

Anyway, enough of this unctuous, self-indulgent, one-sided psychotherapy. Let's get into some evidence to help minimise the drain on ourselves and understand what we can put back.

The control factor (this is the stress bit)

#dontletthebastardsgetyoudown

The grab: Stress is normal. Distress is not. Nor are chronic, unrelenting feelings of being put upon and having too little freedom to make your own decisions about work and life. It's a sweeping generalisation, but it's better for your mental wellbeing if you're able to feel that you are in control of your life rather than feeling that external forces and events are directing how you live and work and how your future is going to unfurl. It's called our 'locus of control' and the more we're able to bring it home to ourselves, the better. It can be tough, though, if you've no money, lost your job, have three kids while on income support or are under a micromanaging boss in a high-pressured work environment.

*

My first memory of stress was of the kind that many people are addicted to, but for me then and ever since it's been very unpleasant, to the extent that my children, whenever we're in a funfair or theme park, call me a 'feartie' ... Scottish for a wimp or 'wuss'. The cause of that unpleasant experience is in fact at the intersection of where healthy stress can be very unhealthy indeed. And it's also about control.

When I was a kid, every Christmas in Glasgow they had an indoor fair in a huge Victorian barn of an exhibition centre called the Kelvin Hall. The Kelvin Hall had all the rides, stalls and excitement that you might experience at a fair. I must have been about four years old and my father, who rarely did anything with his children and hadn't a clue about child rearing, triumphantly announced that he had a friend at the Kelvin Hall who could 'get him in' and my dad was going to take me to the carnival. As a complete aside, Jews in those days considered it a crime against the Laws of Nature to buy retail. You had to know someone who knew someone in wholesale, which was why my clothes were pretty ugly and never what I wanted to wear until I started earning my own money. Anyway, getting free tickets to the fair was like a Jewish wet dream. Actually (another aside), Jews generally only have wet dreams about food.

Where was I? Oh yes. I'm four and going to the Kelvin Hall with my well-meaning but gormless dad. We found his friend amid the crowds and it turned out that he was a 'carnie' running a popular ride that was a high-speed open carousel which had you sitting on life-sized motorbikes, whizzing around, going up and down a bit like a mini big dipper. Since peak excitement for my father was sitting down to matzo ball soup and potato kugel (pudding), there was no way he was going on this ride but he wasn't going to deny his four-year-old the pleasure. So against my wishes, I was plonked onto a saddle, told to hang on and away I went. My father stood on the side talking to his friend and as I flew by every few seconds screaming in terror and waving to him to get me off, he waved back thinking I was having the time of my life. Took me years even to trust him to take me to the shops after that and to this day, fairs and theme parks are places of terror where the roles are reversed. My kids used to beg me to go on rides with them but I refused, retreating to the solace of an ice cream and waving at them, confident they – in contrast – were having a good time. Their mum was a much better sport.

The source of my terror was having no choice and needing to trust that it was safe and I wasn't going to die. My preschooler self's locus of control had dramatically become externalised. Locus of control refers to the extent to which people feel that they have control over the events that influence their lives. If you believe you have control over what is happening you have what's known as internal locus of control. If you have no control over what is happening and that external variables are to blame, you have external locus of control. In my case my life-long response at any fun-park when seeing a ride of death has been to think NO F..KING WAY. But imagine if that loss of control were to happen in a steady, low-key way every day of the week. It can be erosive and profoundly affect the way your body works. For some reason, whether it be genetic or as a result of my Kelvin Hall horror, whenever I've even sniffed at being in a situation where that sense of lost control is likely – usually at work – I try to do something about it and bring that locus back inside. It's a deep-seated need and has nothing to do with not liking to be told what to do or being given direction. People who resent that get nowhere in life. No, it's being told what to do constantly and microscopically and giving a person no credit for their skills and knowledge and ability to be a collaborator in deciding how the job might best be done. Some entrepreneurs get away with 'my way or the highway' but most successful leaders have vision, get others to share it, set clear goals and let smart people get on and achieve them. In so doing, probably unknowingly they reduce this most erosive form of chronic stress.

The word 'stress' just trips off the tongue as does 'burnout'. We need some stress in our lives to provide the oomph to get things done and improve our performance. The people who love the rides of death are hooked on the adrenaline high of acute, short-lived stress. Those same people, however, if ground down by a workplace or a life circumstance, such as trying to bring up three kids by yourself on a low income, and feel that life is doing stuff to you rather than you are the one with the power, may experience the unremitting stress which can lead to psychological and physical ill health. With chronic stress we trade adrenaline for high levels of cortisol (hypercortisolaemia) which affects almost every organ system including the immune system. Anxiety and low mood from chronic stress are obvious effects but so are heart attacks, strokes and maybe even diabetes and cancer.

The word

Before I go on, a word about the mind and body. The word is 'one' and it's the main message you need to take away if your goal is physical and psychological wellbeing.

The idea that the mind and body are separate is deep-seated and goes back centuries. Four hundred years ago, the French philosopher René Descartes argued that the mind (particularly consciousness) was a thing in its own right, independent of the physical stuff that we're made of. A bit like a puppet master, which makes perfect sense because your arm doesn't lift your morning coffee in its own right, you've got to tell it to. Actually that's not a good example. My arm would have to be cut off not to lift the coffee to my mouth but you know what I'm saying. While a physiological explanation of consciousness eludes scientists, to state the bleeding obvious, when you die, consciousness dies with us unless you believe in an afterlife, which of course is up to you. All I can deal with is the here and now and the here and now is that the mind, brain and body are a single entity.

That takes away a lot of mystery and allows you to focus on causes and solutions.

We get tied up in paranoia when it's suggested to us that our psychological state is contributing to physical symptoms like pain and fatigue. People who profess to believe in holistic medicine and the power of meditation and nutrition rise in anger because we think the doctor is telling us it's all in our mind. Get over it. Complex problems have complex causes and complex solutions.

Chronic stress is impossible to understand unless you accept that the mind and body are one.

The implications of That Word – there are more curves to flatten

One liner: The effects of chronic stress on the body can be huge and it starts in the brain. The big question is what flattens the epidemic curve of the problems caused by chronic stress and lack of control?

Let's start broad before zeroing in so I can show you the deep impact of chronic stress.

Health isn't evenly spread

There's a concept called the health gradient. It's like a hill where some people get stuck at the bottom and some people are at the top. The hill exists for just about everything in health, from depression and anxiety, to cancer, heart disease, diabetes and even the age at which you die. The people at the bottom of the hill get all these things – including premature death – and the people who reach the top live longer, healthier lives. But with the health hill, the gradient or steepness can be changed. What you want to do is flatten the hill so there's no gradient. It's a bit like flattening the coronavirus epidemic curve. While what flattened the COVID curve wasn't easy, it was pretty straightforward, namely social distancing, masks and hygiene, and, later on, vaccines. What flattens the health gradient is far less apparent. The first thing you think about is income and it's certainly true that rich people live longer than the poor and disadvantaged but it doesn't explain everything. In fact, far from it. For instance, wealthier people may live in suburbs with better facilities and schools and less polluted air. There's some evidence from the United States that local government spending is associated with longer lives but even then there's still more to the story.

If you want to study health gradients, it's best to follow the health and wellbeing of groups of people who are already in a hierarchy that is a gradient in its own right, from the low to the high and mighty, then see how that translates – if at all – into a health gradient. That's why three generations of UK researchers have been studying people working in the Civil Service – a highly circumscribed set of organisations where you know your place according to your job classification, from the cleaners to the mandarins who run the departments. It is named the Whitehall Study, after the Civil Service's HQ.

You won't be shocked to hear that the health gradient in the Civil Service maps closely, although not perfectly, a person's place in the hierarchy. The heads of departments tend to live longer and healthier lives than those below them.

So what causes this gradient? If you know that, then you can go about flattening the curve so more of us have a fair share of health and wellbeing. That was the challenge expatriate Australian Professor Sir Michael Marmot and his team set themselves at University College, London. In fact, Michael has spent his life trying to abolish health inequities and in so doing has found several factors which make a difference. More on that later.

The traditional risk factors for heart disease and cancer, like cholesterol, high blood pressure and smoking, didn't seem to be the cause of the gradient in their own right. Something else was going on. Income didn't make much of an impact nor did use of health services. The level of education did matter but not as much as they'd expected.

Then they factored in locus of control. In fact, they adapted it to something they called 'job strain', defined (crudely) as how much pressure you felt under at work to perform and how much freedom – or latitude – you felt you had to decide how best to achieve the targets being set for you. Job strain was strongly linked to the health gradient and the more job strain, the further down the hill you found yourself, and the reason wasn't necessarily that high job strain made you smoke, eat badly and get no exercise. The poor locus of control was in itself unhealthy for some reason. It was doing something to your body.

Around the time of these findings, Professor Len Syme, a public health researcher at the University of California Berkeley, USA, was also looking at the causes and effects of health inequalities. He thought there was more to it than job strain or having too external a locus of control. What, he wondered, were the practical effects on people when they lost that sense of personal control? He was studying disadvantaged populations in the Bay Area, specifically Oakland, on the same side of San Francisco Bay as Berkeley but much poorer. He was struck by what a low locus of control did to people. It took away their belief in themselves and their confidence to make decisions or take action. Some call it 'loss of self-efficacy'. Others call it 'learned helplessness'.

Many years ago, Professor Martin Seligman, of the University of Pennsylvania, USA, and a founder of the positive psychology movement, reached a turning point in his thinking when he was doing conditioning experiments on dogs using light electric shocks. The shocks were administered in an enclosed environment from which there was no escape. When the dogs were then put in a box where they could escape shocks easily, amazingly, they didn't. The psychologists hadn't realised they'd conditioned the dogs to believe that escape wasn't possible. They lay down and accepted what the psychologists doled out. They had learned to be helpless and accept the adversity, whereas when dogs which hadn't had the first round of shocks were put into the box from which they could jump out, they didn't accept the light shocks and scarpered.

Len Syme found that a single mother of three on income support having to phone a social service for help would, if faced with a recorded voice offering press-button options for services, hang up rather than make the decision to press button 2. It's well recognised in the demoralised, long-term unemployed that they sometimes find it hard to take even simple actions like getting dressed for a job interview. Prolonged adversity does this to us. This loss of self-efficacy has also been seen in women with cancer while they've been undergoing chemotherapy. The medical system, when it takes decision-making and power away from their patients, however unintentionally, can remove decision-making capacity about life in general. There's no escape, so what's the point? It makes us vulnerable to trauma and post traumatic stress disorder (PTSD), with all the physical symptoms that go with it, and probably fatigue as well.

This control thing isn't some namby-pamby, squishy, lefty idea. There's hard science behind it.

In addition to the work by Professors Marmot and Syme, biologists have found extremely potent physical effects on our brains and genes.

Overload and the brain

The late Professor Bruce McEwen, a neuroendocrinologist at Rockefeller University in New York, USA, led the way studying the impact of chronic stress on the brain and the rest of the body. (Rockefeller, by the way, is one of the world's leading research universities with many Nobel Laureates in its history.) Bruce McEwen studied chemical messengers such as stress hormones. His name for the burden on the brain from chronic stress and loss of internal locus of control was 'allostatic load'. Allostasis is the natural balance of stress in our bodies (including mind and brain). Acute stress from, say, a threat to our lives or a near-miss car crash creates a surge of adrenaline and other acute stress hormones to allow us to fight the threat or flee it (fight or flight). Most of us recover quickly from this kind of stress and largely stay in control. We all need some of this allostatic load to gee us up to meet deadlines and perform well but, as I said, it's a balance. The second kind of load which disrupts this allostasis of brain function and hormones is just what we've been talking about here, namely a dysfunctional environment which loads us up day after day and which we find hard to change. This can tip us into allostatic overload and here McEwen observed troubling consequences affecting stress hormones as well as centres in the brain involved in mood, memory and how our immune and cardiovascular systems operate. There's no flight response – no escape by running away – from this overload. We're like those dogs in the box. The solution is to change the way we live and work, and preventing and dealing with life-sapping disadvantage. McEwen and others argued that exposure to this kind of stress in early childhood could mould kids' brain function and make them additionally vulnerable as adults. In other words, there's a risk that the brain becomes less plastic and the person more prone to anxiety.

The story then is of many factors coming together to increase our vulnerability, from the genes we were born with, to traumatic life events, to lack of opportunities, to poverty and deprivation, to a badly managed or designed workplace.

Stress and shoelaces

There are also important physical effects of chronic stress on our chromosomes. Those are the structures in our cells which contain our genes. These findings come in part from research by Tasmanian Nobel Laureate, Professor Elizabeth Blackburn, who's based in the USA. Professor Blackburn and her colleagues discovered telomerase, an enzyme that preserves the telomeres – the protective ends of our chromosomes – a bit like the plastic on the end of a shoelace to stop it fraying. You don't want your chromosomes which contain your genes to fray. That's what causes ageing. The shorter our telomeres, the more likely we are to age prematurely. And what shortens our telomeres? You've guessed it. The disadvantage and life circumstances that produce allostatic overload as well as the unhealthy behaviours that go along with it and which in turn generate oxidative stress. So it's no surprise that damaged telomeres are associated with cancer and other age-linked diseases. In fact, Elizabeth Blackburn and her colleagues have found that women with high levels of perceived stress can have telomere shortening equivalent to ten years of ageing.

The good news is that Professor Blackburn's research and others have shown that diet and lifestyle changes can lengthen and protect telomeres. The damage is reversible.

We humans value freedom because it's hardwired into us. It explains why older people resist going into residential aged care – even before COVID-19. It's the fear of loss of control. It also helps explain why indigenous communities value control above almost all else, because from that control comes freedom to express culture and identity and change destiny. It's why education has such a potent effect on our health, wellbeing, longevity and even whether we get dementia, because knowledge and understanding allow greater resilience and control. It's why government departments like finance, employment and justice have far more impact on our allostatic load than health departments.

What to do about it and where anxiety fits in

In short: Don't jump prematurely to the conclusion that it's your job which is causing you to feel chronically stressed. You might think that work is the problem when it's actually a build-up of control-sapping life events such as relationship breakdown, a parent who's unwell, financial difficulties, or all of the above. There's quite a lot you can do for yourself to reduce your allostatic load. Taking control of what you can in your life is the first step, but many people need help to go through the issues and that's not a sign of weakness or a cause for shame. Seeing a psychologist can be incredibly useful and there are online psychotherapy programmes for the anxiety and depression that often go along with it. Many of these online programmes have good evidence behind them. People who are in work are healthier than the unemployed and no workplace is perfect. That's not to downplay the fact that you might be in a workplace that's badly organised or chaotic with a boss who doesn't know how to manage people, but that will seem a heck of a lot worse if there are other things going on in your life at the same time.

*

There's a blurred line between anxiety and perceived stress. While I have my anxious moments, I don't see myself as a generally anxious person. When faced with a crisis, my family and others know that I'm the one who stays cool. If something unexpected happens on air, my producers know I'll handle it. When there are toxic incoming texts from listeners on the studio screen, I say to myself, 'F..k the lot of them,' and get on with it. Yet there have been periods when I've been repeatedly paralysed by stomach-churning anxiety that's so bad I want to double over in a crouch position. The most recent lasted more than a year and started with my mother in Scotland being put into a locked ward because of aggressive behaviour, then a short illness on my part, then my daughter having a terrible bicycle accident and a life-threatening brain injury, then a relationship falling apart, then my mother dying. And everyone was looking to me. At one point just after the accident, explaining the situation to my other kids in the cafeteria in an Italian hospital, I broke down and started to cry. With horror, I saw the horror and fear in their eyes as they filled with tears and

I immediately realised I couldn't do that. I couldn't let them see my pain. They were relying on me. Later that day on the phone to a close friend who was a professor of psychology in Glasgow, she reminded me of the saying, 'Keep your shit wired tight'. When in a crisis or emergency, there's usually little to be gained by opening up. It's a bit of a myth that having a cathartic conversation is good for you psychologically. It can make things worse if you feel pressed into doing it and that has a lot to do with creating maladaptive memories. If you are distressed and want support, then that's a different matter.

The most extreme form of anxiety is post traumatic stress disorder (PTSD). It often occurs after an event which you felt at the time seriously endangered you and that you might die. I know all about PTSD because I had it for most of my adolescence. I was 14 years old and on a coach with a group of kids my age, when the bus unexpectedly exploded into flames in the middle of the countryside. Those flames are seared into my memory. My coolness under fire (so to speak) worked against me. When the fire started I stayed in my seat a second or two too long by which time the exit door was engulfed. Everything was on fire and there was no air to breathe. Luckily the bus had windows you could pull down, but not by much. A girl was by my side and after getting the window down I pushed her out. Then I shoved myself through the gap but overwhelming pain made me black out. I came to, lying on the road, and got up to walk away, dazed. Someone pointed at me and I looked down. I was almost naked below the waist. My pants had burned off as I'd hung upside-down outside the window. There are worse memories of what followed which I won't share with you but for years after I would get flashbacks, nightmares, mood changes and a fear of enclosed spaces which only dissipated when I worked out how I'd escape if there was a disaster. No-one understood PTSD at that time and eventually it dulled, although I still automatically look for a way out in new, confined places. It came back a bit after my daughter's accident because I'd got to the scene just after it happened and it was ugly.

It won't have eluded you that I can still describe these events in full technicolour. The theory behind PTSD is that the trauma lays down abnormally strong memories which can swirl in your brain rather than being parked for future use like most memory. It used to be thought that when a disaster occurred, like a bushfire or a train wreck, the right thing to do was send in counsellors to debrief survivors and first responders. It's now known that acute debriefing can cause PTSD or at the very least make it worse. The reason is that debriefing makes you talk through what happened and in so doing reinforces the memory in your brain. Professionals should be on hand to provide support for those who ask for it, but the support that people want may not be psychological.

After the 2004 Indian Ocean tsunami, which killed hundreds of thousands of people, a friend of mine who's a professor of psychiatry in Tamil Nadu argued with the Indian government, which wanted to send in counsellors to the Tamil Nadu coastline. He had been to the area and when he asked survivors what they wanted and needed, it was carpenters, electricians and builders to restore their homes and lives. Some would go on to experience PTSD and needed to know that when they wanted help for that, a few weeks or months later, it would be available.

The vast majority of people who have anxiety that interferes with their lives do not have PTSD nor indeed have had much trauma in their lives. Some will have inherited the tendency from one or other parent but whatever the reason, if it is affecting your life, then it needs to be dealt with. For some people, all they need is to understand anxiety, its causes and how it can be helped. That's sometimes called bibliotherapy – knowledge as therapy – and of course the reason it works is about being able to take back your locus of control and not assuming that anxiety rules your life. For many that's only part of the solution and there are various psychotherapies which can help by readjusting your thinking and responses to events around you, which, by the way, might include looking for another job or career. And if psychotherapy doesn't work, then some antidepressant medications which affect the serotonin system in the brain (serotonergic) are good at controlling anxiety. What doesn't work is drinking, smoking, sniffing or injecting your way out of it. Moderately intense daily exercise and trying to get unbroken sleep are my therapies. Mental Health UK has great resources and can direct you to the right place: mentalhealth-uk.org.

The bigger picture and what it means for living younger longer

The gap: You might recall that when I was talking about nutrition, what counted was far more than the nutrient content of your food. It was the whole package of our lives, about culture and cuisine and identity and the people around you. When I was talking about the control factor, you'll have quickly realised I was again talking about our lives as a whole and the importance of bringing a strong sense that we have some control and agency over our lives and decisions. But one of the most potent causes of loss of control is bad or neglectful government policies. They have an enormous influence on how long we live and the gap between those who live long, healthy lives and those who live short, unhealthy ones.

*

The west of Scotland, where I grew up, had one of the highest rates of coronary heart disease in the world. The life expectancy gap between the richest and poorest suburb was 15–20 years. External observers put this down to smoking, deep-fried Mars Bars, haggis and chips, and no physical activity. Glaswegian researchers knew better. Some call it 'The Glasgow Effect'.

When there's a life expectancy gap, it's easy to assume that it's because fewer 70-year-olds reach 80 or 90. While there's some truth to that, it's far from the whole explanation. Most life expectancy gaps occur because younger people die and in so doing lose – tragically – many more years of life than an elderly person and therefore can have a disproportionate effect on the statistics. Young people by and large don't die of heart disease and cancer. They die of drug use, preventable accidents, crime and suicide, and those are caused by disadvantage, poverty, cultural alienation, fragmented social networks and loss of identity.

Glaswegians didn't actually smoke a lot more or eat a lot worse than people in similar British cities. Paradoxically, their life expectancy started diverging when Scottish authorities – with the best of intentions – knocked down the worst slums in western Europe and relocated people to vast council house (social housing) estates. In an attempt to give people a better life, governments inadvertently destroyed community cohesion and identity and the supports which went with them. There was nothing romantic about a Glasgow tenement slum but everyone knew everyone else and there were safe courtyards for the kids to play with each other. Yes alcoholism, domestic violence and smoking rates were high, but that didn't stop when people moved to high-rise council blocks in poorly designed, one-class suburbs distant from the facilities of a city. Drug use ran rampant and people died relatively young of preventable causes which didn't affect richer communities nearly as much.

The biggest life expectancy gap in Australia, when you compare the longest-lived postcode to the shortest-lived, is an astounding 45 years, according to research by Professor John Glover in Adelaide. In the UK, according to the Office for National Statistics (ONS) report for 2017–2019, the biggest gap is between London and the North East and is 11.3 years for men and 8.7 years for women.

In Australia, according to data from the Australian Bureau of Statistics (ABS), the leading cause of years of life lost (YLL) in 2019 was suicide plus intentional self-harm and it was by a long way, with heart disease trailing a distant second. Dislocation, loss of identity and feelings of helplessness drive this with a cycle of disadvantage which starts in pregnancy. First Nations communities in countries like Australia and North America, though, have for years recognised that self-determination and taking control are the solutions they need to pursue.

Communities are stronger than families and individuals when it comes to acting for change.

Acting as a community is what's needed to encourage employers and governments to develop policies which are good for young kids, families, schools and workplaces irrespective of gender, ethnicity and disadvantage. Housing and education have more long-term impact than health services, important as they are.

We tend to think that money can solve all problems but that doesn't play out when, for instance, you try to find out why how long you live – life expectancy – varies from country to country. It's what a nation does with the money it has.

While people in very poor countries tend to live shorter lives, once you get past a gross domestic product (GDP) per capita of just over $5000–7000, there isn't a strong relationship between how much a nation earns and how long its citizens live. How rich your country is isn't much of a determinant. Cuba, Chile and Costa Rica have a third to half of the GDP per capita of the United States yet their people have a similar life expectancy. The UK, Canada and Australia also have a lower GDP than the US, yet a higher life expectancy. It's also not closely related to how much you spend on health care. Australia and Canada, for instance, spend a lot less on health care as a proportion of GDP, yet on average, Australians, Canadians and the British live longer than Americans. The World Bank's World Development Report 'Investing in Health' found that one of the key determinants of a nation's life expectancy was not how much a country earned but the gap between rich and poor. In other words, how the income was distributed and how fair a nation was. The attributes of a longer-lived nation tended to be investment in areas of social infrastructure where the market fails such as housing, education and health care.

The word 'average' hides many sins.

Successful governments invest in what builds successful communities and are not hung up on unproven notions that markets will solve everything or that the power to change rests on individuals. There's a place for enterprise and the drive of commerce. Planned economies generally fail but that is different from governments recognising where they need to intervene in partnership with communities.

Professor Marmot suggests six things individuals, communities and governments can do, based on scientific evidence:

1. Give every child the best start in life.
2. Enable all children, young people and adults to maximise their capabilities and have control over their lives.
3. Create fair employment and good work for all.
4. Ensure a healthy standard of living for all.
5. Create and develop healthy and sustainable places and communities.
6. Strengthen the role and impact of ill health prevention.

History and your health (this is the pandemic bit)

Takeaway: We've just lived through the worst pandemic to hit humankind for more than a hundred years, caused by a new virus that's probably only existed for a year or two. COVID-19 has killed millions of people and will now likely be with us for eternity. History in the making but it's not the first time that a germ has made history and changed human destiny. History is important for our health in a couple of ways. Firstly, our genes reflect our personal history going back centuries. They've been handed down to us from ancestors we'll never know, who often lived in faraway places and who survived privation and disease partly because the genes they themselves inherited helped them survive. History also matters because it's a description of human behaviour through the ages. Changes in human behaviour, the environment and the way we live, create new diseases or thrust old ones back into the spotlight. Cigarettes brought lung cancer and heart disease. Political, social and sexual revolutions in Africa and around the world brought HIV-AIDS. Travel, trade and environmental change brought the Black Death. A voyage of discovery then warfare brought syphilis. The market for cheap, manufactured food, along with motorcars and television, brought obesity.

*

The message? Don't be beguiled by modern medicine or politicians who distract us with dramatic announcements of new cancer drug funding or peddlers of simplistic and therefore always wrong solutions. Bigger forces determine our health and wellbeing and we need to be aware of them so we're not mugged by reality.

Pandemics: what we know and don't know

So far in history, pandemics have usually started in animals and passed to humans when there's been social change, war, new technologies, environmental disruption, or all of the above. I say 'so far' because with gene editing (CRISPR), it's only a matter of time before a terrorist with a biology degree and a small lab produces a novel organism that sweeps the world. That's if they haven't done it already.

But back to what we know or don't, as the case may be.

It's curious how some patients remain in your memory.

It was 1977 and I was a medical resident in Aberdeen Royal Infirmary in northeast Scotland. It was winter and we were accustomed to elderly people being admitted with pneumonia. But this man was different. He was young – in his 40s – and came in for tests for a history of odd infections. He had travelled a lot in his job and his white cell count was a bit low. He started off in the general ward but soon became very ill, though it wasn't at all clear what was actually wrong. All our tests came back negative and he died shockingly quickly. The autopsy found nothing to explain it. A few years later as a medical journalist covering the HIV-AIDS pandemic, I often thought about that man and wondered, could HIV (human immunodeficiency virus) have been the cause?

Stick to veggies in the jungle – what can happen when you eat animals from the 'wild'

When AIDS (acquired immune deficiency syndrome) became headlines in the 1980s, people thought that this was the first new virus to infect humankind. Well, it wasn't the first and it certainly wasn't the last, just as the COVID-19 virus won't be the last. At the time of writing, the AIDS pandemic has infected 75 million people directly and had an impact on many times that number in terms of families, children, friends and economies. Thirty-three million have died and it still kills large numbers because of inadequate access to testing and treatment.

Researchers now know that HIV has been around for at least 100 years. So in fact it wasn't at all new when it emerged globally as a pandemic. Genetic and chimpanzee studies have pieced together the story. For centuries in Central Africa, in the Congo and Cameroon, chimps and small monkeys have lived with versions of what's called the simian immunodeficiency virus (SIV). Chimps are carnivores and eat the small monkeys and at some point – just like the coronavirus in bats – their viruses mingled. Around 1920, a new version of SIV emerged in chimps which was contagious and could infect and cause disease in the hunters who killed and butchered the chimps for bush meat. This SIV was pretty much identical to HIV. It's likely the first person with HIV was in Kinshasa around that time. This happened after a period when Christianity had made inroads into traditional life with the effect that it was harder for young men to find sexual partners in their family group. The result was growth in the sex trade.

Getting the picture?

The origins of HIV are about how we live, make a living, what we eat and what we believe. HIV spread to other parts of Central Africa but, in those days, travel was difficult and in some communities, HIV would have reached a bit of a dead-end because of the high prevalence of male circumcision – which is known to reduce transmission. It took another 50 or 60 years for HIV to go global. Kinshasa was already a transport and trading hub but became an HIV epicentre just as sub-Saharan Africa had opened up with easy and commonplace international travel. The virus spread globally, finding vulnerabilities among intravenous (IV) drug users and gay communities, which it ravaged. However, HIV-AIDS is not a 'gay disease'. In sub-Saharan Africa and many other places, the spread is primarily heterosexual. HIV has no brain. Its only biological drive is to survive and reproduce. It's our behaviour which allows that to happen. Luckily, while there's no effective vaccine yet, we have effective treatments.

Once a new disease has arisen, it almost never disappears.

Smallpox – a dreadful viral infection which killed children in vast numbers – was a scourge that probably made the jump from monkeys to humans thousands of years ago. It was the first virus to be mass-immunised against around 200 years ago and its spread was eliminated after a huge global effort which, in the end, focused on cluster outbreaks (sound familiar?).

Farming made lives hard and created new diseases

One of the greatest technological changes to affect humankind was agriculture, because it allowed our ancestors to stop being hunters and gatherers and settle into villages and cities. We know this was the period when measles and chickenpox would have become pandemics. Once they made the jump from animals, they became exclusive to humans so they needed enough people living together to survive and spread. Agriculture allowed that to happen through increasing population numbers and density. Studies of skeletons pre-agriculture and after showed that we became shorter – a proxy for ill health – and people didn't regain the height of their Stone Age ancestors until the beginning of the 20th century. When you see paintings of Indigenous people at first contact, say in the New World and Australia, they were tall and strong.

That changed within a generation or so.

Agriculture, while a huge innovation, brought its own miseries.

The Black Death

This is a bacterial infection not a virus. The bug is called *Yersinia pestis* and mostly lives quite happily with rodents and other mammals until, for some reason, it mutates to become more deadly and contagious. Some think that happens when there's environmental disruption such as a flood or earthquake. That may be what occurred in Central Asia in the 14th century when the plague spread via the Silk Road trading routes and landed in a war in Crimea. The Mongols laid siege to the port of Caffa, which was part of the Genoese trading empire. There is some evidence that the Mongols used plague as a weapon by using catapults to fling plague-ridden corpses into the city. It worked, and the Genoese and others fled around the Black Sea coast and back to Italy, taking the plague with them. Once the disease landed, it spread quickly, killing maybe 30 per cent of the population of Europe, ending serfdom, creating wage labour and setting the scene for the Reformation. Daniel Defoe's *A Journal of the Plague Year* reads familiarly to all of us who've lived through the COVID-19 pandemic.

The Black Death lasted for 300 years and re-emerged in the 19th century in China, again at a conjunction of environmental change and social unrest. It spread around the Pacific, including Australia. But in the USA, something disastrous happened when the plague landed. *Yersinia pestis* clearly liked what it saw in North American wildlife and became endemic in those animals as it had for thousands of years in Central

Asia. And here's the horror scenario. Plague is endemic in wild animals around San Francisco. If there's a massive earthquake along one of California's major fault lines and a mutation in *Yersinia pestis*, you could see a plague outbreak in the domestic animals of the city, and then to humans. If it became pneumonic plague, passing directly from person to person, thousands could die within hours before getting access to antibiotics.

Trans-Atlantic travel has a lot to answer for

Syphilis is a nasty sexually transmitted disease caused by a bacterium called *Treponema pallidum*. It can affect most organs of the body and pregnant women can transmit it to their foetuses with devastating consequences. There is no evidence that syphilis existed in Europe prior to the first voyage of Christopher Columbus to the New World, where there is considerable historical evidence of it from skeletons in South America. What seems to have happened is that sailors on his 1492 expedition caught syphilis or a related bacterial disease called yaws while on Hispaniola. They brought it back and fought as mercenaries for the French at the Siege of Naples only a year after they returned. The victory 'celebrations' may have been the 'super spreading event'. When it first appeared syphilis was a ghastly skin disease which eroded bones and cartilage anywhere on the body including the face. Many died. This is the first recorded outbreak of syphilis. By 1520, only two decades later, it had become a pandemic. Syphilis had gone global. Over the subsequent centuries it has become less aggressive but is still dangerous.

President Trump called coronavirus the 'China virus'. In the early days of syphilis, it got the name of the country which someone in authority thought he could blame for it: the French Pox, the Neapolitan disease, the Polish disease, etc. etc. Men thought they could get rid of syphilis by having sex with a virgin. Which is what happened again centuries later in Africa, with HIV-AIDS.

The next pandemic

Pandemics are no surprise to people who know this history. Prior to December 2019, when SARS-CoV-2 took off in Wuhan, China, the two viruses that people were expecting to cause a pandemic were influenza and the coronavirus family. Bats are incubators of new viruses and they live in huge colonies with no social distancing. Domesticated pigs and fowl are incubators of new influenza viruses. New viral diseases are emerging all the time. Most come to little, mostly because they're not very contagious, which is a good thing since quite a few have terrifyingly high death rates. But ... the time has come for the experts to be surprised because of technological change and a bit of history.

One of the persistent stories of the COVID-19 pandemic has been that the virus is an escapee from the Wuhan Institute of Virology. We'll probably never know the trigger but this was not a mad theory. The lab had a scientist who's a world authority on coronaviruses and had predicted a bat-sourced outbreak from an experiment which manipulated a coronavirus in the lab. It's called 'gain of function' where genetic engineers can make a virus behave more or less aggressively. No-one knows how many labs and scientists around the world have this capacity to manipulate life forms and all it takes is one rogue lab for humanity to be threatened in a much more profound way than the COVID-19 virus.

On 5 July 2019, two leading Chinese Canadian researchers and their Chinese students were marched out of Canada's highest security lab for the study of viruses. One of them had been instrumental in developing a treatment for Ebola. The Royal Canadian Mounted Police had been carrying out an undercover investigation since May of that year. The researchers were married and restrictions had already been placed on their travel to China. The laboratory said that it was an administrative matter. This was despite Ebola and Henipavirus samples supposedly having been sent to the Wuhan Institute of Virology in March. The Henipavirus family are considered to have high biowarfare potential. Two of their members, *Hendra* (first discovered in Australia) and *Nipah* can have mortality rates above 50 per cent.

Over the past 20 years or more, while the world has been dazzled and obsessed by the technology revolution which has allowed smartphones and invisibly powerful computing in our living rooms, there has been a quiet, incredibly powerful revolution in the technology of synthetic biology. For a few hundred thousand dollars, biologists can manipulate and even create life forms in labs. The technology and costs of gene editing are such that a member of ISIS with a PhD and a relatively cheap lab could produce a unique and deadly version of the smallpox virus along with its own exclusive vaccine.

Pandemics are like global hurricanes where the shock of their force is amplified by a sense of our vulnerability, the surprise that a microscopic organism with no life of its own can do this, and the uncertainty about how they began and where and when the next one will emerge. Because it could be perilously soon. It's not likely but equally not impossible that the COVID-19 virus came from a lab and for the first time in history, the next pandemic could be made by humans. The answer is global vigilance for emerging diseases and urgent detective work to ascertain where they came from and international checks on raw materials going to labs working on gene editing.

Never forget that as we change our behaviour, we can expect new diseases.

Your genes as history in the making – but they're not destiny

Takeaways: Our genes drive 20–70 per cent of how we behave, eat, love and generally make decisions. That leaves a lot of room for us to change the way we live and learn and the extent to which people are able to have choices. Yet again – don't be beguiled by biology, no matter how fancy.

*

When I was a lad, genes were a political battlefield. Some on the extreme right argued that genes were destiny and if you were Black, Jewish or Asian, then that meant you had inferior genes. Eugenicists used that to justify racial segregation aimed at avoiding the mingling of these genes with the 'superior' ones belonging – usually – to white Europeans. At its most extreme, this view of genetics justified genocide – the deliberate elimination of a race. Slightly more subtly – again on the extreme right – there was nothing you could do to improve the lives of disadvantaged people because they were, in fact, disadvantaged because of their genes. So social policies in education, employment and housing, for example, were a waste of money. You couldn't change genetic destiny. These wrong and toxic beliefs provided sustenance to the Australian and North American history of neglect and persecution of its First Nations peoples.

Those on the left had an equal and opposite reaction. Any suggestion that genes could decide a person's fate was anathema. The environment was everything and if you gave families better housing, access to health care and education, then they could pull themselves out of disadvantage. Genes played no role.

Nowadays science has settled but not eliminated these arguments and prejudices.

If you want to stick to genes, skip the next couple of paragraphs but it might pay to stay with me, because I want to take a small but important meander. It goes directly to this tension between our biology – our physiological make-up – and our social and physical environments.

The idea that germs cause disease is so deeply understood by us all that it's hard to appreciate that this wasn't known until the 19th century, when Louis Pasteur in Paris brought together evidence that had been gathering for decades thanks to the invention of the microscope. Now, you'd think that doctors and the public would have embraced this. Well, they didn't for another 30 years or so, despite scientific discoveries such as finding tubercle bacillus, the bug that causes tuberculosis (TB). One reason for that resistance is that doctors are generally appalling at taking up evidence into practice and a 25-year delay isn't unusual, even now. But the other reason – and again was from the left – was the intuitive belief that the social and economic environment drove disease and disadvantage.

One of the proponents of this view was a giant of 19th-century medical research, Rudolf Virchow. Like Pasteur, Virchow used the microscope to investigate human disease but, rather than germs, Virchow traced it back to the various cells in our body. This is the basis of modern pathology. Virchow described leukaemia and had insights into the origins of cancer which have held up to this day. But Virchow rejected the germ theory of disease because his political observations drove him to conclude that it was far more complicated than a simple germ. Virchow believed that medicine was a social science. In the late 1840s he had studied a typhus epidemic in Upper Silesia which was then in Prussia. Now it's mostly in Poland. It was a desperately poor region and there were food riots among the impoverished coalminers there. What Virchow saw confirmed his belief that epidemics are social in origin and require political action.

The thing is that both views were – and are – right. Germs do cause disease but not in a social vacuum. The theme in this book is that much as we'd like to, we can't dissect out individual variables and give them significance they don't deserve. We humans come as a package in the world in which we live, with the people we live with and next to, the state of the physical environment and how fair our society is, especially when free markets can't supply all the answers, as they can't in education, housing and health, not to mention policing, justice and defence.

Anyway, having got that off my chest, back to germs, disease and society before I revert to genes.

The scientist who discovered the tubercle bacillus, that's the bacterium which causes tuberculosis, was Robert Koch in Berlin in 1882. While Koch proved that the tubercle bacillus caused TB, what he couldn't have known is that a significant proportion of the population of Berlin had the bacillus in their bodies, but far from all of them developed TB. Tuberculosis was quintessentially a social disease whose incidence was affected by gender (women seemed to get it worse than men), disadvantage and poor housing and nutrition. The point is (I'm sure you've got it by now) if you drill down to just the biology, you're risking, as I said before, being mugged by reality.

Meander over. Back to genes.

Two research techniques have produced overwhelming and challenging evidence on the influence of genes on almost every aspect of our lives. One is scanning for thousands of mutations at single points across the genome. They're called single nucleotide polymorphisms (SNPs) and they're like markers where researchers generally know what genes are nearby. Researchers use such maps to do what are called genome-wide association studies (GWAS) – massive exercises in huge numbers of people to see what genes light up in association with all sorts of things. For instance, heavily addicted smokers are linked to genes which speed up the breakdown of nicotine; and people who use cannabis tend to have genes that give them an owlish sleep pattern, namely staying up late at night and sleeping late into the morning. Whereas people who actually become cannabis dependent tend to have genes which increase the risk of alcohol use, tobacco dependence and mental health issues such as schizophrenia, ADHD and major depression. There are also associations with genes which seem to influence risk-taking behaviour.

But these are associations – links – not proof of cause and effect, and such findings don't buy health professionals or governments a way out by blaming genes.

The acrimonious and ideological gene versus environment debate has cooled down in recent years for a couple of reasons. One is that the human genome study showed that the genetic differences between individuals are greater and generally more meaningful than the differences between ethnic groups. The second reason is that studies comparing identical to non-identical twins and, less commonly, twins who've been separated and raised in different households, have been clear that the environment plays a huge role. Identical twins have very similar sets of genes whereas non-identical twins are no different from normal brothers and sisters, so you can start to compare the effects of genes and environment. The influence of genes varies anywhere between 20 and 70 per cent. Even at 70 per cent, there's still a lot of room to change the social and physical environment for the best.

Your destiny can affect your genes

The message: Your genes are susceptible to good and bad environments and that can make a difference to your kids when you have them. It used to be thought that our genes change incredibly slowly over centuries or thousands of years. Recent research has shown that genes are exquisitely tuned to the way we live, whether we have money, have had the benefit of a decent education and live in a nice house. And some of the changes induced by a poor environment can be passed to your kids.

*

Earlier on, I mentioned the effects of chronic stress and disadvantage on the telomeres. These are like the plastic tip protecting a shoelace, whereas telomeres guard the ends of chromosomes. The longer they are, the better; and the shorter, the greater the likelihood of chronic disease and early death.

Another effect of our environment on our genes is on their shape and function. In the early days of genetics, researchers were pretty much solely focused on mutations – physical changes in the genetic code. But as techniques for studying DNA have advanced, it's been realised that genes don't need to mutate to change the way they work. It's called epigenetics. What appears to happen is that there are changes to the links which hold the spirals (the double helix) of DNA together. As the shape of the helix changes, so does the ability of the gene to do its job.

There's growing evidence that how we live and the environment in which children grow up can induce epigenetic changes in our genes which may last for life and some believe can be transmitted between generations.

The good news is that there's also growing evidence that epigenetic changes are not necessarily permanent and might be reversed or at least slowed down by lifestyle changes and, in diseases like cancer, perhaps with medications.

Gobsmacked – gene testing your spit

Any value? It's far from clear what the value is in having one of the commercial online consumer genetic tests, either for checking out your origins or disease prediction, and there are risks. These tests are not a sequence of your whole genome and the results can vary according to which company you use. Be very wary of nutritional genetic tests. They can be a scam or, at the very least, scare you unnecessarily and get you to buy a nutritional product you don't need.

*

Let's start with where your genes and maybe you have come from. In general, these companies compare your genetic pattern with the samples they hold from other people they've tested. So you might initially find out you're 2 per cent Greek (which one of my brothers did) but another company might find 14 per cent or not at all or revise their findings as time passes and they're able to use a bigger population for comparative analysis. There's no such thing as a Greek gene, it's more like shared genetic patterns. So it's fun which can turn out to be disturbing if you find out you're not who you think you are – say, if your siblings get tested and are very different from you (I've chosen not to, but have taken it as explanation for my addiction to spanakopita and moussaka).

If you want to know whether you're at risk of having inherited a susceptibility to, say, heart disease or cancer, the best indicator is still knowing what close relatives in your family have died of and at what age. A few close relatives being diagnosed younger than usual or more frequently even at an older age is a warning sign that might be explained by gene testing but there's still a lot that's unknown about genetic patterns of risk. Similarly, a consumer test that turns up a risk which doesn't match what you know about your family may not be real.

You see, the way they're doing these saliva tests at such a low price is to look for the single nucleotide polymorphisms (SNPs) I mentioned earlier, the single point changes that can indicate there's a particular gene nearby. So it's about patterns rather than detailed genetic analysis for diagnostic purposes. When it comes to your ancestry, the SNP patterns tend to reflect the current genetic pattern of, say, Greeks, rather than what truly might have prevailed at the time of your distant forefathers and mothers.

If a consumer genetic test gives you some health information you find troubling, you really do need to have it double-checked with your GP and maybe a genetic counsellor. For example, with the broad range of breast cancer genes, consumer tests don't often actually tell you that the gene is present, they only indicate what might be a worrying pattern, which may not be a worry at all.

The interpretation of real gene sequencing, as opposed to £150 SNP patterns, is complex. It's not like a cholesterol level which is either high or low. It's nuanced. When someone has genome sequencing – that's what I'm calling real gene testing – it sometimes needs a panel of experts to judge what's really going on. Some answers are easier. Do you have the breast cancer gene BRCA1 or not? Do you have the risk gene for Alzheimer's disease (APOE4) in a single or double dose or not? But the significance of many of the findings thrown up by genomics are ahead of the ability of medical science to understand or act upon. There are still relatively few medically 'actionable' genes but that will change as knowledge deepens.

To give you an example from non-gene testing how complex it can be, you'd think that if your cholesterol comes back raised then that's something to worry about. Well, yes, if it's raised a lot then it is a concern. But if it's only a little bit high, then what you do about it depends on other risk factors such as blood pressure, your age, whether you smoke and if you have high sugar levels. You couldn't get a more simple read-out than a chemical like cholesterol in your blood, but the interpretation of even that and whether you need medications or not is complicated. How much more complex then is the genetic read-out of thousands of your genes and squillions of gene combinations on top of your lifestyle and environment? We've a long way to go.

The other warning about consumer gene testing is that in some countries it has the potential to affect your ability to acquire life insurance. In the UK, insurance companies cannot ask for, or take into account, the result of a predictive genetic test unless the insurance is for more than £500,000 and you've had a genetic test for Huntington's Disease. The irony is that gene testing might uncover a risk that you can get rid of with a lifestyle change and your siblings could too.

Also ... beware nutritional genetic testing. A lot of it is complete bullshit. You'll obviously do what you think is best, but me? I wouldn't touch it with a barge pole. One day it might come into its own but not yet. A popular but notorious test is for the MTHFR polymorphism related to folate metabolism. MTHFR is a gene that helps the body utilise a substance called homocysteine, a chemical that your body uses to make proteins. The gene test is sometimes pushed to sell unproven therapies by scaring you with grossly overstated associations of certain versions of this gene with disorders like autism. The general view is that there are few reasons for doing MTHFR testing in a healthy person.

And finally, do you trust a commercial company to hold and protect your genetic information? I'm pretty relaxed about privacy when it comes to government and believe that secure sharing of, say, my electronic medical records in the health system can improve care and make it more efficient, but I'm not so sure that a gene version of Google is where I'd want my genetic data to be stored no matter how much they guarantee security and anonymity.

Having said all that, some of these companies now have vast stores of genetic information which is starting to inform medical research. The bottom line when you decide to do an online genetic test is to know its limitations and don't panic when a result arrives that looks scary. Get advice.

PART 3

Living younger longer

Staying young as old as possible

The messages: You can, in your 90s, have the health and vigour of someone many years younger. What you do to keep yourself healthy can be more important than how long your mother and father lived. Your genes don't play as big a role in your destiny as you might think. The things which take years from our lives hunt in packs. That means we have to hunt them in packs. The causes of longer survival are more than just a low cholesterol and flat abdomen. Life-shortening and life-lengthening factors aren't equal. Some are more potent at losing and gaining years than others. There's no waiting period for a return on your investment in changing how you live and eat. Conquer fatalism. There are always surprises around the corner out of your control, some of which will add years and some of which will subtract them, but we can still make our own future to a significant extent.

*

Let's get something straight right from the start. Life's a fatal condition and scary as it is to imagine a world without you or me in it, that's going to happen one day. I can't speak for you but I'm in the business of staving it off for as long as possible and what's surprising when you look at the evidence is that the limits of life expectancy are more elastic than many of us imagine. We've been told for years that the best way to live long is to have or have had long-lived parents. Don't knock it, that's a 'nice to have' but you don't need longevity genes for long, high-quality survival.

It's not so much about living to 120. It's about aiming to be alive and healthy in our 90s. Around 80 per cent of us reach the age of 65, although only 20 per cent get to 90. What you want to be by age 90 is what's called an 'exceptional survivor' – people who reach old age with minimal physical or mental impairments. Even if you've had bad habits all your life and now you're looking down the barrel of ageing and mortality, it's nowhere near hopeless. The trick is to focus your time, effort and money on what's going to make the biggest difference.

Don't know your limits

The experts argue a lot with each other about the limits of human survival. After years of adding years to our lives since the 19th century – actually around 18 months of extra life every decade for 150 years – improvements in life expectancy in some rich countries are levelling out, perhaps due to obesity and being overweight with too little physical activity. The thing is that life expectancy is an average, which means some people will live young a lot longer than others. The solutions do, however, need to follow the broad theme of this book, which is that there's more to health than individual risk factors or nutrients. It's about how we live, how fair our country is and how much chronic stress some of us experience because of loss of control, which includes cultural dislocation.

Some believe that in the US, life expectancy is maxing out and won't go much beyond what it is at the moment. They say that even though we've been doing well, it can't and won't last. In other words, sooner or later life expectancy will plateau and these researchers believe sooner, given the dual threats of body fat and pandemics. In addition, they claim that humans evolved to reproduce and then die. Our bodies weren't designed for all this ageing stuff and therefore we're genetically programmed to hit a brick wall at what they think is an average of about 85. Our bodies simply fall apart.

In fact there's untold potential to gain years of healthy life.

Bending your genes

As I mentioned, a common misconception is that the best way to live long is to have long-lived parents and it's true that being part of a family where people survive to a healthy old age does help. No-one's too sure, though, how much of that's fixed in your genes and how much is growing up in a home where parents teach or model good coping strategies so their children can deal well with stress; where people learn healthy habits from an early age and where life-enhancing food such as a Mediterranean diet has been on the table since infancy.

An example of how weak genes may actually be in determining life expectancy is Russia, where health and wellbeing were thrown into reverse after the collapse of the Soviet Union. The social degradation and economic chaos following the end of the Communist regime resulted in a tragic reduction in longevity, with Russians dying younger than in previous generations and indeed younger than in some developing countries. If genes were as strong as people assume, they'd have resisted this environmental pressure better. You'd have to say our DNA's doing a lousy job combating economics and poor access to education, healthcare and decent nutrition.

Another test of how tightly genes determine our survival is the difference in life expectancy between men and women. Most scientists say the male–female survival gap is because of the genetic make-up of the sexes, meaning men are programmed to live, eat, work and play more dangerously than women. Fascinating research, however, in cloistered communities, such as monasteries and convents, where the living environments are fairly standardised, has found that the differences between men and women become narrower. They don't go away but the chasm is smaller. Studies of centenarians – people who live to be 100 – also suggest that lifestyle is at least as important as having long-lived parents.

We've got to make the most of our genes and not be overwhelmed by the thought that they'll defeat us in the end. Me, I plan to be defeated by them at 105 rather than 75.

Life-shorteners hunt in packs

Most people who have a heart attack or stroke don't have blood thick-shaked with cholesterol, skull-lifting blood pressure, a waist circumference the size of the Equator or smoke 40 cigarettes a day. It's unusual for someone to have just one risk factor. They have a bit of everything: a tummy that's more out there than you'd prefer; an LDL cholesterol (the bad form) that's modestly raised; an HDL (the good form) that's lowish; and blood pressure that's a bit higher than it should be. Risk factors don't understand maths. They don't add up, they multiply. So having several working together is bad news. Which is how come …

One and one can make three, which means immediate and disproportionate benefits: It cuts the other way. You can make the multiplier effect work for you on the upside by working on the risk factors you can change.

Life-shortening factors aren't equal

There's no doubt that smoking is bad for you. Very bad. A woman smoking 20 cigarettes a day when aged 20 who doesn't quit will lose 14 years of life. But with the other risk factors, there isn't good information on their relative toxicity, meaning how they compare to each other. That's partly because medical researchers tend to be down one foxhole or another – for example, heart disease, diabetes or cancer. So they rarely lift their heads to see the whole picture. In addition, the risks of obesity, high cholesterol and high blood pressure tend to have been studied in whole populations and not brought down to what it means for you or me as individuals. The other problem is that researchers are just as prone to fads as you and me and often only study what's 'in' at the time. Nonetheless, it is possible to construct a league-table.

Top of the league for all causes of death is our age. The older we are, sadly, the more likely we are to die. But there isn't much we can do about that. Next comes smoking because it's a factor in so many life-threatening diseases such as cancer, heart disease, stroke, dementia and chronic obstructive lung disease. High blood pressure is pretty bad for heart disease, stroke and dementia. Lack of physical activity cuts across several conditions as well, increasing the risk of heart disease, cancer, and poor outcomes when you already have cancer, diabetes and probably dementia. Bad nutrition also cuts across most conditions. It makes you realise why they say that a high proportion of cancer is preventable if you take a broad, multifaceted preventive approach. Obesity is harder to measure but it does affect the risk of heart disease, diabetes and cancer. Happily, having regular sex seems to be life lengthening.

For rich countries like the UK, the league-table for years lost to both death and disability looks something like this:

Risk Factor	Effects
1. Dietary risks – low fruit/vegetable intake	Heart disease, stroke, cancer and diabetes
2. Smoking	Heart disease, stroke, respiratory disease and cancer
3. High blood pressure	Heart disease, stroke and dementia
4. Overweight and obesity / High body mass index	Heart disease, stroke, diabetes, musculoskeletal problems and cancer
5. Physical inactivity	Heart disease, cancer, diabetes and musculoskeletal problems
6. Alcohol use	Heart disease, mental health issues, stroke, cancer and injury
7. High cholesterol	Heart disease, stroke, vascular dementia and cancer
8. High fasting plasma glucose (blood sugar)	Heart disease, stroke, cancer and diabetes
9. Illicit drug use	HIV-AIDS, mental health issues and injury

But remember this isn't a risk factor league-table for individuals. It's for populations and takes into account the prevalence of these factors in the community. Which means the table does show, for example, how incredibly toxic smoking is. It's the number-two killer even though there are fewer people smoking than there are people who are overweight and obese.

There are blood tests which indicate you might be heading in the wrong direction: like for LDL, the bad form of cholesterol; your sugar levels; and maybe uric acid, which is the substance which if high can suggest you have gout. But a cost-free test of risk is your waist circumference, which tells you crudely how much fat you're carrying inside your abdomen. That's the most dangerous kind of fat. A woman's waist circumference should be 80 cm or less and a man's 94 cm or less. Mental wellbeing is important too and some argue that depression is as bad for your heart as a high cholesterol.

There is a trap in considering each of these factors separately because remember they hunt in packs. For instance, smokers tend to drink alcohol excessively, eat badly, have more problems with impotence if they're male, and not take as much exercise as non-smokers. On the other hand, heavy people aren't necessarily as unhealthy as you think because they actually might be eating quite well – as they have done in the past around the Mediterranean – and getting exercise.

A global picture

If you take a global perspective and look at causes of years lost and gained including both years lost to early death and healthy years lost (i.e. years of life which would have otherwise been free of disability), the global league-table for risk factors (including poor nations) is:

1. Childhood malnutrition (underweight)
2. High blood pressure
3. Unsafe sex
4. Smoking
5. Alcohol use
6. High cholesterol
7. Unsanitary environment
8. Overweight and obesity

9. Indoor smoke from solid fuels (cooking on open wood stoves inside)
10. Low fruit and vegetable intake

How risk factors work together

Take stroke, for example. It accounts for roughly one in ten deaths. High blood pressure can explain about 60 per cent of strokes, high cholesterol is the reason for about 25 per cent, followed by overweight, obesity and smoking, then lack of exercise and low fruit and vegetable intake.

For heart disease, which takes about one in six lives, the story is similar, although cholesterol rates more highly.

Cancer also involves multiple risk factors but because each cancer is different, you can't generalise about the mix. The level of ignorance about the causes of cancer is huge, although in addition to genetic susceptibility, what is known according to reasonable evidence is that:

- Cervical cancer is related to unsafe sex and being unimmunised against HPV.
- Lung cancer is related to smoking.
- Stomach cancer is related to smoking, low fruit and vegetable intake, and poverty.
- Colon cancer is related to obesity, low fruit and vegetable intake, and lack of exercise.
- Breast cancer is related to obesity, alcohol intake, lack of exercise, and affluence.
- Non-Hodgkin's lymphoma is related to occupation to some extent (e.g. farming and meat workers).

◉ Melanoma is related to sun exposure.

The impact in terms of years of life lost in rich countries annually equates to:

Risk Factor	Total Years of Life Lost Each Year
Smoking	15 million years
High blood pressure	11 million years
High cholesterol	7.7 million years
Overweight and obesity	6.6 million years
Physical inactivity	3.6 million years
Low fruit and vegetable intake	3.3 million years
Alcohol use	2.4 million years
Illicit drug use	860,000 years
Unsafe sex	600,000 years

These figures come from a large body of research done by a group of collaborators in the US, Switzerland, Australia and New Zealand who, over the past 15 years, have revolutionised thinking about the burden of disease in nations and globally. While dramatic, their figures, however, don't tell you much about what you stand to gain or lose as an individual, but I'll get to that soon.

Conquer fatalism and fear

There are always surprises around the corner out of our control, some of which will add years and some of which will subtract them and many aren't immediately and obviously related to health. As a respected medical historian once said, whenever we change the way we live, new diseases arise. Perversely, that's actually good news because it shows how malleable our destiny is.

All we can do is give ourselves our best chance rather than take a fatalistic view that we might be hit by a truck so why bother? If we're fortunate to have the resources and knowledge to be in control of how we live, we can still create our own futures to a significant extent, even though some of us might be unlucky crossing the road.

It's also important to inject a dose of reality here. Pushing out our survival by lowering our risk of the common causes of lost years will mean revealing rarer illnesses in some of us at older ages. They'll have been uncovered because heart disease would normally have got us first and would have kept the curtain drawn on unusual conditions. As our healthy lives extend, it's going to be easy to be panicked into thinking there are new diseases emerging – rare cancers, for instance – when all that's happening is that we're living long enough in large enough numbers, in good enough health, to experience them. We'll be entering an unknown zone if two out of three of us reach our 90s.

Exceptional survivors

This is what we all want to become. There are various definitions but essentially it's about reaching ripe old age in good shape. Exceptional survivors are people who arrive at the age of 85 with little or no disability, minds fresh as daisies, and little or no chronic illness. Some would argue that a person who's 85 with heart disease, high blood pressure or diabetes yet is still fit, active, not demented and spry also qualifies as exceptional.

One study used information from a 40-year follow-up of Japanese American men mostly born in the US and living on Oahu, Hawaii. It's a study that's been productive in showing what matters when it comes to health – particularly heart disease. Anyway, when the men were 85, the researchers looked back and asked whether there was anything in the men's middle age at age 55 which predicted who were destined to become exceptional survivors defined as not having any major chronic disease and no impairments in their thinking or physical abilities.

And there was.

The things that made exceptional survivors stand out at 55 were being lean, having lower than average blood pressure, less likely to have ever smoked or drunk too much alcohol, having lower blood sugar and triglyceride levels (a blood fat), having a stronger grip strength which could mean better fitness and greater physical reserve, and higher levels of education. Being married also made a difference to overall survival.

A man who fitted this bill at age 55 had a 40 per cent chance of getting to 85 in good shape. If he didn't match any of these categories in middle age, his chances were less than 1 per cent. It's sobering, but note that almost all of the factors were amenable to change. The factors are similar for women although not being married appears to be better!

Be critical of percentages – look for numbers

Most times you read about risk factors for your health, the statistics are expressed in terms of percentages. Reduce your cholesterol by this amount and you'll reduce the chances of a heart attack by 30 per cent. Get your blood pressure down and your chances of a stroke will drop by 20 per cent. While figures like that look dramatic and allow pharmaceutical companies to sell more drugs, they're meaningless when it comes to us as individuals: 30 per cent of what? 20 per cent of what? If you're fit and healthy, your chances of a heart attack or stroke in the near future are low anyway, so reducing the risk by 30 per cent might mean you go from a three in 100,000 chance in the next five years, to a two in 100,000 chance. It's not something to get worked up about. Marketers love big but meaningless percentages. It's called relative risk reduction. They fire us up emotionally and charge us into action which may not be worth the time, money and effort. What you need is a number for you as an individual, but it's harder to discover. A starting point is an assessment from your healthcare professional – what's called your QRISK. They measure BMI, blood pressure, cholesterol, physical activity and look at lifestyle issues, then calculate your risk of developing heart disease or a stroke.

So what counts?

There are tools around which try to predict your future but most are limited to heart disease, diabetes and stroke and guide whether you should be on medications like statins and blood pressure lowering drugs. The risk scores usually only look forward five or ten years and don't tell you about your personal risks of, say, cancer or dementia. There are tools for some other diseases but they have reliability issues. The time frame is also an issue. A low risk in the next five or ten years doesn't detract from the fact that we've a 40 per cent lifetime chance of dying of a heart attack or stroke. What use is knowing there's not much to worry about in ten years but a lot to worry about in 30 years? Actuaries aren't much help because they're mainly interested in predictions up to the age of 65, which is when some life insurance policies stop coverage. You and I want to know the long-term returns on an investment today in a lifestyle change or a preventive medication like a statin.

Common variables which are plugged into these predictive tools for heart disease are age, gender, total cholesterol, HDL cholesterol, whether you smoke, your systolic blood pressure (that's the top number) and whether you're on treatment for high blood pressure. But they leave a lot out. For instance, while depression might be as strong a risk factor for coronary heart disease as cholesterol, most tools don't take depression into account. Central adiposity (your waist circumference) is important for the risk of heart disease and type 2 diabetes and again many tools miss that out. Exercise makes a big difference to survival and some argue that going from sedentary to active is at least as good for your health as quitting smoking, yet exercise isn't in many equations. There's also debate about the impact of blood tests for inflammation (C reactive protein – CRP – is one of these) in risk assessment tools.

Then there's just plain ageing itself, the wear and tear of life.

Inflammation may count

This goes back to the earlier sections on diet because, for example, the way of life of elderly Greek Australians produces low levels of inflammation in the body. It's an add-on to the free radical and oxidative stress story because inflammation can speed up tissue damage and ageing.

A clue to the potential importance of inflammation came from a surprising and mysterious finding. In the first large trial of cholesterol reduction using a statin medication, researchers in Scandinavia found themselves with almost unbelievable results. The reductions in deaths from heart attacks and strokes were significantly better than they'd calculated based on what they thought they knew about the benefits from lowering cholesterol levels. In other words, more people survived than should have.

There are several theories to explain this phenomenon, which has since been noted in other studies. One is that a low cholesterol level, or statins themselves – or both – produce a calming effect on the lining of arteries making them less twitchy and less prone to spasm and blockage. And this in turn probably relates to the role of the immune system in atherosclerosis. You see, it's not sufficient to have a high LDL cholesterol (the bad form) for your arteries to silt up. The immune system is needed. In fact, some people argue the problem *is* the immune system.

The pattern of events is thought to go something like this. A high LDL cholesterol and/or a low HDL fire up the immune hormones and white blood cells which control inflammation. Inflammation is the way the body deals with wounds and infections by triggering the production of chemical messengers which in turn whistle up hungry white cells called macrophages which chomp up foreign material. Now that's a great response if what you have is an infected cut but it's maladaptive when you have too much LDL cholesterol in your blood. In this instance it's not an infection causing the problem. It's metabolism gone wrong. Maladaptive inflammation inside our bodies where we can't see it, is linked to premature ageing, heart disease, strokes and dementia, and is made worse by LDL cholesterol, diabetes, smoking and obesity.

For cholesterol to do its damage, it needs to be brought inside the artery lining and changed chemically. Blood with too much cholesterol irritates the artery lining and damages it a little. The artery lining responds by producing sticky molecules which act like flypaper catching immune cells passing by in the hope of helping the lining heal itself. The trouble is that it catches more than that. Blood fats like LDL get caught up and the inflammatory reaction starts to spread deeper into the artery wall, taking cholesterol with it. Subsequent oxidation or biological rusting – the interaction of oxygen free radicals with LDL – makes LDL really toxic to arteries. This is the beginning of what's called plaque – the stuff that years later blocks arteries, attracts blood clots, and causes heart attacks and strokes. On top of this, high levels of inflammation make blood more prone to clotting, and these damaged arteries more twitchy and liable to heart attack–inducing spasm.

Then there's the potential link with premature ageing. Once you've stoked up the immune system and its rusted-on partner, oxidation, they're all dressed up to party but since it's maladaptive, there's no party to go to. Like frustrated toddlers on a rainy Saturday afternoon, they get to work on the rest of the body. This is increasingly thought to be one of the fundamental processes causing tissue ageing.

The sad news is that, for some reason yet to be discovered, anti-inflammatory drugs don't influence this much and antioxidant vitamins may make it worse. The good news is that this inflammation seems to respond very quickly to changes in our lifestyle and may be the reason why eating less, eating more plant-based foods, reducing cholesterol, increasing exercise, and consuming fats which might reduce inflammation may have quite rapid benefits.

It's about being young at heart, at brain, and even at your kidneys as long as possible.

How old are you really?

It's all very well saying you're 39 or 69 but all of us know people in their 30s who look decrepit and people in their 70s who look young, are so bursting with wellbeing they put the rest of us to shame and can climb Kilimanjaro before breakfast. It makes a mockery of chronological age. Our biological age – how old you are on the inside – can, to a significant extent, defy time. But how do you know how old you are on the inside?

The kidney clock

People tend not to think about their kidneys unless something goes wrong with them and research is suggesting that's a mistake. In fact, our kidneys may reflect our real age. It's also known that by the time the standard test of kidney function – the creatinine level in your blood – is registering as abnormal, you've already lost 30–40 per cent of your kidney function. At that point – and it's probably a tipping point – your kidney damage starts to multiply your risk of heart disease and stroke. If someone has reduced kidney function, they're probably a lot older biologically than their last birthday would indicate.

It looks as though the activity levels of certain genes in the kidneys correlate with our biological age better than the time we've had in our mortal coils. Researchers are finding that it has a lot to do with how energy is made in cells and the tissue-damaging oxygen free radicals produced as a by-product. This ties in with the inflammation story because that, too, has a link to free radicals. It's not that our kidneys control how we age, it's more that they may be clocks – windows through which we can see what's truly happening inside ourselves. How these energy pathway genes work in muscle may also be a good indicator of ageing.

There's also a possibility that a simple blood test can give advanced warning that our kidneys might be going over the hill. The test is called cystatin C and is showing promise although there's lots of work to be done to see if it's reliable enough to be widely used.

Preserving kidneys

The common things that damage kidneys are: your mother's health when she was pregnant with you (if it was poor or she smoked, then you could have been born with small kidneys with less reserve for ageing); smoking; high blood pressure; and possibly inflammation from being too fat, having diabetes or not getting enough exercise.

What you can do is: keep your blood pressure low by

losing weight; exercising; limiting salt and alcohol intake or taking medications if necessary; not smoking; possibly avoiding advanced glycation end products (AGEs, see Brown Isn't Such a Good Colour); and adopting a Mediterranean style diet.

There's no such thing as normal

The fact that there's no such thing as normal is one of the most important messages for living younger longer. Smoking's the simplest of all the life-shortening factors and it's unambiguous. You either smoke or you don't and any smoking's bad for you.

Most of the other risk factors are nuanced because they're part of our biology – the way our body works. No blood pressure, you drop down dead. No cholesterol, no nutrition, no fat on or in your body: same. No exercise? We all move a bit unless we're under anaesthetic in an operating theatre – or dead. No depression? You'd have to have iron in your soul never to have felt low at some time or other.

These are what the statisticians call 'continuous variables'. Line up any thousand people at random according to their blood pressure – low to high, left to right – and you'll find no break in the line where there's a sudden jump to hypertension. Line them up again according to their cholesterol levels, degree of cheerfulness or waist circumference, you'll find the same phenomenon: an even spread of low cholesterol to high cholesterol, happy to sad, or flat to fat tummies. For each of these, some group of experts somewhere has drawn a line in the sand and said this is where normal is and to the right it is relatively bad and to the left is relatively good.

A word of warning though about continuous variables. You've got to be sure who's drawn the line in the sand between health and disease. You see, there's money to be made from that decision through selling drugs and treatments to people who are now defined as sick. Notoriously, some expert panels who have decided on where the line should be drawn have been sponsored by the pharmaceutical industry. It's called disease-mongering and it's being increasingly called out, with expert panels having to declare conflicts of interest.

Going back to our line of a thousand people, though, while it might be unbroken, where certain groups of people stand along it is a different matter. Those who didn't complete high school, or who are poor will tend to group on the right hand side – the relatively bad end.

It makes nonsense of the idea that there's such a thing as a normal blood pressure, cholesterol, state of mind or tummy.

That's why you should think in terms of personal targets rather than aiming to be normal because, on average, the more to the left you can move on the line, the better. In fact, one of the most significant findings of medical research in recent years is that if you have more than one risk factor you need to aim further to the left on the line than the official targets would suggest. Remember, risk factors hunt in packs so if you can weaken a link or two, you'll weaken the pack. For example, if you've diabetes or heart disease or high cholesterol, even if your blood pressure seems to be 'normal', most times you'll benefit from taking an antihypertensive medication.

So to extend your life, aim as left on the line as you can on every dimension unless your doctor advises there are reasons not to.

Under pressure

Your blood pressure is measured in your arm using two numbers. The top one is the systolic pressure – the peak pressure generated by the heart pumping – and the bottom number is the diastolic, which is the pressure between heart beats – the background blood pressure in your body, which reflects in a sense how 'tense' your arteries are. The unit for blood pressure measurements is mmHg (millimetres of mercury).

The headline numbers for blood pressure are that:

At age 50 or 60, a blood pressure of 140/90 or over reduces:

- life expectancy by five years
- life spent free of a heart attack or stroke by seven years

If you have other significant risk factors, then these numbers will be worse and the level of blood pressure needed to bring on a heart attack or stroke will be lower.

If the average adult's blood pressure could drop by 5 mmHg, then about one in three strokes would be avoided and one in five heart attacks.

If a 50-year-old man or a woman has a blood pressure of 120/80 or less, then compared to someone of the same age whose pressure is 140/90 or more, the person with the 'normal' blood pressure will live on average five years longer. When you look at the quality of that life, then the person with the lower blood pressure will spend seven years more of their life free of a heart attack or the effects of a stroke. For people with, say, a blood pressure of 130/85, the gap in years lived and lived free of heart disease is about midway. In addition, when the analysis was done for 40-year-olds or 60-year-olds, the gains and losses according to level of blood pressure were similar.

That's just part of the story, because high blood pressure (hypertension) isn't just a risk factor for strokes and heart attacks; also linked are heart failure, vascular dementia (dementia due to arterial damage), Alzheimer's disease, and possibly osteoporosis and glaucoma (damage to the optic nerve in the eye). So, like quitting smoking, reducing your blood pressure is very likely to extend your life with good-quality years.

The reason high blood pressure can be so pervasively bad probably has a lot to do with pummelling.

While blood pressure depends in part on how forcefully the heart pumps, a more important factor on a day-to-day, hour-to-hour basis is how much resistance the arteries put up to the push from the heart – the push-back, if you like. If the resistance in the arteries rises, so does the blood pressure; if the arteries relax, the blood pressure tends to fall. The word 'hypertension' often makes people think that stress is the thing that's behind high blood pressure. In fact, it's not the main factor but there is evidence that chronic life stress (see The Control Factor) – such as having a job where your boss orders you around and doesn't give you much chance to decide how to do the job or set your own priorities – is linked to high blood pressure. The level of stress hormones (adrenaline and noradrenaline) and the sympathetic nervous system (the network of nerves that prepares the body for emergencies by, among other things, constricting arteries) help to control blood pressure. So physical and psychological stresses are not to be ignored but solely focusing on them is a mistake because there's a lot more going on.

Which brings us back to the kidneys. The kidneys and the adrenal glands, which sit on top of them, control water and salt balance in the body through a family of hormones called the renin-angiotensin system. For instance, if you consume too much salt, the kidneys retain fluid to dilute the sodium in your blood. That means a bigger blood volume and increased blood pressure. People with hypertension often have a badly set renin-angiotensin system which chronically raises their blood pressure.

Biological ageing is speeded up by high blood pressure earlier in life. If you have raised pressure in your 40s or 50s (which is a common time to develop it), then the battering received by arteries throughout the body stiffens them up prematurely. Just like being supple in your limbs as you age is a good thing, you want the same kind of elasticity on the inside. The combination of excessive inflammation and the pummelling from the high pressure causes scarring and fibrosis. Then you're into a vicious cycle: accelerated arterial ageing, which then leads to reduced blood supply to various organs like the brain, lungs, kidneys and heart, which then start to age faster under the stress of being relatively starved of blood.

Like the kidney tests for biological ageing, another measure of ageing is arterial stiffness. The stiffer your vessels, the older you are regardless of calendar age. One of the signs of this is a larger than average gap between the systolic and diastolic blood pressures. In other words, you might have a blood pressure of 165/85 mmHg. This is called a raised pulse pressure.

Preventing the pressure rise

The main thing is not waiting until your blood pressure's up before doing something about it. Having said that and given how important a life-shortener high blood pressure is, we should know our level.

Take the pressure off

- Know your blood pressure accurately – don't jump to conclusions on inadequate evidence. Ask your physician when was the last time they had their blood pressure machine professionally calibrated. Blood pressure measurement at home is more accurate.
- Weight loss of about 10 per cent has been shown to have a similar effect to a blood pressure medication.
- Exercise that raises your pulse significantly for about 40 minutes most days of the week is associated with lower blood pressure and more elastic arteries. It's likely that High Intensity Interval Training (HIIT) has a similar effect.
- Cut your alcohol intake – this has good evidence for blood pressure reduction.
- Reduce your salt intake.
- If you can – and it is hard – reduce chronic stress from a job or a personal situation where you feel pressed and seem to have few choices available.

Now, while measuring your blood pressure might seem straightforward, it's not. It's probably rare that doctors and nurses take readings which accurately reflect a person's true blood pressure. If physicians don't regularly have technicians calibrate their blood pressure machines, they can both over- and under-diagnose high blood pressure. You shouldn't have taken any caffeinated drinks or smoked for a couple of hours beforehand. You need to have been relaxed and settled for a while rather than rushing in and having it done straight away. Blood pressure should be measured twice in the same arm and the cuff needs to be big enough for the size of your arm and kept at the same level as your heart. If there's much of a difference between the two readings, the nurse or doctor should wait for a few minutes then take a few more readings. If it's the first visit, then the other arm should be done too. A difference between arms suggests there may be an abnormality in the large arteries near the heart.

If the pressure's high in the physician's office, there's about a 30 per cent chance it'll be significantly lower at home and there's evidence that home measurements are more accurate than surgery or clinic ones. If you do take readings at home, it's increasingly thought that a blood pressure which is up at night is a sign of hypertension.

Is your blood fat?

Despite all the headlines about the evils of cholesterol, there's not a lot of research quantifying the impact of lowering blood fat (lipid) levels on extra years of life, although people with genetically high cholesterol levels do die early unless they get it under control. There's plenty of information on relative risk reduction but as mentioned before, saying that reducing your cholesterol lowers your risk of a heart attack by 30 per cent is meaningless because it's '30 per cent of what?'

First of all, you've got to define what high is, and just having a high total cholesterol is a pretty crude measure of risk. So you need to know your high density lipoprotein (HDL – good cholesterol), low density lipoprotein (LDL – bad cholesterol) and triglyceride levels. Some experts argue that if they're abnormal, you should have them measured on two occasions to make sure they're accurate.

The headlines on blood fats (lipids)

- If you're aged around 20 with a low cholesterol, and things stay that way, you can live up to nine years longer than a 20-year-old with high levels.
- The lower your LDL cholesterol, the better – even below what's recommended.
- If you have modestly raised blood lipids with no other risk factors (not very common, actually, since they hunt in packs), losing weight, exercising and a Med-style diet might be all you need, but that's for you and your doctor to decide.
- Blood lipids, when part of a raised 'risk package', are strong healthy-life shorteners and reducing them may be easier than other factors and still gain you more years. This is the commonest circumstance in which people find themselves.
- Since what you do about your lipids depends on your total risk rather than just the lipid levels themselves, active reduction should begin at what might seem 'normal' levels especially if you have diabetes, heart disease already or are in a high risk group such as those with South Asian ancestry. If you're in a high risk category, then you need to drive your LDL cholesterol under the recommended level and your HDL as high as possible through exercise and weight loss. Just how much you should exceed targets is debated among cardiologists.
- Triglycerides are important, not least because if they're raised they can make your LDL cholesterol more toxic.

> - At the moment, raising HDL by anything other than natural means, such as exercise and weight loss, is inadvisable since there may be risks for reasons which are yet to be explained.
> - Lipids are associated with dementia but it's still unclear that reducing them makes your brain work better.

Does size matter?

Some doctors will try to tell you that to really know your risk, you need even more sophisticated lipid tests, such as knowing your LDL particle size and your numbers of LDL particles. These tests are expensive and still largely research tools rather than something that makes a difference in real life. They don't give a person or their physician much more information than they already have from the standard lipid tests of LDL, HDL, total cholesterol and triglycerides alongside other measures of risk such as waist circumference, fasting blood sugar and blood pressure. A study of 25,000 people with a raised LDL showed that HDL and triglyceride levels gave as much predictive information as LDL particle sizes and numbers.

There is a little evidence that if you have the metabolic syndrome (fat tummy, high blood pressure, high triglycerides, low HDL, high fasting blood sugar – see The Metabolic Syndrome) yet your LDL is 'normal', measuring the numbers of LDL particles may give an added idea of your risk but the added benefit of knowing that is very unclear.

The fact is that if you have the metabolic syndrome you should probably be on statins and blood pressure lowering medications regardless, even if your LDL levels aren't high. The situation where particle size and number may count is in someone with a strong family history of heart disease at a young age yet who seemingly has normal lipids.

Some cardiologists measure 'very low-density lipoprotein' cholesterol (VLDL) because they believe it's a better marker of risk than LDL, but it's harder to measure and there isn't convincing evidence that in most people it's any better than measuring your triglyceride level. That's because VLDL contains a lot of triglyceride and when you lower your triglycerides the VLDL seems to follow. Refined carbohydrates like sugar seem to be bad for VLDL levels and could explain why they increase the risks of heart attacks and strokes.

HDL – not simply good

HDL is involved in taking cholesterol away from arteries and for every mmol/L (millimoles per litre) your HDL goes up, your risk of a heart attack or other cardiac event goes down – but paradoxically, very high levels of HDL seem to increase your heart risk. That means it's best only to use natural means to raise it.

Like LDL, HDL is a mix of particle sizes, which largely depend on whether they're on their way back to the liver loaded up with cholesterol which they've taken from the arteries. So on current evidence, measuring your total HDL seems just as good a guide as doing more sophisticated and expensive tests of particle size.

HDL goes up with exercise, weight loss, quitting cigarettes, small amounts of alcohol, reducing your saturated fat intake and increasing monounsaturated fat intake. When it comes to medications, though, statins for cholesterol lowering are not good at raising HDL. Older drugs like niacin and fibrates do it to some extent but with side effects, although there's a little evidence of heart disease reduction when used in conjunction with statins.

Degreasing your blood

- Be sure your blood lipid tests are accurate if they come back raised.
- Focus on HDL, LDL, total cholesterol and triglycerides.
- Even if your risk profile is good, aim low with LDL and triglycerides and aim high with HDL.
- Follow the Mediterranean-style dietary pattern.
- Lose centimetres from your waist, especially through exercise and smaller portions.
- Eat oily fish once or twice a week and don't waste your money or the environment on fish oil supplements.
- If your overall risk profile isn't good, especially if you have diabetes or the metabolic syndrome, get your LDL as low as possible and make sure your triglycerides aren't raised.
- Plant sterols in, say, margarine, do work.
- Know your total risk by asking your GP or healthcare professional for an QRISK assessment.

Triglycerides

These are the least straightforward of all the blood lipids because they form part of LDL, and VLDL in particular. In addition, they go the opposite way to HDL. When HDL levels rise, triglycerides fall and vice versa. Triglycerides can be high when the other measures of cholesterol are low and seem to be more important in women than men. In men, for every 1 mmol/L rise in triglyceride levels, there's a 14 per cent rise in the risk of heart attacks and other coronary problems, whereas in women the increase is 37 per cent. These risks rise with age.

If you want to see triglycerides in the flesh, just look at the fat on and in meat. It's oozing with them.

Triglycerides go up with excessive alcohol, some medications like steroids and the contraceptive pill, abdominal fat, pre-diabetes and diabetes, and some diseases like kidney failure and autoimmune diseases like SLE (Lupus).

It's often quite easy to reduce your triglycerides with lifestyle changes. Weight loss, reduced fat diets and exercise get most people to where they need to be. Medications can work too but that needs a discussion with your GP. Older medications like niacin and fibrates (for example, gemfibrozil) all bring down triglycerides, although the evidence isn't absolutely solid that this actually contributes to the survival advantage from cholesterol reduction and they have side effects.

Fish oil and survival

Over the years there's been hope and hype about fish oil (omega 3 fatty acid) supplementation. An Australian survey of 45-year-olds and older found that around 45 per cent were taking fish oil supplements. The accumulated evidence shows almost no benefit for heart disease or much else. In fact, at the time of writing, the latest trial showed an increased risk of an unpleasant heart rhythm abnormality called atrial fibrillation which is associated with heart failure and stroke.

Eating real fish, on the other hand, is good, at least in part because it displaces red meat.

This is a case where what I say and do are the same … I eat lots of fish and not a single fish oil capsule passes my lips.

The polypill

A few years ago, two respected British researchers looked at the available evidence on medications and vitamins to reduce risk factors for heart disease. After examining trials involving half a million people, they concluded that if anyone aged 55 and over took a single pill containing a cocktail of a low dose statin, two blood pressure lowering drugs (a beta blocker and an ACE inhibitor), folic acid and aspirin, in theory you could cut the risk of heart disease and stroke by nearly 90 per cent.

Theoretically, one in three people who took this 'polypill' would benefit and in them on average it would delay the onset of heart disease or stroke by 11 years. Up to one in six people, though, would experience some kind of side effect.

This paper caused an enormous furore partly because many

people were outraged at the thought of medicating normal people, but research continues into simpler forms of the polypill in high risk populations and trials are showing some benefit.

Living longer with more sex

An analysis of a 20-year study of men in Wales found that having sex twice or more per week was associated with reduced chances of dying from coronary heart disease. Sudden death from sexual intercourse was rare and didn't seem to affect the results. The benefits from sex (if they were real) were in the earlier part of the study and lessened as time went on – possibly because age brought greater risk from other things which swamped sex. Or maybe what swamped the sex was ageing itself.

To be serious, though, sexual dysfunction in men is linked to obesity, diabetes and cardiovascular disease so less sex may be caused by being less healthy. In women, several of the medications associated with these conditions can create sexual problems such as dryness.

Living longer with less salt

Societies with low salt intakes have lower rises in blood pressure as people age. Populations with high salt intakes tend to have higher rates of stroke and heart disease after adjusting for other risk factors like cholesterol and smoking. In addition, several trials of reducing salt intake have shown that it can lower blood pressure. (See Our Salt Addiction.)

Life and your abdomen

Hardly a day goes by without someone talking about obesity and how we're getting fatter and fatter and how this epidemic's already slowing the gains in life expectancy over the past 100 years or so.

The headline numbers for obesity, overweight and your life expectancy are:

- If you're middle-aged, overweight and don't smoke, on average your weight can trim three years off your life.
- Middle-aged, non-smoking women who are obese can expect to lose seven years off their lives.
- Non-smoking middle-aged obese men lose about six years.
- Obese middle-aged smokers compared to normal weight non-smokers lose between 13 and 14 years off their lives.
- In terms of years of life lived free of the effects of heart disease or a stroke, obese men live six years fewer than normal weight men free of cardiovascular disease, and obese women live eight years fewer free of heart or stroke problems.
- More disturbingly, obese men live 2.7 more years with cardiovascular disease than normal weight men, and obese women live 1.4 years more. In other words, obese people get heart attacks and strokes earlier than they should and even though they die faster of them, they still spend more years of their lives with the after-effects than normal weight people.
- Obese men die of or have their first heart attack at 65 years of age compared to 71 for normal weight men, and obese women at 69 years of age compared to aged over 77 for normal weight women.

- You should be aiming for a waist circumference of 94 cm or less if you're a Caucasian man and 80 cm or less for women. If you're ethnically Chinese or Asian-Indian, then the target for women is the same but men should aim lower, to between 85 and 90 cm based on international thresholds for the metabolic syndrome. Basically, if you're male, regardless of your race, if you take a size 34 in jeans then you're significantly more likely to be in better shape and have a longer life than the guy next to you at the rack who's trying on a size 40.
- The rot begins in your 20s, if not earlier, but can be reversed.
- If you have the metabolic syndrome, then compared to people who don't have it, you've triple the chances of having a heart attack or stroke, double the chances of dying of one, and five times the chances of developing type 2 diabetes.

Why waists waste more years

The trouble with measuring obesity and overweight is that none of the methods are very accurate at predicting your risk of developing other diseases or dying prematurely.

Measures of fatness include body mass index (BMI), waist circumference, waist to hip ratio, and even having a CT scan of your abdomen to see how much visceral fat you've got as opposed to subcutaneous fat. What you decide to use depends on what risk you want to know about. If it's diabetes, then there's probably not a lot of difference. But if you're after a predictor for coronary heart disease, stroke and total mortality including cancer, then waist circumference and waist to hip ratio are probably better than BMI. In fact, according to one study, waist to hip ratio is a better predictor of heart disease and stroke than blood pressure and cholesterol. BMI tends to pick up all fat and there's actually evidence that subcutaneous fat is protective for diabetes and a lot of evidence that the fat inside your abdomen is toxic. It's metabolically very active, seems to charge up your level of inflammation, squirts out unhealthy fats into the bloodstream and reduces the effectiveness of insulin at handling the glucose – sugar – in your blood.

Your waist circumference expansion

This is mostly a man thing – but far from exclusively – with the greatest growth in the 50s. And here's the trap for both men and women. If you're focused on your weight on the scales you might miss the shift of fat to your tummy. It can happen in the absence of overall weight gain and that means you shift from relatively benign to toxic fat.

Calculating your fatness

BMI

A body mass index (BMI) of 30 or more is the definition of obesity, whereas overweight is defined as a BMI between 25 and 29.9. You calculate your BMI by dividing your weight in kilograms by your height in metres squared.

Waist circumference

Get a tape measure. Stand up. Take off your top; loosen your pants or skirt; feel for the highest point on your hip bone at the side of your waist (the iliac crest) then feel for the lower edge of your ribs just above the hip bone. You circle your tape measure approximately at the midpoint between the two.

Breathe out and make sure the tape measure is snugly around you but not tight. At this point, you're allowed to cheat. You should find the smallest circumference just above or below the midpoint and take that as your waist circumference. Either way, it doesn't really matter as long as you always use the same technique.

The waist circumference targets outlined above are those defined by the International Diabetes Federation (IDF).

Waist to hip ratio (WHR)

Take your waist measurement and divide it by the widest circumference around your buttocks. People disagree on the ideal target but it probably should be 0.9 or less in men and 0.8 or less in women. This is the strongest predictor of heart disease and stroke but it does have problems. Take, say, a woman who's 20 and thin. She might have a terrific WHR of less than 0.8. Then over the years she puts on weight around both her hips and abdomen and her BMI is now in the obese range. It's possible that her WHR has stayed the same even though her waist circumference might have gone from 66 cm to 91 cm, which means she's in the risk zone.

So what's best?

For the purposes of living longer healthier, it's your waist circumference. Although, the fact is that if you've a BMI of over 30, unless you're all muscle, you're not in good shape regardless of what your tape measure's telling you. BMI, while not bad at estimating the risks attached to being overweight or obese, is not as good as waist circumference at determining visceral fat – the dangerous stuff.

The metabolic syndrome

Research is showing that in many people, waist expansion is the first event which leads to a progressive elevation in blood pressure, blood fats and fasting blood sugar. This is the metabolic syndrome and it predicts developing diabetes, having a heart attack or a stroke or all three.

To know whether you have the metabolic syndrome, you need three out of the five criteria below. I've used the European and Australian definitions of an unhealthy waist circumference. They're so fat in North America that they've made their cut-off higher, presumably because it'd be embarrassing to admit that an eye-watering percentage of their population have the metabolic syndrome.

Let's start with waist circumference. It's a bit complicated because what qualifies as unhealthy depends on your ethnicity. Some groups are much more sensitive to the fat in the abdomen and may look thin but be at increased risk. So …

An unhealthy waist circumference is:

- Europeans (Caucasians), people from the Middle East and Eastern Mediterranean, and probably sub-Saharan Africans:
  Men   more than 94 cm
  Women   more than 80 cm

- Japanese, Chinese, Indian, Pakistani, other Asian, Central and South American:
  Men   more than 85–90 cm depending on ethnicity
  Women   more than 80 cm

The other criteria are:

Triglyceride level high:	1.7 mmol/L or more
HDL cholesterol low:	1.03 mmol/L or less in men or 1.29 mmol/L or less in women
Blood pressure high:	130/85 or more on the top or bottom number
A fasting blood sugar that's:	5.6 mmol/L or more

If you have metabolic syndrome, then compared to people who don't have it, you've triple the chances of having a heart attack or stroke, double the chances of dying of one, and five times the chances of developing type 2 diabetes. If you already have type 2 diabetes, the risks mostly apply already.

You need to aggressively get these measures down. Weight loss of even just 5 or 10 per cent can make a big difference. Blood pressure lowering is helped by eating less (which will usually mean less salt as well), reducing alcohol intake and moderate exercise, and you need to talk to your GP about whether medication, for example metformin, will give you a helping hand.

Laying waste to your waist (this is the weight loss bit)

Before you bought this book you were probably, like me, eligible for a PhD in fad diets. Diet writers make millions out of them and none work for much more than a year. So here's my take on waist loss (and, of course, this is yet another example of do as I say but not as I do).

It isn't easy but you can maintain significant weight loss for many years. You know this already, but it's worth reminding you that exercise won't get you there by itself. You have to change how much you eat and if you can control your eating and increase your physical activity as well, the centimetres will fall off your waist. First, though, you need a realistic target because if your aim is to look like Paris Hilton or have a washboard abdomen like Brad Pitt, it's a different story than making yourself healthy. If living longer younger is your aim, then even a 10 per cent reduction in weight and waist size can help enormously.

The seven things that successful long-term weight losers tend to do:

1. Weigh themselves daily.
2. Keep food diaries when they need to lose weight.
3. Restrict their calories.
4. Don't change their diet at weekends.
5. Exercise fairly vigorously, tailored to their own capacity and health, for about an hour a day.
6. Eat most of their calories before dark.
7. Eat healthily.

To lose weight successfully, you need to discover something that may be entirely new in your life: hunger. And learn to like it, because when you're hungry you're losing weight. To achieve hunger – and this insight will amaze you – you've got to eat less: a fraction of the quantities you've been used to. One carbohydrate portion of cooked rice is about half a cup and with dinner you probably shouldn't be having more than three carb portions in total. Daytime eating is better than at night since you've a chance to burn some of those calories before bed.

You don't actually have to give up anything, although you'd have to think twice before blowing a day's calories on a plate of fries, a pizza or a few beers or Negronis. Learn to live with hunger and only eat when you really need to and then in small portions. Learn to leave something on your plate. When you have a chocolate craving, ease it with savouring a single mouthful rather than a whole bar. Only eat at the table with food on a plate and don't hoover up other people's leftovers. If you start exercising on top of that, you'll be on the right path to meeting your target weight and waist circumference.

Losing weight for life

Learn to like being hungry
To do that, you need to become hungry in the first place. And to do that: eat less.

Know your calories and portion sizes
Know what carb and protein portion sizes truly are and what you should have each day. If you can afford it, get a down-to-earth, non-faddish dietician to give you a portion prescription.

Monitor your weight daily
Weigh yourself daily after your shower in the morning. You can lie to your friends and even to strangers but be honest with yourself. Understanding your calorie and weight patterns gives you a much better feel for what will and won't affect your weight.

Keep a food diary
Again, don't kid yourself and don't blow out at weekends or when you're at home.

Only eat what's put in front of you
Don't hoover up the rest of the family's leftovers. You're not living in a famine, so it's not the end of civilisation to leave food on your plate or on the table. You want to save the planet? Serve small portions to minimise food waste, save leftovers for lunches, replace meat with plants, donate to a science-based development charity and take public transport.

Eat most of your calories during the day
Most overweight people consume most of their calories during and after their evening meal and most of these calories are excess to requirements. Night-time calories are bad. Start with a good breakfast (although in a weight loss phase, missing breakfast reduces your daily calories), have a decent lunch and with a healthy mid-afternoon snack, you should be able to get home in the evening not feeling like your first stop has to be the fridge.

Aim for an hour of real exercise a day
That means getting your pulse up and feeling as though you're exercising moderately.

If only you could bottle exercise

There is no pill, no micronutrient and no magic diet that equals exercise in its effects. Physical activity (including muscle strengthening) reduces heart disease, stroke, diabetes, probably dementia and certainly some cancers, especially bowel and breast. If you're diagnosed with cancer, you live longer and better by taking exercise and maintaining or building your muscles.

High intensity interval training (see HIIT and Living Longer) may provide added metabolic stress which is good for nerve growth in the brain, but exercise has to be at least moderate for maximum benefits, particularly its antidepressant effect. Having said that, the biggest gain you'll ever make is to go from being sedentary to taking regular exercise of any kind.

Incidental exercise counts. So take the stairs and leave the car at home as much as possible.

The headline numbers for physical activity

- At age 50, moderate activity gets you two years extra and heavy activity four years and can also deliver you several more years of healthy life.
- At age 80, there are still around two extra years to be had from exercise.
- If you've participated in sports at a high level, you can gain up to six years of life and the diseases you'll eventually die of come on ten years later than in people who haven't played sports to a high level, especially if your alcohol consumption is low. The figures are similar for non-elite sports participation.
- People who exercise reduce their chances of premature death by 34 per cent.
- Middle-aged women who have an hour or less per week of physical activity have a 50 per cent increase in the chances of dying prematurely from any cause and twice the chances of dying young of a heart attack or stroke compared to women who exercise.
- The biggest gain is from going from sedentary to some

exercise. Nothing you do again in your exercising career will come close to that first step away from the couch.

- More is better. Increasing the intensity and amount of physical activity increases the gains but intensity for a fit person is different from someone who's just getting going.
- Being fit is better for you but the amount of exercise is almost as important.
- The fitter you are, the lower your risk of dying of cancer.
- Many of the benefits from exercise accrue over the three or four days after you've taken it. Physical activity drops your blood pressure, your triglycerides and level of inflammation, and raises your HDL cholesterol. All good news but it means it's better taking exercise every day or second day rather than waiting until the weekend and suffering a 'benefits gap'.
- Exercise which builds muscle can prevent type 2 diabetes.
- There is a belief among researchers that, bizarre though it may sound, our hearts have just so many beats in them and once that number has been reached, our number is up. So the slower your heart beats the longer it takes to clap out. The other measure is something called heart beat variability which is a natural and healthy variation in the space between beats. People who are fit tend to have a slower pulse and healthy variability.

Support the METs

A MET (metabolic equivalent task) is the amount of energy you burn doing a particular exercise. A MET is about 1 calorie per kilogram of your body weight per hour while you're at rest. For people between 20 and 65 years of age, around 5 METs per hour is moderate exercise and 8 METs per hour is fairly vigorous exercise. That declines with age, so at 80 years of age, moderate exercise is between 2 and 3 METs and vigorous is between 3 and 4. Brisk walking is around 4 METs, swimming's similar and jogging is about 8 METs. The aim is to burn at least 1000 calories per week by exercising, ideally aiming for up to 3500 calories over seven days. If you're 80 kg, then brisk walking burns about 320 calories an hour, whereas jogging burns around 640 calories an hour.

Having said that, what seems to count most is what you yourself perceive as light, moderate or hard exercise, not necessarily what the textbooks say you should burn. If you've not been physically active and are overweight, then just taking a walk will puff you out and seem like pretty heavy activity. Take that message seriously and don't overdo it too soon. If it feels moderate, it probably is. You can take your time to build up your fitness – if you're anxious about it, or have pre-existing conditions, take advice from your physician in case there any risks you need to be aware of. The key is to gradually and safely increase your effort because as you become fitter, the bar for what constitutes moderate exercise is raised. The other bonus is that if you can speed up your walking then you'll burn more in less time.

Speaking of time, it's short for most of us and if you're told that you need to walk briskly for 2.5 hours a week, then it's tempting to save it up for the weekend. The evidence is that 'weekend warriors' – if they don't have any risky behaviours like smoking – do derive benefits from their exercise but not as much as if they'd spread it out during the week. Those who take daily or semi-daily exercise reduce their risks far more even if they're smokers or have other risk factors for, say, heart disease. One reason for the added benefit is the short-lived nature of some of exercise's effects on the body. That's good because like quitting smoking (see What You Need to Know About Smoking) you don't need to wait months to gain benefits but you do need to keep going on most days of the week.

The burn

Rules for safety: If you feel that exercise – even just walking – is moderate or hard, then it is moderate or hard for you, no matter what someone else tells you. Build up how much you do, slowly and steadily.

The biggest gain you'll ever make is getting up from being sedentary and most heart association guidelines suggest that's safe as long as you start slow carefully and build up.

- Aim to burn 3500 calories a week and start with 1000 a week.
- Walking burns about 320 calories an hour.
- Jogging burns 640 calories an hour (but note the safety rule above).
- As you become fitter, it'll take less time to burn the calories.

HIIT and living longer

High Intensity Interval Training (HIIT) aims to get your heart rate to 90 per cent of maximum in short bursts followed by slightly longer bursts of lower intensity, often lasting as little as four minutes overall. The suggestion is that maybe as little as two sessions a week can equal moderate intensity continuous exercise for 30–45 minutes almost every day.

There's pretty good evidence that HIIT can achieve similar

levels of cardiorespiratory fitness which is a measure that predicts a longer, healthier life, although whether HIIT can also help with weight loss is not clear.

As to comparing moderate exercise on most days of the week to HIIT for their effects on living longer, there has only been one randomised trial in a general, real world population. This was in Norway – the home of HIIT – in a large sample of fairly healthy elderly people aged on average around 73. They compared a control group who were asked to adhere to Norway's guidelines on physical activity to two groups, one of which had supervised moderate intensity continuous training and the other had HIIT.

The control group, in a sense, stuffed up the experiment because they were really good at following the activity guidelines. That meant there were no statistical differences in the chances of dying over five years when compared to the combined training groups. However, the HIIT group had a slight advantage when compared by itself and indeed the control group drifted towards HIIT over the five years of the study.

So … the data that being physically fit helps you live longer are solid while exactly what kind of exercise is best is still open. HIIT may have some advantages, particularly if you have days where you're short of time and need to compress your training.

A warning about getting ripped

Quick rip: Be self-aware and try to have insight into when this is getting out of control or when you notice it in friends or workmates. It can be toxic and a sign of poor mental health.

*

You already know that body image can be toxic but that doesn't make you immune to overwhelming media (and usually touched-up) images of idealised male and female bodies. These contrived ideals drive women to overvalue thinness and men to overvalue being lean and muscular, especially if the images they have in their minds are largely unrealisable for all but the obsessed. While we think of eating disorders primarily affecting young women, it's likely that a third of people with abnormal eating patterns are male. The male pattern tends to be more about bulking up and having low body fat so you can show off those oversized muscles. At the extreme, the result can be very high protein diets, synthetic foods like shakes, low carbs, high fats, constant states of ketosis apart from blow-outs on a Friday night, and sometimes anabolic steroid abuse.

Male pattern anorexia nervosa hasn't been well researched, but it does seem that other mental health issues like anxiety and depression can go along with the eating disorder. Finland, like the UK and Australia, keeps a register of twins which allows them to study the influence of environment and genes on people's health and wellbeing. It also allows a way of accessing a group of people about whom they know a lot already – like their BMIs, for instance. They targeted males aged around 25 with low BMIs and found that the average age of onset was around 17. Obsession with musculature was common as were depression and anxiety. These twins also had mental health issues. While the eating disorder was often short lived, the mental health issues weren't. Another feature of these Finnish men is that they tended to have been overweight when younger.

US data suggests that 60 per cent of young men say they've changed the way they eat to help build more muscles, and when this is getting worse, things like compulsive exercise and regular weighing start to appear. What's become known as muscle dysmorphia is an important driver. Body dysmorphia is when you can't stop yourself thinking that your body has flaws. It causes a lot of distress and can lead to eating disorders and even potentially harmful overuse of cosmetic surgery. Muscle dysmorphia is a subset of this, usually in males where they become obsessed that they look puny and under-muscled – even when an independent person looking at them will say their body seems normal and well proportioned. The dietary pattern can oscillate between an enormous focus on protein intake with the aim of bulking up then once that's happening, they feel fat and go into 'cutting' to reduce their subcutaneous fat even further. Then there are the 'cheat' meals when they blow out on hamburgers and chips or their equivalent – a binge. You don't need a PhD in nutrition to realise this isn't normal and potentially both physically and psychologically unhealthy.

Treatments have been better researched in young women but family therapy, which helps the family deal with this behaviour and respond appropriately, has been shown to have an effect and there's some support for evidence-based psychotherapy. If you or someone you know has this pattern of behaviour, encourage them to seek help. They are likely to be distressed and unhappy beneath it all (see Distress and Depression: Two Sides of the Same Coin?).

Can my mum blame the menopause?

Doctors have a history of blaming the menopause for stuff that it has nothing to do with, like dementia and heart disease. This is more about getting older than any hormonal changes in our bodies. There's no doubt that protein metabolism changes with age and that means unless we keep up protein intake and muscle strengthening, we will lose muscle mass and with it the tissue that keeps diabetes at bay. Muscle is very good at using insulin and losing the ability to use insulin is at the heart of the metabolic syndrome and type 2 diabetes. Muscle burns a lot of energy. So if you lose muscle you're less able to take exercise as well as burning fewer calories per day. That means unless you step up the muscle-building exercise and step down the calories, it can spin out of control.

As people enter middle age, they tend to take less exercise and eat more but what happens before the menopause or middle age probably counts more. The most rapid rises in weight gain occur earlier in life and there's some tantalising evidence from following women through the menopause that the heavier they are prior to the menopause, especially in the abdomen, the greater the loss of muscle and protein. This is for complex metabolic reasons which aren't fully understood.

Oestrogen is part of this story but there isn't much evidence that oestrogen replacement therapy makes women thinner or fitter.

What you need to know about smoking (vaping comes later)

If you're 70 and still smoke, you've only a 7 per cent chance of getting to 90. If you don't smoke, then your chances could be as high as 33 per cent. In middle age, smoking doubles your chances of dying soon.

There's no doubt that smoking is bad – very bad – and allowing for all other factors in people's lives, smoking's generally worse for women. A woman who smokes 20 per day at the age of 20 and doesn't quit is likely to die 14 years sooner than a woman who's never smoked and the chances of premature death rise with the number of cigarettes smoked. Women smoking two packs a day lose 19 years of life, whereas male heavy smokers lose 15 years compared to never-smokers. A female never-smoker is 40 per cent more likely to reach the age of 70 than a female moderate smoker. So, on average, female never-smokers have a 9–14-year gain in life expectancy at age 20 compared to women of the same age who currently smoke and in males it's 7–10 years.

There are 30 causes of death related to smoking and thousands of excess deaths each year attributable to cigarettes. That beats terrorist attacks and plane crashes hands down – each and every year.

The impact of quitting on our life expectancy has probably been underestimated and some people believe that one of the causes of the expansion of life expectancy at middle age has been low smoking rates. As people drift into their middle years and see the brick wall at the bottom of the hill, they tend to quit. So the chances are that by chucking away the death sticks, you can catch up on many of those years which otherwise might have been lost.

Quitting at age 40 restores men to the life expectancy they'd have had if they'd never smoked – in other words, about a ten-year gain. Quitting at 50 adds six years to your life and halves your chances of a fatal smoking-related event.

The benefits of quitting are pretty much immediate:

- In minutes – your blood pressure and heart rate fall.
- In hours – your carbon monoxide levels begin to stop looking as though your mouth's been over your car exhaust pipe.
- In a day – the carbon monoxide's gone.
- In two days – nicotine's gone from your blood.
- In two weeks – your arteries are beginning to settle down and blood flow is improving through them.
- Not long after that – your risk of a heart attack falls significantly, halving within a year, and your risk of lung cancer progressively falls too, albeit at a slower pace.

Not just lack of will

Smoking's a classic example of how risk factors cluster. Smokers are more likely to be poor, have less education, be socially isolated, have other medical problems, work in more dangerous situations, drink alcohol excessively, take less exercise and not wear seatbelts. Smokers are also far more likely to have depression or a major mental illness like schizophrenia and use other substances. According to one study, an astounding 44 per cent of all cigarettes consumed in the United States are smoked by people with psychological problems. Research in Australia showed that people with schizophrenia have very short life expectancies and while suicide is one reason, the main causes are physical illnesses like heart disease and cancer often brought on by smoking and not helped by poor medical care.

School and university education are important variables. If you take people aged 25 or over with at least 16 years of education as the benchmark, people aged 25 or more who only completed high school are up to four times more likely to be smokers. At age 55, Americans with the lowest education levels have more than double the smoking rates of those with the highest years of education (28 vs 13 per cent based on 2002 figures). And even just comparing smoker with smoker, lower education levels predict shorter lives. Education is a potent life extender and that lack of education, probably through associated relative poverty and deprivation, is a life shortener which cuts across almost all known risk factors.

The implications of these social, psychological and economic factors coexisting with smoking are enormous. It means that just telling people to stop smoking isn't going to be enough – although there's strong evidence that if a GP identifies a patient who's a smoker and spends just five minutes talking to them about quitting *and* importantly, offers support, a significant percentage will actually stop their cigarettes. Helping people out of their depression will make a difference too. But, say, for a woman who didn't complete secondary school, who's a single mother with three children, and is struggling day to day financially and psychologically it might not be so easy to convince her that her highest priority is to stop smoking.

As with many risk factors, the temptation is to think that medicine has most of the answers when it hasn't.

Stopping smoking before it starts and beware vaping

This is about preventing teenagers taking up the habit. If you're not smoking by the ages of 18 or 19, you're unlikely to start. The key factors here are price, regulations, advertising and role models.

Price means taxation which increases the cost of cigarettes. Teenagers are extremely price sensitive. Regulation means not being allowed to sell to teenagers. Advertising and role models mean restricting forms of encouragement to teenagers which give them the idea that smoking's cool. With bans on most forms of advertising, the tobacco industry has long focused on Hollywood. Studies have shown that a significant percentage of children who smoke have been influenced by smoking on the movie screen. Advertising also means having well-researched campaigns which discourage smoking in young people. Promoting good role models involves parents not smoking.

Vaping (E-cigarettes): In the UK, E-cigarettes can be bought in specialist shops, some pharmacies as well as online. They are not available on prescription so you can't get them from your doctor as a means of smoking cessation, for example. In the US, where regulation has historically been light, there has been significant growth in nicotine vaping and associated switching to tobacco and vice versa. While debate rages about whether nicotine vaping is a gateway to tobacco and also about the long term safety of inhaling overheated flavourings, what is clear is that inhaling nicotine has the potential to be addictive regardless of how you inhale it. So if you're a non-smoker and start vaping nicotine you could end up addicted. If you're a smoker and want to quit, there are other less addictive ways of replacing nicotine and overcoming your dependence.

What to do about your smoking

- You can quit by yourself if you want to – most people do.
- Don't worry about failure – it's common and persistence pays off. It doesn't mean you're a hardcore nicotine addict, it just means you're an average quitter. Ultimate failure is rare. But there is no shame in seeking support. It makes a difference.
- Counselling works.
- Medication and nicotine replacement increase quit rates.
- Smoking does affect your energy-burn and stopping can increase your weight. So, combining an exercise and diet plan with quitting can minimise that impact.
- Support politicians and others who want to prevent you inhaling other people's smoke at work and at play.

Many, if not a majority of people who quit smoking, do so by themselves without much help. Not a lot is known about how they do this or what tricks they use. So don't feel you have to attend a clinic or take something to help you along but equally, don't throw in the towel if you go back to smoking after a few weeks or months because several attempts is a common experience even in people attending clinics or receiving anti-smoking medications. While that sounds depressing, the setbacks are clearly surmountable since the 2019 figures for the UK show that the proportion of ex-smokers is at its highest level since 1974 – and there are more ex-smokers than smokers.

According to an authority on cessation, Professor Simon Chapman at Australia's University of Sydney, around 3 per cent of unaided quitters have long-term success each year. Nicotine replacement therapy (NRT) can increase this by about 70 per cent – in other words, NRT might increase the background rate to about 5 per cent. Counselling aimed at problem-solving and giving you skills and tips on quitting works, especially if it's given on a regular basis. Then there are medications like bupropion and varenicline, which increase success rates further in people who have no medical or other reasons not to take them. The best-case scenario with evidence-based treatments triples the background rate. Medications such as varenicline (Champix) and bupropion (Zyban) are available on prescription only from your GP or a quit smoking clinics.

The other piece of information you need to have is that just cutting the number of cigarettes you smoke each day isn't enough. For reasons researchers don't fully understand, the first ten cigarettes are the most dangerous. So quitting means quitting.

Just remember the prize: it's several years added to your life and those are likely to be good years. And don't forget the Quit lines which can provide a lot of support.

Smoking versus weight gain – which matters most?

Look, I'm vain and you probably are too. I forlornly hope that one day I'll have a six-pack like Brad Pitt, rather than the bottle of pinot noir that's described my abs for years. If you're a woman, you might yearn for narrower hips and thinner thighs. So I don't want to sound naïve here and assume that health's all that matters and we don't care what we look like. Smoking does increase your calorie burn and quitting can mean putting on weight. If you scale up your exercise level at the same time as quitting, the effects of not smoking on your metabolic rate should be minimised.

Speaking personally, the body beautiful for me includes the quality of your skin, the colour of your teeth, the smell of your breath and the smoothness of your voice.

Your life and other people's smoke

It's not clear what effect inhaling other people's smoke has on your life expectancy but it's likely that about one-tenth the number of people die prematurely from passive smoking compared to people dying from active smoking.

What you need to know about alcohol

Alcohol consumption is a major cause of preventable premature death and lost years of health in people aged 15–49. If you think you're drinking for your health, you're mostly deluded. Enjoy alcohol for its taste and as a social lubricant but don't ever think it's benign.

The trouble is that while we're told that we shouldn't exceed 14 standard drinks a week, spread over at least three or more days, most people aren't too sure what exactly a standard drink is and once you've released your inhibitions with a couple of drinks, more follow.

We've been sold a pup on moderate alcohol use. It's been credited with the 'French paradox' – the supposed reason why the French live longer despite croissants and Gitanes. When you observe populations, it looks as though people who don't drink and those who drink too much have higher than average premature death rates, while those in the middle taking two or three standard drinks a day have the lowest death rates for their ages.

It turns out that this so-called 'U' shaped curve is a mirage, the main reason for the delusion being that people who don't drink are actually sicker than average. This means that being an abstainer isn't a risk factor for anything. In studies of alcohol consumption, abstaining tends to be a sign of the people in the study being unwell, which means that the 'U' curve isn't a curve at all. Rising risk is a straight line. The more alcohol you drink, the more harm you do yourself.

Moderate amounts in people with heart problems probably do help the heart a little through effects on HDL, but it's a fine line which has to be balanced against the risks of injury, violence, raised blood pressure, breast cancer and all the other problems alcohol use can bring. The trouble is that we tend to think that if a little is okay, more might be better; and if we assume that moderate use is healthy (albeit for one thing only –

your heart) then our total consumption will drift upwards.

The good news is that small amounts of alcohol are not particularly harmful assuming you're under 65, not pregnant or trying to conceive, you don't drive or do anything requiring skill afterwards, and you don't mix alcohol with other drugs. So enjoy that beer or glass of wine. Just don't delude yourself it's necessarily extending your life and remember, alcohol equals calories. If you're obese, you're likely to have excess fat in your liver and every drink you have has a significantly increased risk of causing liver damage which could lead to cirrhosis.

Tips for a Friday night after work: Start with a soda water, not an alcoholic drink, and take your time over it. If you get ribbed about it, say you're feeling dehydrated. Doing that will result in you drinking less during the evening and then try to alternate alcohol with something like lemon, lime and soda.

What is it about turning 40?

What's the problem?

Do you know the story about Tabitha the cheetah? The wild animal who once roamed the African savannahs, but now sits caged inside an American zoo providing entertainment for school kids.

Tabitha is the brainchild of American blogger and author Glennon Doyle. Doyle's book, *Untamed*, became a sensation in 2020, and Tabitha a metaphor for what happens to modern women in their early 40s. Now … stick with me here. I don't want you to think that I've suddenly become a spin doctor for the American self-help industry.

Over the years – as both a doctor and journalist – I've seen a shift in the public commentary and experience of women aged 40 and over. They're working harder, earning more, but not necessarily feeling more carefree. Phrases like the 'mental load' and the challenge of the 'double shift' (i.e. work at home and in the office) populate women's conversations.

These observations seem to mirror the message at the heart of Glennon Doyle's thesis.

Doyle argues that women in their 20s and 30s have the freedom to live life the way they want. Then along comes marriage, family and responsibility. Their carefree spirit is replaced by permanent sacrifice and women become hidden and overlooked. At 40-ish, with usually small but not tiny children roaming around the house, women confront feelings of restlessness and frustration.

Doyle urges her followers (and there are many) to break out of this lethargy and 'stop pleasing, start living'.

She took her own advice and did 'break free', out of a troubled heterosexual marriage into a more fulfilling lesbian relationship.

Social science seems to offer more to this cohort of women than medicine. Women tend to access formal medical help during their child-rearing years and tend not to see doctors much (well, except with their children or older parents) until they reach menopause. And what happens in between? Women take their kids to the doctor, nurture their partners and elderly parents, often at the cost of their own wellbeing. And in the meantime, they turn to novels or podcasts as a safe space to discuss what constitutes a good life.

Which leads me to wonder: is this just the 21st century

version of the mid-life crisis, where women are suffering the crisis, not just men.

History of the mid-life crisis

Can I pause for a moment in defence of medical science?

It's hard to measure a period of life without easy parameters. The Economic and Social Research Council in the UK says mid-life refers to the zone between 37 and 58, which is very broad.

Where did we get the idea that with 'mid-life' comes a slump?

In the 1930s, Swiss psychiatrist Carl Jung described mid-life as the afternoon of life for linking earlier (the morning) and later (the evening) periods. A period of the day that lends itself more towards rest and reflection rather than cutting loose.

Jung wrote: 'The afternoon of human life must also have a significance of its own and cannot merely be a pitiful appendage to life's morning.'

It's a notion of mid-life as a step back from the rapid growth and change in adolescence, that in order to free yourself from this period of stasis, one must do something pretty radical to keep living, or perhaps live a more colourful, broader life.

What do the stats say?

The latest data in the UK and around the world go a long way to explain why some women in their 40s are deeply frustrated with their lot.

The gender pay gap in Britain is around 15 per cent over all employees and 7.4 per cent in full-time workers, so there's still room for improvement. Our FTSE 100 company boards remain dominated by men. Women occupy 34.5 per cent of directorships and only 6 per cent of these companies have female CEOs.

More than half of UK employers still provide no access to employer-funded paid parental leave (that's on top of the government's mandatory paid parental leave scheme). Of the companies that do offer it, women still account for more than 90 per cent of all primary carer's leave.

Relatively few British employers offer onsite childcare, although the government does provide some financial support towards child care costs for nursery-age children.

But it's not just childcare. The Pew Research Center, a US think-tank, has looked at the 'sandwich' generation. These are people aged between 18 and 44 and spending three hours a day looking after elderly parents. Compared to people aged 45 and over, this group is also raising young children. So they're sandwiched in the middle of these two responsibilities, while their male partners go off to work, eat lunch with two hands, make time for a run after work before rejoining the family unit just as kids are happily tucked up in bed.

Fantastical?

Actually, data does show that men are now doing more at home but women are still doing the lion's share. According to a study conducted by Australia's University of Melbourne in 2018, women are falling into the trap of the 'double shift' by increasingly doing more in the office but not cutting back on work at home. Their data shows that the 'mental load', as is now so commonly discussed, is real.

The researchers investigated what happens in a household

after children are born. Around the time of the first birth, women's share of employment decreases markedly from equal in the years before birth down to 14 per cent in 'year zero' (that is, right after birth).

Meanwhile, women's share of care increases strongly, to 72 per cent in the year after the birth, and their share of housework, which was already higher than that of men's, increases further, to 64 per cent in the year after the birth. This pattern reflects the fact that in Britain most new mothers take at least several months off work to focus on full-time caring.

Locked in: The Australian research goes on to show that this gendered division of labour is not renegotiated as the first child grows older. Women's share of gainful employment increases only very slowly over time. One year, three years and also five years after the birth of the first child, it still amounts to only 23 per cent, and even ten years after the first birth it only reaches 30 per cent. This increase is accompanied by a small decrease in women's share of care time, but even ten years later, women still contribute an average of 66 per cent of the couple's care time.

The University of Melbourne report concludes that the birth of the first child is a turning point in couples' division of labour towards a gender-specific, long-term pattern. And that's only reinforced by the arrival of more children.

All of which American blogger and author Glennon Doyle would see as a vindication of her thesis that women become 'hidden' in the home without proper recompense for their hard work.

So what about divorce?

The crude divorce rate in Australia, which measures the number of divorces per 1000 people, rose in the 1960s and peaked in the mid 1970s with the introduction of no-fault divorce. In the 2000s, it started trending down. The figures are similar in the UK but, according to the latest ONS data, are currently about 8.9 per 1000. In the UK full no-fault divorce will not be introduced until 2023, but it will then apply to marriages and civil partnerships.

In the UK around one third of all marriages end in divorce and on average the duration of a marriage has fluctuated from 8.9 to 12.5 years. The average age of women divorcing is 43.5 years (and 46 in men). However, the proportion of couples divorcing who've been married 20 years and longer has been increasing.

But of course divorce is not the only measurement of a relationship in trouble.

In 2017, a reasearch programme in Australia's University of Sydney investigated the lives of 2000 working women aged under 40. Four in ten of them had at least one child and 50 per cent said they anticipated having another in the future. The women were concerned about earning enough to be able to afford children and childcare in order to return to work.

The research showed that flexibility was essential for women to combine their personal and private lives, but there was also widespread recognition that other colleagues were sometimes resentful of the flexibility offered to working parents.

Women seem to be moving towards the 40+ time of life with a lot of anxiety.

Looking after kids

Australia has also gathered data over the COVID-19 period in 2020, and we get an insight into the typical way Australian families divide childcare at home.

When asked 'who typically cared for the children' *before* COVID-19:

- 54 per cent answered 'mother'
- 38 per cent said 'equally'
- 8 per cent said 'always Dad'

During COVID-19 those numbers shifted slightly, with:

- 52 per cent of women saying that they always looked after children
- 11 per cent of men saying it was always them
- 37 per cent sharing the load equally

So women are still doing the most nurturing in the home, and many are experiencing stress as a result of those parenting obligations.

One of Australia's leading experts on women's mental health is Professor Jayashri Kulkarni, the Director of the Monash Alfred Psychiatry Research Centre, Melbourne. Talking about the challenges of the work–life 'juggle', she says: 'Often the busy woman is extremely good at juggling work and juggling other people's demands at the expense of herself.

'We need to teach women to think in a more mindful way about what's on their to-do list and to reduce the things that aren't critical. Often women are driven by a need for perfection and that can be a terrible pressure to live under,' claims Professor Kulkarni.

She wants women to throw out the endless to-do list and be a bit kinder to themselves.

'So if you're there with your child, then be there with the child and actually get enjoyment out of that. It's trying to decrease the sense of anxiety you get by thinking, "I've got 25 things on a to-do list and I'm only at number two".'

Let's talk about sex

Let's piece together a fictional woman from some of the evidence outlined above. She's got up early to make the school lunches and left work early to pick up the kids from childcare. Her elderly parent is considering elective surgery and will need to be cared for afterwards. As she's bathing her children, she mentally schedules a trip to the craft shop to source fabric for her daughter's Book Day outfit.

Now imagine just how keen she is for some night-time romance …

Sexuality is unique. But it's easy to see how that kind of stress and tension takes a toll on couples.

According to an important study of sexual and reproductive health, The Australian Study of Health and Relationships, while Australians appear to be having sex less frequently, they have broader repertoires of sexual practice. The study is conducted every ten years and was last done in 2012–13. The findings suggest that women's reports of numbers of partners and range of sexual practices are becoming more similar to men's, which the study sees as a reduction in double standards.

But this study didn't take account of the unique factors

associated with approaching middle age. A US report from the Universities of Pittsburgh and Utah sheds more light on women aged 45 and over. According to this study, middle-aged women experience a series of changes and factors at mid-life that may affect sexual function.

These included physical (menopause), psychological (disrupted sleep and mood), sociological (cultural expectations regarding older women's sexuality), and interpersonal changes (loss of their sexual partner or problems with the relationship or the partner's health).

They cite other research showing sexual function declines during mid-life, particularly during menopause, often leading to low libido and vaginal dryness.

The study was solidly binary though, with all but two of the respondents identifying as heterosexual.

Many cited some of these physical problems as the reasons their sexual appetite waned. But they also said that their multiple roles as wife, daughter, mother and worker made it difficult for them to relax and enjoy sex. The result was often that they were turning off and 'just going through the motions'. Many women noted that their partners had the same stresses they were experiencing, and lowering their desire for sex too.

The couples who were bothered by these changes adapted and changed their sexual behaviour. This included lengthening foreplay, trying different sexual positions, and using lubricants and sexual aids. They also placed more importance on feeling connected and intimate with their partner than the physical aspects of sex, such as reaching orgasm.

It was far from all bad news, though. The study revealed lots of positives associated with mid-life.

For some, sex was actually more frequent than when they were younger. Or if they did it less, the sex was better quality. Women cited feeling more comfortable in their own skin than when they were younger, which left them more free to express themselves in the bedroom. They said they better understood their own sexual needs and were more confident of communicating those needs to their partners.

Finally, some explained how, over the course of a years-long relationship, two people can develop a deep and intimate connection, which went along with a deep understanding of each other's sexual needs, making sex more fulfilling.

There are problems with extrapolating too widely from this study given its small size. But several women mentioned that they were interested in participating in the study precisely because they had never talked to anyone about their sexuality.

But it notes how important it is for doctors to explore psychosocial factors, like relationships or stress, as well as medical conditions.

So:

Maybe mid-life doesn't have to be a crisis at all

The divorce memoir *Eat Pray Love* sold 10 million copies and was made into a feature film. Women are buying these narratives in droves and they've a common theme: that out of the darkness comes the light. That these women feel they lose their identity, but when they re-emerge they do so stronger and wiser. With a powerful drive to live better.

So if you look at it this way, it's not a crisis at all.

The thing is that the women in these popular culture accounts aren't necessarily broken. But many women in this group feel lost and stretched to a point that they feel they're likely to snap. At this point I'm feeling uncomfortably close to becoming patriarchal and patronising. Having asked the question 'what is it about turning 40' based on my observations of women around that age, I feel embarrassed that the system and economy are still so male focused and non-conducive to shared family and household responsibilities. And doctors have to pay more attention to these feelings.

Medicine needs to evolve faster than it has.

In 2012, a group of obstetricians and gynaecologists published a paper titled 'Sexuality in midlife: Where the passion goes?'. Their thesis is that very few women's healthcare physicians are adequately trained to monitor a woman's sexual health from the end of her childbearing years, through the menopausal transition and beyond. They argue that doctors fail to properly treat sexual problems that can arise during this time.

But this is a lot more than a discussion around intimacy and sex.

Professor Jayashri Kulkarni from Australia's Monash University prescribes a daily 'prescription of fun' in which women spend half an hour doing something enjoyable just for themselves. She says learning to view this time as necessary for recharging, rather than narcissistic or selfish, is important for mental and physical health.

Men need to 'lean in' and help their partners, sisters or friends find solutions if they're under strain.

Bain & Company, a global consulting firm, looked at men's

engagement in gender equality efforts In Australia. They broke up the group into 'supporters' – who were actively engaged in driving for more equality – and the 'passives'. Passives weren't necessarily against gender equality, but didn't feel it necessary to engage. About one-third of the passives cited a lack of time, but one-fifth said that gender discrimination was no longer a significant issue.

It's telling. As women in mid-life are becoming more professionally empowered, yet more stressed because of the work–life juggle, some men are missing the debate entirely.

A Gen-Y friend of mine suggested that education needs to start earlier. Perhaps the personal development curriculum at high school could be updated with the line, 'There's nothing sexy about picking up your boyfriend's underpants off the floor.'

#whatunderpants

#malepatternblindness

Endometriosis and its curious genetic links

Quick take: Endometriosis is common. It affects one in nine women prior to the menopause, which is around the time when the symptoms tend to disappear. And there are many symptoms – including none at all, when the problem is found when a woman is investigated for infertility (a complication of the condition). But by and large the problem is pain – usually in the pelvis – associated with the menstrual cycle and sometimes heavy periods. The cause is unknown but may be genetic. What happens is that 'nests' of tissue similar to the lining of the uterus (the endometrium) are spread to other parts of the pelvis and abdomen. Women with endometriosis have, for years, noticed they have gastrointestinal symptoms, depression and migraines, but that has often been ignored as a coincidence or a psychological reaction to the disease. Now genetic studies link all this together. Doesn't offer a new treatment yet but it does mean that doctors have to think of endometriosis as more than a gynaecological problem.

*

I won't get too technical but there's a way of surveying people's genomes without needing to sequence every letter of the genetic code. They look for about 700,000 landmarks knowing which genes are nearby each of them. It's like a high level map called a genome-wide association study (GWAS). GWAS analysis isn't perfect but it does let you know which genes come together when someone has a condition – like endometriosis – whose origins are a bit of a mystery, not to mention not knowing whether the depression that goes along with endometriosis is a psychological reaction to having to live with the condition or part and parcel of endometriosis itself.

Long story short, a GWAS in women with endometriosis found a significant overlap between the genes associated with endometriosis and genes linked to being susceptible to depression, suggesting a common genetic cause. But the study didn't end there. Since it was genome-wide, they could pick up other signals that might be around and what they found was a link with abnormalities in the lining of the gut, perhaps associated with ulcers and reflux. And yet another study found a genetic link between endometriosis and migraine.

The net effect of such studies is that they focus researchers on the possibility that the same thing might be going on in all these conditions – the same mechanics – opening up the way to new treatments.

When do my eggs clap out?
And when do his sperm?

Quick one: Unfortunately, age is the most important factor here – for men and women. Women should stop beating themselves up about infertility. Men need to take notice of their own contribution.

*

Words matter: There are two words which are worth thinking about. One is fertility and the other is fecundity. Fecundity is what most people who want to have a baby care about, because fecundity is your capacity to have a baby. So focus on that. There are lots of clinics willing to take your money in the name of fertility (falling pregnant), whereas what you want is fecundity. As women contemplate career, finding a partner and wanting to have a family before it's too late or too medically and financially traumatic, they worry about their biological clocks. The thing is that men should be worrying about their age too when it comes to fathering.

Eggs: Many people think the reason that women in their 30s find it progressively harder to have a baby is that all their good eggs have been used up, leaving only the clapped-out ones behind. That's not true. What actually happens is that the eggs which haven't been shed, age. And eggs age in the same way as all the other parts of our body age – largely through oxidative stress (see Stress and Shoelaces). So that means if you've smoked, not got enough exercise and are grossly overweight, it won't have been good for you or your eggs. It should also mean that the eating pattern at the beginning of this book is better for your eggs too. Research has not shown a significant effect on egg ageing from antioxidant supplements which isn't a surprise since they don't work for anything very much. So stick to the eating pattern. As to the age you're best to have a baby? That's debated but just before you're 30 with the hill steepening after 35.

But it's a couple thing: If you're a heterosexual couple, that is. Couples who have trouble having a baby usually have lots of things going on. The woman is often older which means her fecundity has dropped. The man is often even older which means his sperm are off the pace. And sometimes there's remarkably little sex going on. There are many people in same-sex couples who aim to have children and for whom sex isn't the route, but if it is, then – duuh – it's the starting point for having a baby.

Which brings us to his sperm (and other things): The first thing to say is that if you get off on men who are abnormally ripped, and find it hard to fit their guns into their T-shirt sleeves, then don't be surprised if you have trouble falling pregnant. Steroid use reduces male fertility and increases the likelihood of abnormally developed sperm. Now given that I'm not ripped and my problem with T-shirts is the abdomen not my biceps, you could put what I've just said down to envy. Fair enough, but what's fundamentally true is that, like women, the older a man is, the less fertile he becomes and the more statistically likely to father a child with a congenital or developmental problem. Men's ability to churn out sperm until quite late in life gives them false confidence, whereas women only have the finite supply of eggs which they were born with. Trouble is that with sperm, quality counts, as does the count itself. And both decline with age. So an older man with an older woman (in reproductive terms, that is) means that one plus one could equal 0.5. In other words, infertility is frequently a couple problem. Independent of the age of his partner, a man in his 40s is 30 per cent less likely to conceive than a man less than 30 years old. Men also have sex less often as they age and have an increasing rate of erectile dysfunction, neither of which is terrific for women of childbearing age who want to have a baby. And it's not just the sperm decreasing in quality (more DNA errors) and number. The glands which produce the fluid that helps sperm to survive, they age too. So semen quality declines. The results of all this are longer time to conception, lower fecundity because of increased miscarriage rates, and possibly an increased risk of developmental issues like autism spectrum disorder in the children.

And don't forget your tubes: Sexually transmissible infections, like chlamydia, damage and block the sexual plumbing of both men and women, reducing fecundity.

Makes you wonder how anyone manages to have a baby.

Goldilocks and weight: There is a lot of evidence that the more overweight or obese a woman is, the longer it takes to become pregnant. The research in this area is clouded by the fact that the more obese people are, the more likely they are to have other unhealthy lifestyles such as smoking and inactivity or indeed, in women, to have polycystic ovarian syndrome (PCOS) which is strongly associated with infertility. But BMI does seem to be a factor in its own right. It's been shown by following women from age 18 and comparing their time to pregnancy (when they're trying, of course) compared to increases in their BMI. Weight loss has also been shown to shorten the time to conception. Obesity also increases miscarriage rates.

On the other hand, being underweight also increases the time it takes to conceive when you're trying. You need fat on your body to have normal ovulatory and hormonal function. So weight loss or maintenance should be around a normal BMI.

Weight in men also matters. Underweight men are more likely to have semen abnormalities, and overweight and obese men are more likely to have erectile dysfunction and other issues affecting sex and conception.

So, like Goldilocks, you should try to keep your weight just right.

The flip side … when you still have all your eggs

Takeaway: The message for parents of young girls is that lifestyle changes which may delay the start of their periods (menarche) are a good thing. Delayed menarche in an otherwise healthy girl is associated with a reduced risk of breast cancer later in life, as well as obesity, possibly heart disease and fibroids. The best way to delay the start of periods is a good dose of sport and exercise. Not having smoked in pregnancy is also good. The hard way to delay menarche is to have more brothers (no-one knows why), and the ways you'd like to avoid if you can, are having chronic disease or an eating disorder.

*

When do periods normally start? Early age at menarche is often defined as under 12 years. A study in the UK recorded an average age of girls getting their first period of 12.7 years. Around 4.8 per cent of participants reached the menarche before the age of 11 and around 10 per cent did not reach it until the age of 15 or older. This is a complicated story since factors such as disadvantage (linked to being younger when your periods start) and ethnicity can make a difference.

Breast cancer and age at first period: This isn't about having something else to panic about but it is worth being aware. Age at menarche (older is better), and age at first full-term birth (younger is better) are well-established risk factors for breast cancer. One large study found that for each two-year delay in onset of menstruation, breast cancer risk was reduced by about 10 per cent. Another study found that women with onset of menstruation at or after age 15 years had a 23 per cent lower risk than those with an age at menarche of 12 years or younger.

The mechanism is thought to be that a higher number of lifetime periods and therefore ovulatory cycles exposes a woman's breasts more frequently to hormones which drive the growth of breast cells and from that to cancer risk. Pregnancy reduces breast cancer risk partly because it gives the breasts a rest from menstrual hammering and also the process of preparing the breasts for feeding makes breasts more cancer resistant. That benefit can last many years. The younger a woman is when she first falls pregnant is also protective.

Uterine fibroids: A large study in the US following the health of female nurses found that a lower age at menarche and lower age at first birth was associated with a higher risk of uterine leiomyomata (fibroids).

BMI and the metabolic syndrome: Earlier age of menarche has been associated with increased BMI in childhood and adolescence and may reflect restricted growth in foetal life followed by rapid growth after birth. A study of 6507 US adolescent girls found early maturation (11 years and under) nearly doubled the odds of being overweight. But that doesn't prove cause and effect since obesity and overweight are more common in disadvantaged and some ethnic groups. In the US, significantly higher proportions of African-American and Hispanic girls experience menarche before 11 years of age, and a higher proportion of Asian girls reached menarche at 14 years of age or later. This risk may also translate into an association with the metabolic syndrome later in life.

Heart disease: There is a relationship between earlier age at menarche and heart disease but it's controversial because it could be a proxy for disadvantage and coronary risk factors.

Living long: It is unclear whether early menarche has an effect on life expectancy. Strategies to minimise earlier menarche, such as promoting healthy weights and minimising family dysfunction during childhood, may in themselves have positive longer-term effects on survival.

PART 4

The wellbeing thing

Wellness and resilience:
two annoying words

Feel free to discount what I say here because I'm a dour Scot who's sensitive to bullshit and doesn't care much if I pierce a few bubbles as long as there's good evidence to support my sometimes jaundiced views.

A very large piece of bullshit that we've been led to believe by consumer goods companies and other self-interested parties is that the natural state of humans should be a happy state of wellness. More recently, the psychology industry has underpinned that with one of their current favourite words: resilience. I write this with a sense of impending doom, knowing that my inbox will be full of invective from researchers and organisations who've built careers and income by promoting resilience. Same goes for wellness.

Why do they get my goat? Surely I can't be arguing for unwellness and fragility? Of course not.

You know the answer already. Each day of your life you swing between feeling okay, good, great and not so great, and what sometimes causes those swings is where you're sitting on the pendulum between strong and vulnerable. Our mood and sense of ourselves change according to circumstance. It becomes something of concern if a low mood and negative feelings persist or the highs are abnormally high, but my point is that it's normal to be a bit up and down. The risk with using words like wellness and resilience carelessly is that you open up to oversimplification, unrealistic expectations and maybe even blaming individuals for their predicament rather than the context of their lives.

Let's start with resilience

It's the extent to which your psychological struts help you to withstand adversity, adapt and bounce back. The problem is that it's too easy to assume that there are resilient people and weak people because that leads to stigma, a sense of unchangeable destiny and also a misleading notion that resilience is somehow equated to strength or strengths. Looking at your strengths may be more useful when there are issues with adapting to a changing workplace, jobs and relationships. I'll come to strengths later. With resilience, there is such a thing – in fact, there are resilience questionnaires which researchers claim to be validated – but it's not 'on' or 'off', or 'there' or 'not there'. It's on a continuum that doesn't easily map onto an individual's make-up.

I'll give you an example right at the edge. Military recruiters aim to select people who are resilient so they'll turn into soldiers who are more psychologically bulletproof when they go into combat. The recruiters fail at the first hurdle because for some reason – at least in the past – they have overselected for people vulnerable to bipolar disorder. The prevalence of bipolar in new recruits in some defence forces has been around 10 per cent, whereas in the community it's more like 1 per cent. That could be due to the energy and confidence exuded by people vulnerable to the disorder impressing interviewers. Anyway, what every military organisation wants to prevent is post traumatic stress disorder (PTSD) after going into combat. It seems their selection processes are not very good at finding people who are PTSD resistant. For example, studies have found that prior to deployment, US marines who do and do not later develop PTSD have similar levels of mental health issues. The main risk factors for PTSD in repeated studies are your war zone deployment history and whether you've had a brain injury from, say, a roadside bomb blast. There is some evidence that prior traumatic events in your life, such as bereavement, relationship breakdown or abuse, can increase your vulnerability to PTSD. Interestingly, there isn't even good evidence that Special Forces personnel have significantly lower rates of PTSD when they are followed up for long enough. In fact, moral injury, where you're forced to do things that run counter to your values and beliefs, can also add to the risk of PTSD and that applies beyond warfare to other occupations. Sure, there are protective factors such as whether you're an officer and how well educated you are. But what seems to count most when it comes to PTSD resilience is your team, the support around you, the validation by your peers, which in a sense normalises your experiences, and your sense of identity, most of which seems to be true also for first responders such as police, firefighters and paramedics. There's no question that PTSD rates are higher in combat personnel and first responders than in the general population, but the rates really skyrocket a year or two after people leave the forces or first responder organisations. That's when they've often lost the sense of belonging which built up their resilience and their idea of who they are. The friendship and support people were used to as a soldier or frontline police officer were what allowed them to draw upon that resilience. On top of having to find a life away from the identity, there's sometimes the loss of treatment services provided by the defence forces.

Resilience is a more useful concept describing groups than individuals and it's about context more than individual strengths. Who's around you, how much control you have over your life, your education level, whether you have a stable job, do you have somewhere decent to live, has someone close to you died or had a major illness recently, have you had a significant relationship breakdown? If these are negative, then bounce back is eroded. If positive, then resilience is strengthened. However, if what you're focused on is resilience, you may miss what counts such as job training, housing or working on friendships. What's probably true is that compared to focusing on the negatives, zeroing in on what's positive and strong in our lives gives a better basis for building the psychological struts we need for whatever the future might bring.

One of the mysteries in families is why, especially in the face of the same adversity, some kids turn out to be better at getting through life than their brothers and sisters. One suggestion is that in the preschool years, they've experienced more support for a while, say, from a grandparent. It's also about the genes that a child has inherited which, for example, may have given them a temperament which makes adaptation to adversity easier or harder.

Then there's wellness (at least as defined by advertising and the media)

I'm fine, thanks. I don't have a fatal disease (yet), I exercise and eat healthily (too much and too often, mind you), have a good job, great kids, and strong friendships and relationships. So I should be a pin-up for the wellness industry. But do I feel 'well'? Am I bursting out of my skin with the energy that's associated with 'wellness'? Despite my blessings and objective reality, if I think about it (I usually don't and I advise you not to either), I feel a bit crap a fair proportion of the time. By a bit crap I mean a little tired, sometimes anxious about a deadline, feeling blaaahh because I've yet to have my extra strong latte or daily exercise, I've given in to the panettone sitting in that box in the kitchen, or I have a few sore muscles from yesterday's session. Wellness has the potential to be an oppressive concept that assumes you have to be fit and beautiful and constantly happy. There are people with serious illness or disability who feel fulfilled and happy and give as well as receive, yet who struggle each day with pain and uncertainty. They put my feelings of crap-ness to shame. The common concept of wellness does no-one any favours apart from consumer-focused companies and the odd chef who push it. Humans tend to be optimistic but research has found that people who are a bit more on the depressive scale are more realistic even though it can sound like pessimism.

So what replaces wellness?

It's not so much replace as being clear what it means, namely feeling good about yourself and your place in the world and whether (and this comes back to bounce back) you have good relationships at work and outside work, feel able to make decisions and to adapt to change and the slings and arrows that life throws at you. Wellness is not on the same continuum as sickness or mental illness where wellness is at one end and illness or mental health issues are at the other. It's a thing in its own right but not what you've been led to believe by what's commonly portrayed.

Mind you, you could have a rating system like TV shows and movies. My vote would go to GE: Good Enough. Won't sell the latest paleo diet or exercise program or win any advertising awards but it's realistic.

And what determines whether you're GE?

It's having enough money to have a roof over your head and buy the basics; it's having food and job security. It also helps to be sufficiently educated or trained to have future choices. It's about feeling connected to your family and community, having people you can call upon when times are tough, being married (if you're a man, that is … less so if you're a woman) and it's about giving back to others when you can. Physical health does make a difference but people with major illness can be GE because of all the other pretty good things in their lives.

Work–life balance: yet more annoying words

#morebullshit

Again, a declaration: I'm not good at this but there are some fundamentals that are worth thinking about.

Work is good for you. It gives you purpose, human contact, a sense of identity and a better chance at financial stability. There is more than a century of research to show that being out of work is bad for your health, shortens your life, increases the risk of psychological distress, suicide and family breakdown, throws you into poverty and makes bringing up kids really tough.

The phrase work–life balance is based on a false assumption, namely that life is somehow different from work. It's the same thing and there are huge contradictions built into this phrase, not to mention hypocrisy and entitlement. One reason is that it's assumed that when we talk about work–life balance we're talking about people in paid work and that people in these jobs are somehow more entitled to a balance than those who don't earn salaries or wages. No-one seems to care much about work–life balance for the millions of people doing unpaid work – mostly women who work many hours a day caring for children and elderly parents. Or the wage-earning women who come home and then do an unfair share of domestic work.

I can't locate reputable research that finds getting a balance between work and life, as an aim in its own right, is beneficial. We want different things from our work depending on our life circumstances and personal preferences. Some see work as a means to an income, nothing more, and that could as much apply to an investment banker as a casual worker in a cafe. If you're supporting a family, then you might not risk chasing the job of your dreams compared to when you were younger. In that circumstance, work can be a source of conflict, when someone is working long hours while their partner is taking the load of childcare and home duties.

It's all about what I spoke of at the beginning of the book: our goals and the insight into how these change. The 'life' bit is, of course, about the four 'F's – fun, family, friends and freedom – and there's nothing I can write which will assist you to set priorities. I'll leave that to the self-help gurus who manage their own work–life balance by making bucketloads of money out of being a self-help guru. For the rest of us, the 'balance' thing usually arises when work becomes oppressive, which in turn makes us feel there's no freedom for the other three 'F's. And work becomes oppressive when it feels relentless, unrecognised (e.g. domestic work or unpaid caring) and badly managed and the system doesn't allow you to do your best (see The Control Factor). That's when you start thinking, I'd be better off playing with the kids, having a drink with friends or lying on a beach with a good book. Work and the four 'F's are a constant dialogue between aspiration, the expectations of others, recognition from the people you report to and the stability of our relationships. When that fragile equilibrium is upset, then stress and perhaps distress (see Distress and Depression) may set in.

Freedom is much more about control than being able to hit the beach or binge-watch *Bridgerton* whenever we fancy. There's often no control when you're poor and unemployed. As mentioned earlier (see The Control Factor) control is also critical at work and lack of it can colour your non-working life.

So should we be talking about burnout?

Happy to.

Quick take: Burnout isn't a mental health disorder in its own right. It's a state of mind strongly associated with chronic job strain of the kind I spoke about earlier (see Health Isn't Evenly Spread). There are lots of definitions but there are three main things you feel: exhausted; cynical about work and detached from it; and not feeling very effective in your job, dissatisfied with it and sometimes wanting to avoid it. The solutions are not so much about individual therapy but more about how an employer needs to change.

*

Burnout might be a relatively new word but the problem has probably been around as long as workplaces. It's another in a group of issues where the condition is very real for people who experience it, yet psychologists and doctors have had trouble getting a handle on burnout (other examples include chronic pain and chronic fatigue). Anyway, one of the more reliable and validated descriptions of burnout comes from a detailed questionnaire and scale invented by social psychologist Professor Christina Maslach and her colleagues at the University of California, Berkeley, USA. It's called the Maslach Burnout Inventory and measures three areas: feelings of exhaustion and being overextended in relation to your work; the degree of cynicism that you have about work as reflected by a sense of indifference or feeling distant from it; and the third is what Professor Maslach calls 'professional efficacy', which is really about being down on yourself; not feeling you're doing your job very well and the extent to which you think you won't in future. It's mostly about your perception of yourself in the context of your work, independent of the objective reality of your job performance.

The sources of burnout have different patterns but generally involve feeling overloaded without the freedom to make decisions which would allow you to work more effectively, not being given clear and consistent work goals, interpersonal conflict in the workplace, and a lack of time, information and physical resources to do the job that's being asked of you. Feeling you're failing – which may be true – reinforces loss of control and a fear you'll lose respect from your colleagues and become trapped. An important causative factor is being put into a job which doesn't fit you well.

There are rarely simple solutions to burnout but organisations need to take it seriously, since for every person who verbalises it there are probably others feeling burnt out without saying so. And if a boss only focuses on one aspect – say, exhaustion – and gives the person a holiday, then the fundamental issues will remain when they get back. It's a bit like my argument about resilience. It's less about the 'weakness' or vulnerability of an individual than an organisational problem. As I write this, I'm seeing a lot of burnout in my own organisation, the Australian Broadcasting Corporation, as managers and staff struggle with federal government-imposed cuts. Maslach describes burnout as more about '… the situation than the person'. One example is with health workers such as nurses in aged care, who during COVID felt torn by the decisions they were having to make, and the stress and overload which became so bad in some countries that some left nursing altogether.

There are lots of elements to preventing and dealing with burnout. They include being matched to the right job, engaged in defining its goals and how the work is designed, and fairness in the workplace so that the burden and, importantly, the rewards, are evenly shared. It's potentially toxic to feel under-rewarded for your effort compared to others and that's more than money. It includes appropriate recognition. There are also personal strategies which can help, such as setting limits on the number of hours you're going to work, changing what you can in the work environment, or not waiting on permission to do so (Sir Harry Burns, a public health expert in Glasgow, calls this 'proceeding until apprehended'), and finding new sources of satisfaction outside work.

Burnout is a serious issue associated with future mental health and even heart issues, so not something to be shoved under the carpet. What we've yet to find out is whether the COVID and post-COVID trend to working at home reduces, increases or makes no difference to the risks of burnout.

It's usually better to think about strengths

Quick take: It can be very annoying when you're in strife, doing it tough or feeling you're in a dark place, when someone tells you to focus on the positive and count your blessings. People living with cancer, for example, are often oppressed by this from relatives and friends who believe, entirely wrongly, that a positive attitude makes a difference to survival or cure. So when people with cancer feel low, they can also feel guilty that they're not achieving the positivity expected of them. Anyway, this section isn't about cancer, nor is it about counting your blessings, but it is about swivelling away from the negatives towards building on what's strong in your life even though you might at times feel there's not much.

*

First thing I'll say is that if you've had a persistently low mood, not enjoying things you used to, maybe are chronically anxious and especially if you feel you're in a dark place, you should seek help. There are online resources where you can assess yourself and get an idea of what assistance you need. The mental health foundation Mentalhealth-uk.org can provide information and guidance and can direct you to therapists in your area. If you're thinking of harming yourself, call the Samaritans on 116 123 any time of day or night if you're in the UK and if you think someone you know or work with is in distress, ask if they're okay and if they're not okay, support them in seeking help.

I was trained in medicine and it's a training in negatives: disease, risk factors and crises. My specialist training was in paediatrics and after a few years in hospital medicine, it was easy to start to believe – even if you knew it not to be true – that there was no such thing as a normal delivery or a healthy child. Same goes for psychology and other health professions. Sure, we're taught what's normal but every day we see people with problems. So it takes an effort to look for the positive in your own and other people's lives. However, it's worth it because those positives are the building blocks for the future and should be an integral part of the treatment for psychological and chronic physical problems, as well as developing wellbeing.

In certain ways cognitive behavioural therapy does help with this (and I'm grossly oversimplifying) by identifying thoughts which are consistently negative or objectively not true and reframing them: for example, 'I'm hopeless and useless and a failure in life', when there's probably plenty of evidence that's not the case. Guided mindfulness can do a similar thing by noting intrusive thoughts and recognising them for what they are.

But focusing on building strengths is more than that. It's about your social network, who you can call upon for help, your skills and past adaptability, your work and family, your interests and accomplishments, and what you want out of life and your priorities. Not all these boxes will be ticked. Some of them can actually be ticked even though you don't think so. If you're low or feeling traumatised, building on strengths is often too much to expect to do alone. You should feel unembarrassed to seek help, probably best from a psychologist who's been well trained in a strengths-based approach. Seeking help is not a sign of weakness. Getting acknowledgement and validation from someone else about what you're going through can be one of the most important (and first) steps in recovery. This is about moving yourself on the wellbeing scale towards wellbeing, remembering that it can be independent of negative things that might be going on and which are hard to change quickly.

I'm unembarrassed to admit that at a low point in my life with multiple negative things going on, I went to see such a psychologist. In a single session (reinforced at follow-up) with no jargon or deep analysis, he focused me on very practical actions and goals around my social network which had nothing to do with the bad stuff going on but was transformative. Within minutes of meeting me and asking some key questions, he worked out which strengths and aspirations he could build on and helped me set appropriate goals. Within days my mood had improved without a single problem that I went in with having been solved. I soon felt better and strengthened. I doubt that I'd have got there by myself.

Australian Aboriginal communities are way ahead on this one. They've hated the negativity around Indigenous disadvantage and many communities have taken control with services they own and direct. They know their biggest strengths are in identification with country, communities, networks, extended families and the wisdom of elders, and that's what they build upon. It doesn't take away the need for housing, schools and health care but helps to design them for maximum effect.

There's no evidence that strengths-based approaches can replace proven treatments, especially in severe mental illness like psychosis or deep depression, but it's fundamental to recovery and rehabilitation.

Distress and depression: two sides of the same coin?

#Sometimes

Takeaways: Distress is a normal reaction to events like losing someone you love, a relationship breakdown or being made redundant. It might take a while, but most of us get over the feelings of anxiety, maybe hopelessness and not being able to get down to work that are usually associated with the word distress. Distress levels went up during COVID lockdowns, for example. Not everyone who's distressed needs to see a doctor or psychologist, but it's important to know when you might need to seek help and to know that the assistance can be tailored to how your distress is affecting you.

*

There are various definitions of psychological distress and they have different purposes which are often confused in the minds of psychologists and doctors. There are questionnaires where you rate your answers and add up the score. I talk about these only to give you a bit of insight into what distress actually looks like.

One of the early questionnaires which was really designed for GPs to ask patients was called the GHQ-12. It asked about ability to concentrate, loss of sleep, feeling you're being useful or worthless, capacity to make decisions, level of daily strain, ability to face up to difficulties and overcome them, enjoyment from life, your mood and self-confidence. These are things I've mentioned before and they make sense, but the problem with this questionnaire was that it was too easy for a doctor or psychologist to mis-score it and wrongly label someone as okay when they weren't or needing help when they didn't.

There are others such as the Australian K10 (Kessler psychological distress scale), which is more useful for governments and researchers to know the level of distress in the community, and it was the K10 scores which increased during the first COVID lockdown.

The value of understanding the concept of distress is that it can help to know when you should seek care – when you have persistent bothersome symptoms of depression and anxiety.

One useful questionnaire you can fill out yourself on this is the Patient Health Questionnaire (PHQ-9).

It asks about how often you've had certain thoughts and feelings over the past two weeks – from not at all, to nearly every day – and the specific questions are:

- Little interest or pleasure in doing things?
- Feeling down, depressed or hopeless?
- Trouble falling or staying asleep or sleeping too much?
- Feeling tired or having too little energy?
- Poor appetite or overeating?
- Feeling bad about yourself – or that you're a failure and have let yourself or your family down?
- Trouble concentrating on things such as reading the newspaper or watching television?
- Moving or speaking so slowly that other people could have noticed? Or the opposite – being so fidgety or restless that you're moving around a lot more?
- Thoughts that you would be better off dead – or hurting yourself in some way?

You can do this online and your score helps you understand whether you need to see someone about it. Mind you, even if you're at the mild end of the scale, you might benefit from seeing a clinical psychologist for some strategies to get you going.

The GAD7 is an anxiety score and it rates you on questions over the past two weeks such as: feeling anxious, nervous or on edge, how much you're worrying about things, having problems relaxing, being restless or sitting still, being irritable and having a sense that something bad is going to happen.

The problem with seeking help solely based on these questionnaires is that they don't identify everyone who would benefit from seeing a clinician for care. For instance, in some people, distress, depression and anxiety manifest more as persistent physical symptoms like fatigue, disruption of your sleep–wake cycle, pain, headaches and tummy symptoms. The people most likely to come forward are women who are well educated and have above-average income. Those least likely are men and people in disadvantaged or minority ethnic communities where outcomes can often be poorer as well, perhaps because of inadequate or mismatched treatment.

There are also practical ways of deciding whether you need to seek help, such as whether your work is being affected, your ability to complete tasks, the effects on your personal and family relationships, the extent to which you pursue your interests, and involvement in your community.

What's really important is that when you're distressed you should avoid using tobacco, alcohol and other drugs to try to make you feel better. The effects are short-lived while the harms last much longer.

Lifestyle factors can increase the risk of distress in the first place.

For example, in one study, male smokers who were not full-time employed and had only minor symptoms of depression were at a 17 per cent risk of having a major depressive disorder after four years, but if they were full-time employed the risk was less than 5 per cent. Likewise, participants with 4–6 symptoms who were under financial pressure and used marijuana had an 18 per cent risk of depression if they were also using alcohol to a harmful/hazardous extent, but less than 5 per cent for those not using harmful/hazardous amounts of alcohol. That is, there are people with low levels of depressive symptoms who are at increased risk of experiencing a future major depressive episode, but there are those with many symptoms who are 'protected' by factors such as being in good physical health and employed.

How it works with treatment for distress is usually a stepped approach depending on the severity, urgency and preference. The steps aren't necessarily followed religiously but are usually:

1. Simple lifestyle changes – such as sleep, diet, exercise and alcohol reduction
2. Basic problem-solving, stress management and life skills
3. More specialised psychological therapies
4. Medication

Aiming for wellbeing

Quick take: For wellbeing, read overall health, not necessarily a state of perpetual happiness. Remember what I said earlier.

There's no split between the mind and the body. They are closely connected. So it should be no surprise that being persistently depressed or anxious to the extent that it's affecting your life can have profound effects on every system in your body, while if your body is healthy it's going to be good for your brain and mind as well.

*

Mental health issues are associated with the kind of damaging inflammation I talked about in the nutrition section which increases the rate of ageing, and the risks of diabetes, heart disease and possibly cancer and dementia. So ... eating a dominantly plant-based diet which involves healthy cooking with fresh herbs, onions, tomatoes, olive oil and vinegar, not putting on too much weight, and having regular, reasonably intensive exercise, perhaps through high intensity interval training if there are no reasons not to, will all help your wellbeing and the relief of distress.

Folate/Folic acid: There is evidence that folate (the natural form of vitamin B9) levels are low in people with depression – it might be something to do with your genes and how your body deals with it but don't go off getting your genes analysed. It's worth raising your intake as it might make a difference, albeit a small one. A plant-based diet is rich in folate. Supplements contain folic acid, the synthetic form of vitamin B9.

Physical activity: Physical activity has been extensively evaluated as a treatment for depression and the balance of evidence is that exercise does reduce the symptoms of depression and has a preventive effect between episodes. There is a caveat, though. People with moderate to severe depression often find it hard to activate themselves for almost any kind of movement, but if exercise is possible and depending on the intensity and how well it's sustained (also a challenge), exercise can compare favourably to the effects of antidepressants and cognitive behaviour therapy.

Wellbeing does add years to your life because good mental health is associated with lower risks of chronic disease. Conversely, there is lots of evidence that serious mental illness is associated with dying up to 25 years earlier than people without serious mental illness. And that's not explained by suicide but by higher rates of heart disease, diabetes and cancer.

Sleep-iety

The wake-up call: Sleep has become a massive industry, there are apps to send you to sleep or keep you asleep. There are sleep clinics which wire you up to find out which sleep disorder you have. And then there's the sleep research industry, much of which has convinced the world that if you're not getting eight hours a night, then boy, do you have problems, risking all sorts of outcomes, from dementia to obesity to diabetes, not to mention poor performance. The message with sleep in this book is the same as for many other sections. Having a sleep disorder is defined by you or your partner who might be going up the wall. If your sleep pattern is causing you problems, then it needs to be sorted out. If you have sleep apnoea and fall asleep at the wheel or in meetings, that's a problem that needs expert attention. If you feel you have insomnia, then you should deal with it. But it might be reassuring to note that insomnia is really self-defined. In fact, a lot of insomnia research in the past has been experiments where healthy people are deliberately woken up during the night to see what the effects are. Now that is truly designed to piss anyone off and make them feel crap. There are plenty of people getting exactly the same amount of sleep as you and aren't too bothered by it. That doesn't mean you're weak or silly if you feel you have insomnia, but it might relax you a bit to know that it isn't a medical condition. It's a lot about perception; what you've been led to believe is expected of a night's sleep. Sleep deprivation is a thing, though, and is linked to increased deaths and accident rates (on the roads and in workplaces) for people who are not getting enough sleep. The degree of impairment for someone who has not slept for 17 hours is equivalent to having had three or four drinks, while mortality rates are increased among shift workers.

There's no question that sleep is a crucial ingredient in wellbeing and improves mental health.

The thing is … I'm not a big sleeper. If you follow my Twitter feed, you'll have guessed that from the times I post (and probably shouldn't but that's another story). And I don't think that's going to change.

But that's okay because you actually don't have to sleep eight hours a night. You've just got to sleep long enough to meet your needs. While seven to nine hours seems to be the quoted range for a healthy night's sleep, there's significant variation.

When you work in breakfast radio, which I sometimes do, it's almost impossible to get eight hours in a row. The one-time king of Sydney breakfast radio, Alan Jones, used to brag that he needed only about three hours a night.

I googled Jones and his sleep to check if my memory served me right, and sure enough I heard an excerpt from his radio program in 2019. When responding to a global health survey by one of the big corporates which stated that eight and a quarter hours was the optimal night's sleep, the breakfast radio host joked, 'What … is that a week?'

Jones has always worn his sleep pattern as a badge of honour and an example of his work ethic. Former British prime minister the late Margaret Thatcher was the same, as was the US president Ronald Reagan, reportedly, and Winston Churchill. Maybe it's a thing in conservative politics.

Napping works: I don't sleep that much longer than Jones (claims). The difference between us is that I don't generally talk about it. I should sleep a bit more but I do nap. In fact, I'm infamous for it at work. I'm not sure about Jones, but anecdotally, Thatcher and Churchill napped too.

The point I'm trying to make is that sleep isn't a transaction that affects my sense of wellbeing too much, which makes me one of the lucky ones. People with mental health issues often have sleep disruption which then feeds back on itself making treating the sleep problem a high priority. For those who do struggle with their sleep, there's nothing more vexing than not being able to get the amount desired. I know I'll be able to plough through the next day, particularly with a 15-minute nap, and sometimes that knowledge alone can be the difference between feeling dogged by your lack of sleep versus just feeling a bit sleepy.

When I'm tired – and I should add that for long periods of 2020 during the pandemic, I was a wee bit tired. But I believed that it was going to be okay, and that I'd eventually catch up. And I did (well, again, a wee bit). I also just came to terms with the fact that during this particularly busy period in my professional life, I wouldn't be getting quite as much sleep as I'd have liked.

That's how I found a way to distance myself from anxiety that can creep up when you regularly fail to get what people think is a 'normal' night's sleep. I'm also very tired when I eventually fall into bed, which is important too (see How Much Sleep Should You Be Getting?).

Sleep is restorative: It's not a waste of time. In fact, it's the opposite. It takes our body on an important restorative journey, which is why you'll never hear me crowing about my fewer-than-eight-hours shut-eye existence. Sleep allows the brain to re-process and probably even clear out the build-up of certain chemicals, which is why some researchers believe there is a link with dementia (see Sleep and Dementia). The thing is that there may be a difference between the amount of sleep that you want (i.e. lots) versus the amount you need (less than lots). Another important factor is how much uninterrupted sleep you get.

Our lives are a patchwork quilt of experiences. As we grow and mature and take on different responsibilities, our ability to sleep at the volume we want changes too.

How much sleep should you be getting?

Human beings have, like most animals, their own timekeeping system to adapt to the 24-hour day, known as circadian rhythm. It's generated by a 'clock' in the brain which responds to light. This internal clock if left to itself in a dark environment would run at around 25 hours.

It's tuned to two distinct parts of the cycle – night and day. Light from our eyes is turned into electrical signals in nerves which pass near the pineal gland which produces the hormone melatonin when it's dark. Melatonin goes up at night before sleep and is a reason you want your bedroom to be really dark and shouldn't be using screens (see Screens), the light from which can confuse the pineal into thinking it's daytime. It's why you sometimes see the bedrooms of newborns decked out in blackout curtains and even foil in the windows to help facilitate daytime sleeps.

Our circadian rhythms intersect with our 'chronotype', which means the times of day we prefer to be active or like to rest. You might be a morning person, or a night-owl, or hover somewhere in the middle.

Our chronotype reveals a lot more than the time of day you like to go to bed. Research shows that our chronotype influences our diet. Those with an early chronotype prefer to wake early and feel most active during the earlier parts of the day.

Night-owls tend to peak in the late afternoon to early evening and have a habit of skipping breakfast. They also don't eat as much fruit and vegetables, while morning people tend to drink more alcohol.

A delay in mealtimes, particularly for dinner, might also cause circadian misalignment because if you eat late it can make it harder to go to sleep. Eating a big meal close to our natural 'rest phase' can throw out our internal rhythms and can be linked to obesity and other metabolic problems.

The genetic make-up passed to us from our parents influences our preference for operating best early or late in the day.

A study published in the journal *Sleep* in 2017 looked at three major genome-wide association studies (GWAS). GWAS studies look at complex genetic patterns involving multiple genes. These studies showed that our tendency to be a morning or evening person is influenced by our genes. The researchers concluded that genetic factors explain 50 per cent of differences in circadian timings. The rest of the difference might be explained by being raised in a household that ate dinner at 6 p.m., versus later, or an entrenched lifestyle learned in adolescence.

Age matters too

Broadly speaking, we need less sleep as we grow up.

Newborns and children need a lot of sleep. There's a whole industry of books with advice about getting little people to sleep, but sleep for adolescents is just as important as for toddlers. Canadian researchers found that teenagers have shown the greatest rate of decline in sleep over recent decades, especially on school days. In response to this, there's been a push to make sure school doesn't start before 8.30 a.m. for high-school students.

The reasons teenagers seem to be sleeping less has been blamed on increased use of electronic devices, decreasing rates of physical activity, and no bedtime rules in the household, but biology does play a role. Adolescents' circadian rhythms are set differently from adults'. Their highest melatonin levels occur an hour or two later than adults, which means melatonin is still higher in the morning which is why they have difficulty in getting up early. Some schools are adjusting to that.

It's hard to police your teen's sleep particularly when they're using electronic devices for their school work and they often have computers in their bedrooms. What makes it trickier is that hormonal changes can change your chronotype. So your toddler who used to jump out of bed at 5.30 a.m. (despite pleading and bribery to keep them asleep) as a teen, may not surface until mid-morning at the earliest if left to themselves to wake up. Their social 'clock' also tends to run counter to the circadian clock, which might be another reason they go to bed late and wake late.

Sleep patterns vary in elderly people, who in general sleep the least. Older people tend to have a harder time falling asleep and more trouble staying asleep. This period of life is often accompanied by a shift in their circadian clock back to an early setting, as opposed to adolescents who become night-owls.

The research cited by the Canadian study suggests that elderly people may still have the same need for sleep but find it harder to fulfil. This may be a result of sleep-related disorders and other factors like not working anymore, physical inactivity and fewer social interactions.

Sleep deprivation

Sleep and dementia

It may be just coincidence but Thatcher and Reagan did develop Alzheimer's disease. There is a fair bit of evidence that short sleep durations of less than six hours are associated with an increased risk of dementia and the build-up of tau and beta amyloid, the two substances that accumulate in the brains of people with Alzheimer's disease. What's not known is whether that is cause and effect. More and more research is showing that subtle signs of dementia can be detected earlier in life and it's well known that dementia can play havoc with sleep cycles.

So short sleep may just be a marker of dementia risk, which if true would mean that intervening to try to have longer sleeps may be both hard to achieve and not make a difference.

If only the body was less complicated.

Sleep problems

The inaugural issue of the *Journal of Clinical Sleep Medicine* traced early milestones in the development of sleep medicine which emerged from research in the 1970s and 80s. They focused on the electrical activity of the brain during sleep, which classified the stages of sleep. This was one of the early attempts to look at the links between sleep and general health and wellbeing. By 2005, scientists and clinicians had defined a large number of sleep disorders.

Since then the pace of research into sleep has taken off, looking at the effects of disrupted sleep on cell development and hormone regulation as well as diabetes, cardiovascular disease and dementia. What's not been proven is that sleeping 'poorly' is a cause of any of this. It may, in fact, be the reverse; in other words, the downstream effect of having dementia (see above) or being obese.

Mental health and sleep

Disrupted sleep patterns are a common physical manifestation of depression and anxiety. Anxiety can prevent you from falling asleep in the first place, but waking up in the middle of the night and ruminating on negative thoughts is a sign that you may need to seek help for an undiagnosed mental health issue, the treatment of which can help your sleep pattern.

Research from the American University of California

Berkeley found a link between gender and sleep, showing that women are more susceptible to the emotional consequences of sleep deprivation than men. In addition, the prevalence rates for insomnia and anxiety disorders are higher in women relative to men.

What these researchers can't work out is why this is happening. The biology of the nervous system is hard to tie down.

Insomnia and refreshing sleep

Over the decades that I've been in health journalism and broadcasting, insomnia has been one of the most popular audience topics.

Insomnia is defined by trouble falling asleep or trouble staying asleep that's been going on at least three nights a week for at least three months. It must interfere with your ability to function normally during the day, leaving you feeling irritable or unable to concentrate. Insomnia may be transient (less than a month), short term (less than six months) or longer term. It can be due to factors such as changed life circumstances, loss or other adverse events, a side effect of a variety of prescribed medications, general medical conditions, and mental health issues such as anxiety or depression.

Crucially, insomnia is defined by the person with it. It's about how much the lack of sleep is dogging you and leaving you unable to function. One important piece of information that many people don't appreciate is that we normally wake up many times each night. It's just that most people don't become aware of the wakefulness, but if a truck goes by during a waking cycle the noise could raise your consciousness and allow you to start thinking of all the world's problems you need to solve or why I was stupid enough to make that offhand remark at work yesterday.

Drugs are rarely the way to treat insomnia. Hypnotic medications act quickly, usually after the first dose which makes them seductive, but they don't give you a normal night's sleep. They also have side effects and some can cause dependence. Cognitive behavioural therapy for insomnia (CBT-I) and other behavioural measures work better and are longer lasting. Just like the CBT used for other problems like depression, CBT-I is about changing thoughts which are counterproductive to a good night's sleep.

Researchers in New York showed in a big study in 2016 that patients who rely on medication to solve their sleeping problems are in trouble when they stop taking their pills. Conversely, those who receive CBT have a carry-over effect once the treatment phase is over.

Dr Judith Davidson is a clinical psychologist and sleep researcher at Queen's University in Kingston, Ontario, Canada. She led a team of researchers which reviewed the evidence on the effectiveness of CBT-I and found that people reported a better night's sleep, even though they didn't actually sleep longer during the night.

Dr Davidson says that the CBT works by making the negative thoughts less catastrophic. The catastrophising about lack of sleep makes the problem worse. But this version of CBT also broadens out to stimulus control therapy, sleep hygiene and sleep restriction. It's all about sleeping better.

Stimulus control therapy is pairing the bed with sleep, so only go to bed when you're tired, don't use it as the venue to work, watch a movie, read on your iPad or chat on the phone.

Sleep restriction therapy is a strict method of setting a fixed wake-up time in the morning and finding a time to go to bed when you're tired enough that you sleep right through to that set time. An unbroken sleep feels more refreshing and is probably more important than the number of hours of sleep. We all have a biological sleep drive that builds up and grows before we go to bed and if we stick to the routine it stabilises our internal body clock. According to Dr Davidson, these two methods combined are the most effective and powerful components of getting people back to sleep. If you're trying sleep restriction yourself, you might need some guidance, as it requires discipline.

Sleep hygiene and stimulus control are important, particularly as electronic devices invade our lives but for people with intractable insomnia it may not be enough (which is why sleep restriction and CBT are often needed). As you probably know already, these techniques involve leaving your phone or tablet in the living room, or in a place you can't hear or see it, making your bedroom dark, not working in bed, and avoiding television when you can't sleep. You also need to reduce drugs close to bedtime, like coffee and alcohol (that glass of wine or three might be keeping you awake or might wake you up early).

Dr Davidson's research concluded that CBT resulted in better sleeping. Participants reported falling asleep faster and being awake for less time during the night.

They felt happier about their sleep but they didn't sleep longer. It doesn't move you from a five-hour a night to an eight-hour a night person.

As technology has advanced, so too has our desire and ability to measure our sleep, usually with wearable devices which provide information on duration and even supposedly on quality. However, research from the University of Ottawa, Canada, showed that such devices tend to underestimate sleep disruptions and overestimate duration and efficiency in healthy people. Overall, these researchers saw the devices as having shortcomings.

Sleeping long may have its problems

The role of long sleep is less clear. It can be associated with health problems like depression and chronic pain. However, excessively long sleep can also be a sign of poor sleep. So you might be asleep, but it's not great quality. Young people need more sleep than adults, but sleeping late may also be a sign of sleep deprivation during the night because of screen use or psychological issues.

Therapy: now probably counts more than then

#carefulwithfreud

Takeaway: Dredging up the past has limits if you're aiming for mental health. Dealing with what's in front of you now and how you're responding to the world and people around you is generally more effective, which is what therapies like cognitive and similar behavioural therapies and guided mindfulness do. This does not excuse or ignore trauma in your past, but the evidence is that working with where you're at 'now' is more effective and productive. That notwithstanding, trauma does affect your mental health and needs to guide therapy, even if it is dealing with the present.

*

Analytically orientated psychotherapy: For much of the 20th century, what a lot of talking therapies were about was spending hours with therapists who wanted to dig up memories and dynamics from the past to allow you to blame your mum for your anxiety, depression, drug use or distress. I'm obviously trivialising, because many people with downstream mental health issues have had serious trauma earlier in life. The question is not whether a therapist needs to know about that trauma; of course they do. What's up for debate is whether it helps for people who haven't had that trauma to dissect the past to discover what might be to blame for your depression or anxiety so you can 'work on it' and become a better person. For those with the money, therapy could go on for years. There was even a scientific literature on the psychodynamic role of the fee in psychiatry and you can still find a small number of analytically oriented (usually meaning Freudian or Jungian) therapists who'll take you on for extended periods. There's a little bit of evidence that extended therapy might help people with personality disorders but that's about it.

Cognitive behavioural therapy and related therapies, such as interpersonal psychotherapy, dialectical behaviour therapy, solution focused therapy and emotion focused therapy, have a better evidence base and some have the advantage that they can be done online. The key questions to ask if you're being referred to a clinical psychologist are whether they have been specifically trained in these therapies and how closely they follow the protocol (the rules). The more closely a psychologist follows the protocol, the more likely they are to achieve a benefit. Difficulties can arise if someone has complex problems which run together, including personality issues, drug dependence, severe mental health challenges like psychosis and bipolar disorder, and gender identity conflicts. In those circumstances, therapies like CBT are just a part of an overall recovery plan which may include non-health professionals like social workers, job training and rehabilitation. Your GP needs to refer you to a psychiatrist who works in a team and is hooked into the broad spectrum of services you might need.

Couple or family therapy: Many of the problems that a person has to deal with are related to problems in their wider family or social systems, especially their relationship with their partner or family issues that are unlikely to resolve just by focusing on the individual. And it's not just therapy. Often, just involving a family member or partner in a treatment plan, providing them with information or guidance as to how to help the person, or providing them with additional support can be an invaluable part of treatment.

Motivational interviewing can be used by psychologists and counsellors to promote behavioural change. It involves non-judgemental understanding of a person's motivations and then using them empathically to drive change.

Counselling can easily be confused with evidence-based psychological therapies. Counselling is hard to generalise but it tends to be more based on the person's past experience and the relationship with the counsellor who may use a variety of techniques to help the person. While there are short-term improvements from counselling compared to usual care from a GP, they don't appear to be sustained long term.

If you want to know which therapies have the best evidence, then sites such as the UK Mental Health Foundation (www.mentalhealth.org.uk), the Black Dog Institute (www. blackdoginstitute.org.au) and Beyond Blue (www.beyondblue. org.au) have pre-sifted that for you and I can't do any better here.

Self-management: This is a critical part of both mental and physical health issues. You can't have your doctor or therapist with you every minute of the day. Once you've learnt some of the skills and strategies, you may no longer need a therapist to guide you. This includes learning to deal with families' and friends' reactions to the problem or the stress that may be generated by the anxiety of living with a chronic condition.

Mindfulness – does it work?

Well, it depends.

It depends on what you want from mindfulness. There are several routes to mindfulness but in essence it uses various techniques to focus your attention and accept what comes into your mind without judgement. Curiosity, openness and acceptance are three words that are used in association with mindfulness. Focusing attention isn't exclusive to mindfulness. Some people get it on a long walk, at yoga, during more intense exercise, listening to music or using relaxation techniques, but guided mindfulness practice does offer a systematic way of achieving that goal.

*

One of the misconceptions about mindfulness is that it's about emptying your mind or stopping it wandering. It's much more about paying attention to the thoughts that emerge into your awareness in a relaxed state. Guided mindfulness should help to reduce rumination or anxiety in response to what's in your mind. One of the advantages of clinician-guided mindfulness is that it potentially allows the process to be more therapeutic and there's a fair amount of evidence that it helps.

There are many studies showing that mindfulness can reduce stress, although the benefits may wane with time. Increasingly, mindfulness techniques are being added to cognitive behavioural therapy even though there is an inherent contradiction, which is that a core principle of mindfulness is being non-judgemental. CBT, on the other hand, explicitly makes a judgement on negative or unproductive thoughts which are causing distress or are linked to depression and tries to reality-check them and refocus on more helpful thinking. Even so, there's a lot of overlap and clinical trials show benefit from the combined approach.

So it's important to decide whether you're doing mindfulness to improve your quality of life or to help a psychological issue. If it's the latter, you probably need expert guidance.

So what about yoga?

It's hard to generalise about yoga because there are a few different kinds of it, some more energetic and physically stressful than others. I've always thought I should do yoga because I'm the least flexible person (that's physical flexibility) you'll ever meet, but like lots of things I think I should do, I haven't (yet).

There's little doubt yoga strengthens your muscles, increases flexibility and for the time you're doing it allows your mind to totally focus on the activity; in other words, there's a mindfulness quality to the exercise.

Bottom line is if it makes you feel better and stronger then do it, as long as your instructor comes well recommended and won't push you too hard too early.

The scientific evidence for benefits is growing but not based on high-quality research. Even so, there are indications that if you are depressed or anxious, adding yoga to your other care can help. It may also assist sleep and symptoms associated with cancer treatment such as fatigue. In the elderly, yoga may help to prevent falls and of course can help with loneliness by offering a regular group activity and social contact.

And pilates?

Like yoga, people who practise pilates tend to love it and the way it makes them stronger. It's another thing I've aspired to do but, like yoga, not yet. There's evidence that in its own right pilates improves cardiorespiratory fitness, and it certainly requires focus, attention and group work.

The evidence that pilates is significantly better than other exercise therapy for low back pain is weak, but it does seem to help pain and disability like other interventions involving core muscle strengthening.

In women with stress incontinence, there is a little evidence that pilates is as good as pelvic floor exercises, and as you'd probably expect, pilates does help to prevent falls in the vulnerable elderly.

PART 5

Dominated by devices

Screens

It's a heading that you wouldn't have read in a health book a generation ago.

We used to talk about the risks of being a 'couch potato'. Now, it's the fear of being a screen 'addict'.

The science on the effects of screen use – especially excessive use, whatever that might be – isn't very advanced but that doesn't stop us worrying, especially about our kids when we have yet another battle to get them away from their iPad or laptop.

Is there such a thing as screen addiction?

Superficially there is but you've got to separate this from moral outrage at new technologies. Television used to be described as addictive – and in some senses it can be. There is some evidence in adolescents and older adults that people can become obsessed with internet and social media usage and actively resist it being taken away. There are associations between excessive screen use and depression, anxiety and other mental health issues but that doesn't mean cause and effect. It could be – just as with alcohol and other drugs – that internet and screen usage is a kind of self-medication for psychological distress. Trouble is – again just like drugs – the content you're exposed to and the lack of human to human contact could make distress worse.

How many times a day do you check your phone? Do you dare to count?

There's some research around mobile phone addiction, but it becomes a problem when mobile phone use moves to being something that you can't control, interferes with your life and work, and is linked to low mood and anxiety.

The more TV and technology you watch when sitting down, the greater the risk of obesity.

Research on the benefits and costs of screen use in adults is limited by the fact that the digital revolution is still underway – and at a staggering pace. The pace of technological change is outpacing researchers.

American psychologist Doreen Dodgen-Magee in her book, *Deviced! Balancing Life and Technology in a Digital World,* agrees that by the time research about the impact of technology has been published, the devices at the core of the studies have been eclipsed by newer ones.

Her central premise is that 'real life' has to be redrawn in order to encompass what happens in digital spaces, from school to work to social life.

Discussions around technology have become the place where broader conversations about life begin. So if someone is asking, 'How much time should I be spending on my screen?' it quickly segues to broader questions about what else is going on in your life and whether that's satisfactory (or not).

Are we wrecking ourselves by using screens?

There's no simple yes or no to this. You've got to make sure you're being honest with yourself about the time you interact with technology and how you react when it's taken away.

The problem for adults is that we don't have anyone whose job it is to keep us in check. It's harder to tell your friend, or more importantly your partner, to put the phone away than it is a little kid.

A 2017 study of US adults found that spending six hours or more a day watching TV or using computers was associated with a higher risk of depression but yet again that's not proof of cause and effect. Social media may exacerbate that. A 2018 study from University of Pennsylvania, USA, found that undergraduates who limited their social media use to ten minutes on Facebook, Instagram and Snapchat (half an hour all up) showed reductions in loneliness and depression over three weeks compared to the control group who were allowed to use their social media as usual.

In a Lebanese study conducted in 2017, researchers investigated whether anxiety and depression independently contributed to smartphone addiction. Their sample was 668 undergraduate students. They concluded that depression and anxiety were a predictor of smartphone addiction. This study also pointed to other work concluding that women are more likely to develop an addiction to smartphone use than men.

Some experts say 'How much?' is the wrong question to ask when assessing screen time. There's expert disagreement about whether heavy screen use is truly the cause of some people's depression, or if people with depression are just more likely to spend lots of time on screens. At the very least, much of the existing evidence indicates that spending many hours a day on a device (on top of work or study time) is a warning sign that a person is at elevated risk for depression or other mental health disorders.

What about the internet?

According to researchers in the USA, there is ongoing debate about how best to understand behaviour which is characterised by many hours spent in non-work environments on computer games and internet searching, for example. Just like excessive smartphone use, it's linked to low mood, pre-occupation with the internet and some withdrawal symptoms when you're not plugged in. And again, just like phones, some researchers and mental health practitioners see excessive internet use as a symptom of another disorder such as anxiety or depression rather than a separate entity.

A 2019 At Washington DC's Pew Research Center poll found 26 per cent of adults report going online 'almost constantly'. That was up from 21 per cent in 2015. A further 45 per cent say they go online several times a day.

The statistics show younger adults are constantly connected: roughly half of 18- to 29-year-olds (48 per cent) say they are online almost constantly, and 46 per cent go online multiple times per day. By comparison, just 7 per cent of those 65 and older go online almost constantly, and 35 per cent go online multiple times per day.

The share of younger adults who say they use the internet almost constantly has risen 9 percentage points since the last survey, in 2018.

Meanwhile, the share of constantly online Americans aged 50 to 64 has risen from 12 per cent in 2015 to 19 per cent in 2019.

You probably have a problem which is worth seeing someone about if you feel anxious or down when you're away from your device; it's a solution to your boredom; the need to check your phone has become more like a compulsion, rather than a true need to be updated with certain information; you feel preoccupied when you're away from the phone or internet; and you feel like you're lacking control and unable to control your moods.

Content and context

Just like kids and screens (see Content is Queen), content matters for adults too. Psychologist Doreen Dodgen-Magee says that it should be *content* AND *context*. If you have a free day and spend it on a YouTube tutorial teaching you a useful skill, or doing further study, that's a useful way to spend your time. If you're stuck in hotel quarantine during a global pandemic, spending a lot of time on your device is fair enough.

But if your need for the internet is so strong that you check it while driving, or during social events where you're meant to be engaging with real people, or you're unable to go to the toilet without logging on to your phone, there might be a problem. Dodgen-Magee cites scores of conversations with young adults who are looking for healthy strategies to deal with porn use. I've covered porn in another section, Is Porn Addiction a Thing?. But Dodgen-Magee is making a broader point about context here. On a free day, it would be healthier for people to interact in the 'real' non-digital world, rather than watching others do it on a screen.

Couch potatoes

The bigger risk of watching too much TV or looking at your phone screen is getting fat. We've spoken before about screens interfering with the normal sleep rhythms, which can see you plonked in front of a TV or a screen longer than you otherwise would, throwing out your sleep and healthy eating patterns. If you're eating and not moving because of screen time, it won't be long until you're buying bigger T-shirts.

Which screen?

The average household these days owns a lot of large, medium sized and small screens. Even though the television is the most widely used screen-based device among adults at home, its popularity is dropping and portable screen-based devices are increasing.

The (digital) 'haves' and 'have-nots'

There is not universal access to digital technologies, which is a problem when work and learning are increasingly dependent on laptops and access to the internet. It's one thing to have the privilege of trying to moderate your use, another altogether to have none at all.

The Pew Research poll I referred to earlier showed that more than one-third of the adults polled with an annual household income of US$75,000 or more use the internet almost constantly. However, this is true for just 23 per cent of those living in households earning less than US$30,000. Adults who live in urban and suburban areas are also more likely to say they go online almost constantly compared to those who live in rural areas.

A reality check

Two questions worth asking ourselves are:

1. What value are we losing when we're staring at a screen?

2. Can we – *should* we – push against the convenience
   afforded by the technology?

No question we come to this with preconceptions and biases:
for instance, that it's better to meet a romantic partner through
mutual friends rather than on an online dating app – or the
opposite, namely that Hinge is a great way to start dating.

It is, of course, partly generational. People who've grown up
with the digital world are more comfortable with this blended
digital and physical reality and can negotiate it pretty well.

The bottom line is that moderation is hard. Devices
make life easier – theoretically – and only *you* know to what
extent you're gaining or losing from letting the digital world
into your life.

PART 6

The sex thing

Sex-iety

Quickie: There are too many things to worry about in life and worry can make them worse. That's true, for example, of being told there's something wrong if you're not getting seven or eight hours of sleep a night (see Sleep-iety). So there's a generation of medically defined insomniacs, some of whom aren't getting enough sleep because they're worried about not getting enough sleep. Child rearing is another (and the worry doesn't end when they grow up, by the way) and the biggest kahuna of them all is sex. What follows from here is not some self-revelatory manual but some questions and issues I'm often asked about.

#noselfrevelation

*

Identity and sex: is this right? … Is that wrong?

The short version: We're in the middle of a generational change in how we recognise sexual identity. In years gone by, 'coming out' to your family, friends and workmates as lesbian, gay, bisexual or transgender (LGBT) was an enormous issue and still is for many, particularly transpeople. Now the question is really 'coming out as what and do you need to bother?' One driver of the change is a resistance to labels which people can see as prescriptive, boxing them into identities which they don't feel accurately define them. The LGBT abbreviation has evolved to encompass intersex and queer (LGBTIQ) among other labels, and people identify now more than ever in diverse ways, and also want their identities to be recognised and supported. But underneath this seemingly more inclusive attitude to gender and sexuality are disturbing data on significant distress among all groups of LGBTIQ identity (see LGBTIQ Wellbeing).

*

Sex plays different roles according to who you feel you are, where you belong and indeed what age you are. Sex is not important for everyone and there are people regardless of identity who feel little or no sexual desire. Sometimes that bothers them and sometimes it doesn't. Despite prejudice and stigma, there's more freedom than ever before to explore sexual and gender identity and live with fluidity, but that can either help or hinder inclusivity. Despite this, there are still contradictions and reinforced prejudices. Popular culture (TV, films ar d music) focuses heavily on straight (heterosexual) and cisgender (a term that describes people whose gender is the same as that presumed for them at birth i.e. people who aren't trans) sexual culture explicitly and implicitly, which excludes others. Yet the labels lesbian, gay, bisexual, transgender and queer assume that those identities are separate from the straight community. But that's not always the case; in fact, there are many straight trans and intersex people, and the term queer can sometimes capture this flexibility because it can reflect a wish to be non-binary i.e. not wanting to identify as a particular gender or wishing to maintain fluidity.

One of the advantages of closely identifying with your sexual identity, as one gay man I spoke to told me, is to find people who are like you. He explained that men and women who identify as gay can belong to communities which are supportive, focused on increasing wellbeing, allow for safe exploration and expression of sexuality and identity, and provide opportunities to find like-minded people.

Gay men and sex: If you're a man who has sex with men, you already know a lot of this but I'm trying not to make too many assumptions about what people know. Men who have sex with men (MSM) are often stereotyped as having large numbers of sexual partners compared to straight people or LBQ women. The culture produces a strong focus on body image, but also a high level of health literacy, which is part of having safer sex. There's also a high awareness of mental health and wellbeing and an environment that emphasises the RU OK? message. One of the issues for MSM but who don't identify as gay is that they may miss out on the community's health and STI (sexually transmitted infections) awareness focus and could risk putting themselves and their partners at risk. That's partly because information from peers is highly trusted and if you don't have gay peers, you may not get that, although some gay men have a tepid relationship with the gay scene because they think it's too focused on looking good and blindly seeking out casual sex. I'm not here to tell anyone what to do but belonging is an important part of wellbeing for all of us.

The nearly 40-year history of HIV in gay men has driven a strong sense of community, mutual care and self-determination – meaning there's been an insistence that research and policy are done with the gay community, not at it. This meant there are a lot of data on sexual behaviour and risk but less on general health, although this has started to change more recently.

LBQ women and sex (both cis and trans): For LBQ women, a significant issue is sexual health where health professionals often assume that there's only risk when a cis man is involved. Human papillomavirus (HPV) and herpes can live on hands and toys. The focus on cis men as the main source of risk has meant that LBQ women are under-screened for cervical cancer and STIs. In addition, survey data suggest that potentially a significant proportion of women who identify as LBQ still have sex with men. Equivalent data for Britain are hard to find. According to Associate Professor Julie Mooney-Somers of the University of Sydney, Australia, a leading researcher into the LGBTIQ community, the most significant predictors of whether an LBQ woman has had a cervical smear is whether they've had an STI screen or asked their doctor about pregnancy planning. This means that LBQ women who are better connected to sexual health services and GPs who understand the LGBTIQ community are more likely to have better health care and better health-seeking behaviours.

Sex is clearly important to LBQ women, yet according to the people I've spoken to for this book, is probably more wrapped up in early and strong emotional connections and perhaps a more intense desire for monogamy than gay men. The reasons for these differences aren't well researched.

The decades-long fight for women's rights and sexual identity led to a generation of women who proudly identified as lesbian. According to some researchers, younger women and indeed young gay men who didn't go through those struggles feel less need to identify as lesbian or gay and, anecdotally, socialise in more mixed straight and gay circles. Data collected in Sydney, Australia, over 22 years shows a decline in the identity 'lesbian'. They found that fewer than half of the women participating in the Sydney Mardis Gras identify as lesbian and are more likely to pick queer or bisexual when asked. Gay men also seem to be increasingly choosing to identify as queer.

LGBTIQ wellbeing: This increased fluidity in identity doesn't mean LGBTIQ people escape psychological distress. Far from it.

The Australian Research Centre in Sex, Health and Society based at La Trobe University has conducted three large national Private Lives surveys of the LGBTIQ community which have all shown high levels of psychological distress. The data within Private Lives also show that LGBTIQ people living further from major cities have higher levels of distress, lower self-rated health, and access services at a lower rate. The survey also showed that coming from a non Anglo-Celtic culture was associated with higher levels of distress and discrimination.

According to Dr Steve Philpot of the Kirby Institute at the University of New South Wales, Australia, a plethora of research has found that same-sex attracted people experience significantly poorer mental health than the heterosexual population. This is especially the case in young LGBTIQ people, 83.3 per cent of whom have experienced high or very high levels of psychological distress and nearly 60 per cent having seriously considered attempting suicide in the previous 12 months. That's five times higher than young people in the general population.

The reasons include discrimination, homophobia, marginalisation, violence and bullying, particularly in unsupportive school environments. According to one queer man of trans experience I spoke to, who works in the field, transphobia and barriers to gender-affirming healthcare are also determinants of poor health for transpeople.

Many young people who identify as LGBTIQ do not see themselves as included or supported in sex education at school because it's dominated by heterosexual experiences. In one study, says Steve Philpot, only 46 per cent of young LGBTIQ people reported good experiences discussing sexuality with health professionals and 41 per cent chose not to discuss it at all.

Julie Mooney-Somers and her colleagues in Sydney, Australia, have survey data going back many years on LBQ women. It's some of the best trend information in the world.

The trends are worrying. Mental health and wellbeing are declining. In Australia they found that nearly one in two LBQ women surveyed report high or very high levels of psychological distress, and the figure is the same in the UK.

That compares to one in five among women in general in the UK. In the previous year, the Australian project found that 12 per cent of LBQ women had deliberately harmed themselves, and around one in three had felt that their life wasn't worth living. In terms of young LGBTIQ people more broadly, they are between five to 11 times more likely than the general population to have attempted suicide. Transpeople are more than six times as likely to have self-harmed and data from Australia's Private Lives 3 report, released in November 2020, found that one in ten trans respondents reported having attempted suicide in the past 12 months. Further, LGBTIQ people are between six and 13 times more likely to have or have had an anxiety disorder.

US research has shown that LBQ women start drinking earlier than other women and it doesn't decline in adult years (although there is a major issue in the general older community of excessive alcohol use). In Sydney, LBQ women also have high rates of problem drinking – with nearly one in two drinking at harmful levels. There are also higher and rising rates of ecstasy and other drug use such as cannabis, ketamine, LSD and cocaine. Such use is similar in gay men including meth, which is more problematic. However, information on actual dependence is harder to come by. LBQ women have also had high rates of smoking and although those have come down quite dramatically, they're still higher than average. The reasons for the fall are not entirely clear but are probably linked to marriage equality, having kids and a targeted, co-designed anti-smoking campaign.

With general health, LBQ women are not coming forward or participating in cervical, breast and bowel cancer screening to the extent that they should.

If you've got this far in the book, you'll know that health and wellbeing come in part from a sense of control over your destiny. Focus groups conducted by Dr Julie Mooney-Somers with young LBQ women have found they could not imagine a 'future self' nor role models which helped. This lack of role models, or lack of 'blueprints' for learning how to live a happy life as an LGBTIQ person as Dr Steve Philpot put it to me, cuts across all LGBTIQ identities and this is exacerbated by stereotypes in the media. Depictions of LGBTIQ people in popular culture remain relatively sparse (although this is improving), and the depictions that do exist often do not portray identities that resonate with LGBTIQ people in the real world. That, along with stigma and a sense of alienation, may underlie raised rates of self-harm and suicide attempts. Sadly, there are no differences in domestic violence rates among LBQ couples compared to the general community, says Julie Mooney-Somers.

The Private Lives survey has also found that mental health issues are more severe for transpeople of all genders (male, female and non-binary) and are linked to discrimination, a lack of trans community connection, rejection from family, faith, work and school, struggles for recognition, and access to timely, non-judgemental appropriate care.

So while the superficial view might be a more relaxed and less labelled world of sexuality and gender identity, serious issues still exist.

No-one should ever have to experience stigma, prejudice or abuse because of their sexual or gender identity.

Make pleasure a principle

Quick take: Negotiation around mutual pleasure can make sex better and safer.

*

So much that's written about sex is negative, pathologising, puritanical or pornographic. The fact is that most people have sex for pleasure and/or intimacy and there's been a line of research for some years that suggests if you focus on that pleasure and intimacy – giving and taking – and how to negotiate it, then sex becomes better, there may be less non-consensual sexual violence and it also becomes safer. This applies to heterosexual and LGBTIQ people.

It's hard to have pleasure when you're anxious about your sexual health, being hurt or embarrassed, or even worrying about telling someone they're actually being too gentle. More generally, though, there can still be a fear that articulating your concerns, desires or preferences will drain the passion and pleasure, or that saying what you want might mean having to make yourself vulnerable to another person, no matter how well you know them. But there's evidence that the negotiation can actually make things a lot better. In fact, if someone refuses to negotiate or have an STI screen – including HIV in heterosexual couples – it's a sign you probably need to move on, even from something quite casual.

For gay men, it might be a bit easier since hookup apps like Grindr allow people to state their likes and dislikes. Even so, the anonymous sex that can happen in gay male culture makes negotiating sexual health tough at times, but that's where you should have regular STI screens and need to know about pre-exposure prophylaxis (PrEP), where HIV negative people take approved antiretroviral medications to prevent HIV infections.

There are various ways to reduce HIV transmission risk and they work together. People who are HIV positive usually get treated to drive their viral loads down to undetectable levels, which means that they're healthy as well as non-infectious to sexual partners. Condom use has the advantage that it protects against other STIs, for which PrEP has no effect. PrEP, as I said, is pre-exposure prophylaxis against HIV. It's designed for people who are HIV negative and is mostly used by gay men. It isn't a standalone treatment and needs to be part of a process which includes regular STI screens, including for HIV, about once every three months, or more if you've been in a high-risk situation. And it can't be stressed often enough that taking PrEP does not prevent other STIs.

Staying safe and fertile

I know you know this but when you have sex with someone, germ-wise you're having sex with everyone they've had sex with since their most recent sexual health screen. To best avoid most STIs, casual sex can be protected with a condom but that's not necessarily a popular message. If sex is going to become more regular with a partner then it's probably okay to ask them to have an STI screen including HIV. In men who have sex with men, in addition to PrEP, other prophylactic medications might in future be proven effective, such as regular doxycycline to reduce the risk of gonorrhoea, syphilis and chlamydia.

Yes, it's a bit like insisting on a pre-nup because it takes away the romance, but nothing evaporates romance like HIV, gonorrhoea, syphilis or chlamydia. Think of it more as protecting each other than thinking about how much of a risk you are to each other. STI screens are common among gay men and straight men who are having casual sex should also have regular STI screens and must ask their GP to include HIV testing. HIV is not a gay disease. It's a sexually transmissible infection. Older women starting back on the dating scene after a marital break-up do need to be particularly careful and are a high risk group, especially if you think the only role of a condom is to prevent pregnancy and you're past that. LBQ women, as I said before, need to be aware that STIs can occur without a man involved and that while the stereotype of LBQ relationships is serial monogamy, casual sex is commoner than the image might convey.

In the past ten years or so in Australian men, gonorrhoea rates have quadrupled, syphilis rates have tripled and chlamydia has almost doubled. The picture is similar in the UK. Since 2018 there has been an overall rise in STIs of 5 per cent, but that includes a 26 per cent rise in gonorrhoea infection and a 10 per cent rise in syphilis diagnoses. So it's best to be careful and don't be offended if a new partner – male or female – asks you to have an STI check before embarking on condomless sex. Easier said than done when you're at the height of passion or are uncertain at the start of a new relationship but see Make Pleasure A Principle. Gay men who are generally much more active and have multiple partners are becoming increasingly used to pre-exposure prophylaxis (PrEP) for HIV protection (see above). Test, trace and treat is often well understood in gay communities, which has probably generated better adaptation to COVID-19 public health measures.

Chlamydia is a common cause of infertility in men, women and non-binary people. Regular testing when you're sexually active is really important and sensible because the infection is often silent or symptoms take a while to appear. Chlamydia increases the risk of ectopic pregnancy, pre-term birth, having a low birth weight baby and newborn pneumonia. Seventy-five per cent of women have no symptoms but when they do it's things like pain on passing urine, vaginal discharge, pain in the pelvis, bleeding between periods and bleeding after sex. People who have anal sex can have anal and rectal symptoms, too, such as discharge and pain in the back passage. Fifty per cent of cis men don't have symptoms but those who do often have pain on passing urine, a discharge from the penis and, when it infects the testicle, pain and tenderness usually just on one side. Chlamydia can also cause conjunctivitis. The shame is that chlamydia is preventable and easy to test for, which should be done regularly if you're sexually active. How regularly? Well, it's a must if you have symptoms or fall pregnant. If you're sexually active and haven't settled down with one partner or your partner hasn't settled down, then annually. If you've had receptive anal intercourse, then a rectal swab should be included. And no, you don't get to be squeamish about that. Men who have sex with men with a high frequency change of partners probably need three-monthly checks along with their full STI screen including for HIV. It's probably a good idea any time you go for a sexual health screen, regardless of whether you're gay, straight, lesbian, queer or something else, to ask for a full screen, including HIV, and for them to take samples from your throat, urine, and bottom if you've had receptive anal sex.

It's worth remembering that HPV immunisation prevents

sexually acquired diseases such as cancers of the cervix, mouth and throat, anus and probably oesophagus.

Is it love? Is intimacy love? And the limerence thing

Writing about 'is it love?' is way above my pay scale.

Intimacy is maybe easier. As a researcher into sexual behaviour told me, intimacy in the context of sex can be described as a 'shared and special connection between people, but one that you can't quite put your finger on'. Of course, that begs the question of how you know it's shared. What you're thinking and feeling might be a world away from what's in your partner's head.

Limerence has various definitions but in essence it's the highly emotional state of feeling in love, where it's hard to think about anything else than this person, your craving for them and what the future may hold for the two of you. It's often felt in newer relationships and is sometimes called the honeymoon period. Limerence may form the beginning of a successful long-term relationship but at other times it's unrequited and can take time to get over. If you've ever been so infatuated by someone you can't think of anything else, that could be limerence, but the key is not to let it affect your work, daily activities and friendships. You don't have a psychological disorder, much as some would like to define it. There's almost no good peer-reviewed research into limerence.

Intimacy, shared interests and an evolution into companionship if it wasn't there before are probably better predictors of relationship success (if that's what you're looking for) than obsessive, disruptive love. Simply having strong feelings for someone doesn't mean you'll be happy together, and, equally, just having someone you like hanging out with may not be enough either.

Consent: What is completely non-negotiable but is often not negotiated in a relationship is consent, which involves being fully transparent about, and asking and agreeing to boundaries. The blur of alcohol and other drugs is often used as a smoke screen to excuse lack of consent. Being drunk or intoxicated by drugs is not an excuse. Pornography is not renowned for its portrayal of consent and if that's where men have received their sex education, they might be more likely to presume it – wrongly.

Watch out for red flags – and don't abandon your friends for love

The risk is that we think we're in love too soon and are so taken with the magic and passion of a new relationship that we see but choose to ignore some danger signals, thinking 'How could this love be bad?'

We can become too attached too quickly, want to move in quickly and start doing 'coupley' things with them very early on. If that means slipping the social anchors that you've spent years building, then beware.

Red flags include someone 'wanting you for themselves', not liking it when you continue to see your old friends and maybe even family, pushing you to change your appearance or what you wear, and being suffocating. These are all things which in the beginning can feel like someone is head over heels about you and thinks about you all the time, when in fact what they need and want is control. If you see this happening to someone you know and care about, it's worth saying something even if it might not be well received initially. Best to say it than regret not saying it later when the person's life is a shambles.

So, as the clinical psychologist Dr Catherine Boland put it to me, 'My advice to people is don't move in during the first week and don't have kids in the first six months and don't give up on your friends and networks.'

Are we on the same page? Negotiating the path from 'dating' to monogamy

This negotiation of monogamy or otherwise doesn't happen often in cis heterosexual couples and it probably should. Even if in most heterosexual relationships, anecdotally monogamy is the assumption, people may have different ideas about how that looks. For example, is perving okay? Does being exclusive mean we are in a monogamous relationship, or is it not technically a relationship yet? What are the consequences if I kiss someone else? And importantly, if you want to be monogamous, then you have an opportunity to do your sexual health testing to make sure you're both in the clear.

Perhaps stereotypically, monogamy tends to be an early assumption with LBQ women even in relatively short-lived relationships but with gay men it might be less expected as a long-term option. Since sex is so celebrated within gay communities, having multiple partners within a stable loving relationship is not unusual, particularly for older men or men in long-term relationships. That can take a lot of trust and talking through, especially when preventing HIV and STIs is a concern. Heterosexual couples generally don't tolerate open breaches of monogamy well.

There isn't an easy script to negotiate around the feeling that one partner wants commitment to exclusivity while not being sure the other is ready for it.

Such conversations are built on transparent, respectful communication in a relationship where you feel able to seek and receive feedback. That doesn't evolve overnight but if you start that way, it makes more scary conversations easier to contemplate and raise. The problem is, how are you supposed to know when it's okay to bring up this conversation? What if it's too soon? It can be difficult to know, but generally the more time you spend with each other and enjoy each other's company, the more confident you can be that the conversation is relevant. And it's better to have the conversation about exclusivity and monogamy, or not, rather than simply 'fall into' a relationship without much discussion about it.

Sex without condoms in both gay male and heterosexual relationships is often where such conversations can begin. Just because you trust each other doesn't mean there isn't risk so talking about getting STI tested at the same time is an opportunity to talk through where you're at relationship-wise. Testing is a means of protecting each other and shows care and concern and perhaps willingness to move beyond dating to something more exclusive.

Insta sex: beware the algorithm

Insta take: This is particularly an issue for gay men but can affect anyone. Instagram is a medium where the image is everything and suddenly anyone can become a model. Instagram is particularly problematic when it reinforces a body image which drives potentially unhealthy behaviour, such as too many hours in the gym for gay men and eating disorders in both men and women. In fact, eating disorders and extended gym use are often part of the same issue. The bottom line is everyone wants to feel like they look attractive and there's nothing wrong with wanting that, unless it directly negatively influences your wellbeing.

*

Your internet and Instagram behaviour tells its algorithm what you like and feeds that back to you. It is truly an echo chamber. So gay men get an idea of the perfect body which is impossibly muscular and ripped with a six-pack. Straight men can get the same feedback and all too soon the lean and muscular becomes seen as the ideal to which all should aspire. Women have had this experience for decades and are all too used to images of female bodies which bear little resemblance to what they are in reality. Just think about traditional depictions of Barbie. People have reproduced life-size models of what Barbie's proportions would be if she were real, and it's really quite distorted. Research is showing that Instagram exaggerates this and encourages young women to compare themselves with others and makes them strive for a beauty ideal that may lower their mood and raise levels of personal dissatisfaction. Gyms are full of people who are body sculpting and in the case of men, under pressure to take testosterone and other anabolic steroids (see Supplements for Big Muscles). There's no question that we can be too judgemental about Instagram when for a lot of people it's just a bit of fun and flirting, but knowing when to stop and where the boundaries are can be challenging.

Food is a popular destination for Instagram users and there are large communities focused on healthy eating, which is great, but some research suggests that there's a group of people for whom healthy eating becomes an obsession and overlaps with anorexia nervosa. This research suggests that Instagram is particularly potent at reinforcing that. Always remember that the people who are health nuts on Instagram, who post their workouts and eating habits online and preach to others to become healthy, those things are not necessarily attainable for most people working 9–5 with other things in life to focus on too. These people using Insta make it seem like it's such an easy thing to do. Remember their full-time job is eating healthily and looking good.

Instagram didn't start all this but it's definitely an amplifier. This isn't a reason for moral outrage from people who don't use Instagram but a reality check now and again wouldn't go amiss.

The algorithm driving your feed will exploit you if you don't watch out.

Is porn addiction a thing?

Let's start with some of the issues that watching pornography can raise. Only a tiny minority of pornographic films portray condom use. Young women feel pressured to have anal sex and some ascribe that to the expectations young men learn from pornographic heterosexual sex where up to 30 per cent of videos include anal sex. Consent is poorly portrayed in pornographic films and frequent use of porn, at least in young people, according to Australian research, is associated with mental health issues, although it's not clear whether that's cause and effect or just an association. Most young men and women report having watched pornography. The first view for boys is around 13 years old. For girls it's at age 16, and there's some evidence that pornography substitutes for formal sex education. Porn can affect how some people envision their sex lives. What happens in porn is not realistic, but young men in particular come into their sex lives having seen porn and assuming that this is how sex works. That's made worse by poor sex education at school. Most porn is tailored to men, and little attention is paid to what women want or if it is, it's often distorted. Even something as simple as the camera angle means that porn is created in a particular way. The actors are likely engaging in positions that would not feel natural in a regular encounter because they have to make sure their bodies look right for the camera.

But that's not addiction. Let's assume we're talking about a compulsive need to watch pornography to the extent that you find it hard to stop and it's affecting your life. Well, it's difficult to find reliable research on this. The Second Australian Study of Health and Relationships (published in 2014) interviewed nearly 20,000 men and women aged between 16 and 69 and found that 63 per cent of men and 20 per cent of women surveyed said they've looked at porn in the past year. Those rates appear to be rising but previous data may have been unreliable or difficult to compare because the questions changed between studies. However, when asked whether they felt addicted to pornography, only 4 per cent of men and 1 per cent of women said they were and even fewer of those felt it had bad effects on them, although worryingly in the sample as a whole i.e. including those who said they weren't addicted, more than one in ten said it had bad effects. It's not clear what these bad effects were but one assumption by the researchers was that guilt would have been an issue, as would their obsession with pornography interfering with their day-to-day activities. More frequent experience of heterosexual anal sex was also associated with pornographic addiction but that could just be a reflection of sexual experimentation in this group. However, even given that this was only self-reporting rather than an objective measurement, it doesn't sound like an epidemic.

Gay men and LBQ women were more likely to view pornography as were people with higher levels of education and income. Being religious, older and living with a regular partner were linked to lower usage. The factors which seemed to predict self-reported addiction included people with higher levels of psychological distress, living in a remote area and being a young male. Among the many issues around portrayal in pornography – consent, unrealistic expectations, male focus – are also distortions around how transwomen are shown.

Moral outrage is easy to generate and there is some evidence that whether you think you're addicted to pornography depends on whether you feel guilty about it. Arguments go backwards and forwards about whether viewing pornography is a cause of sexual violence or actually helps to reduce it by relieving sexual tension, but there are clearly lines in the sand demarcating total unacceptability, as well as potential illegality, when it comes to videos and other material involving child pornography, exploitation, lack of consent, and violence. It's not a great situation, especially with consumption being so high, and perhaps there needs to be some validated, independent ratings around reliably safe and high-quality pornography.

Is sex addiction a thing?

No, if what you're asking is whether what's usually referred to as hypersexuality is currently defined as a mental disorder in its own right. How much sex you have is like most behaviours. It's on a scale from none at all to a lot and where you draw the line on what's abnormally high depends on whether it's damaging your life or the people around you. The most recent version of the American Psychiatric Association's *Diagnostic and Statistical Manual of Mental Disorders (DSM-5)* chose not to define hypersexuality as a psychological disorder. There is a contradiction here because *DSM-5* does define low levels of sexual desire as a disorder which in turn can be linked to hormonal changes, relationship problems and psychological issues such as chronic stress, depression and anxiety. The trouble is that the research base on hypersexuality is pretty thin. Most of the work has come from practitioners who've studied or reported on patients or clients in clinics who've come forward for care, but that tells you very little about what's really going on in the community at large.

That's not to deny that there are people who have troubling

levels of intrusive thinking about sex and sexual activity which affects their lives, their health through unsafe sex and the people they have relationships with. Focusing just on the sex, though, is probably unhelpful since hypersexual behaviour is strongly associated with other mental health issues which could be causing the problem, such as post traumatic brain injury, pre-existing psychological distress, ADHD, obsessive-compulsive disorder, personality variations, bipolar disorders, substance abuse (particularly amphetamines) and even some medications (including for Parkinson's disease). Treatment obviously depends on what else is going on, after a full and expert assessment.

The bottom line is that you should seek help if this is a problem or encourage someone you think is in harm's way to seek help.

For men – cis and trans

Quick one: You can get holier than thou over unreasonable expectations about body image (see Insta Sex). The thing is that it's happening to both gay and straight men and body dissatisfaction can drive them as far as contemplating steroid use and embarking on abnormal eating patterns to achieve an image of a perfect body. If you're thinking about cosmetic surgery, don't take cheap options. See a properly trained and qualified plastic surgeon, not a cosmetic doctor who's basically a GP with some added training. And remember that a six-pack is not a guarantee that you'll transform into a great lover (discount that remark as jealousy if you wish).

*

Porn: (see the previous section for the stats) I won't ask whether you watch porn, only how often? Here's the problem. If you watch porn that's made by straight men for straight men and you think that's sex, then you're likely condemned to be a crap lover. If you have sex with women, I suspect you'll get a better idea if you watch erotica made by women for women. Trite to say it and you've heard it before but our biggest sexual organ is truly the brain. Hard to have good sex beyond a one-night stand if you don't like someone, connect with them and are in tune with their needs. The vast majority of women do not orgasm with penetrative sex alone and no amount of faking in a porn movie will change that.

Gay men's erotica is more integral to gay sex focused culture. There is evidence that it has a positive effect, teaching men about gay sex, but like other pornography there is a risk of unrealistic expectations and an acceptance of risk taking.

The problem with both can be normalising violence and lack of consent and just plain bad sex.

Your sex organ: For men who have sex with cis women, next to the brain the most important organ is not your penis, it's the clitoris.

The clitoris and men's hunt for the G spot

Professor Helen O'Connell is a urologist in Melbourne, Australia, and a world authority on the clitoris and the anatomy of the lower vagina. Helen and her colleagues have shown that the clitoris is actually quite a large organ which is mostly under the surface and goes quite deep. There are many nerves in the area to detect sensation, and the clitoris, the urethra, which carries urine, and the lower end of the vagina are meshed into a single unit. That's probably why the front lining of the vagina near the entrance can be very sensitive but, according to Professor O'Connell's research, men can stop their desperate hunt for the G spot. There's no anatomical evidence for a spot, but it's certainly true that the anterior wall of the vagina is, in most women, where they experience the most vaginal sensation.

The clitoris is usually the source of women's orgasms. It's up to you to find out a woman's preferences in terms of stimulation. By the way, men tend to overestimate whether a cis woman has had an orgasm (stop asking). Intercourse which leads to orgasm in a woman is usually accompanied by clitoral stimulation of some kind and it's not an insult to your manhood if your partner does this for herself.

Are condoms a spoiler?

I assume that no-one would use condoms if they didn't have to, but the reality is, they're your best defence against STIs, including HIV, and are also a reliable form of contraception. Are they a spoiler for sex? Not necessarily. Research suggests that the key variables that affect your perception of pleasure when using a condom are: the quality of your relationship, the quality of your sexual relationship and the quality of foreplay. All of these can encourage the use of condoms; whereas negative attitudes to condoms, and whether you have erectile problems when you're wearing one, can detract from condom use.

What about recreational Viagra or Cialis?

If you worry about performance, then your performance will suffer. The problem with recreational use of erectile dysfunction (ED) medications can be twofold. One is that they can interact with other drugs and reduce your blood pressure to seriously low levels. The other is that you can become anxious about achieving an erection without taking an ED drug in advance. In other words, you can become psychologically dependent on them. A young, healthy man having sex with someone they're attracted to and who isn't taking other recreational drugs which can cause erectile problems (e.g. alcohol and maybe amphetamines) should not have problems with erectile dysfunction. And ... don't believe what you see in sexually explicit media about sexual performance. Erectile dysfunction drug use is reasonably common in men who have sex with men when embarking on intensive sex partying.

Does sex affect athletic performance?

Probably not.

For women – cis and trans

I'm clearly not qualified to write this section. I will, however, answer a few questions that I get asked, by younger women in particular – usually anonymously.

What's the evidence on stress, depression and their effects on sex for women (and probably men too)?

It varies according to age. In adolescence and early adulthood, there is evidence that stress and depression are actually linked to increased rates of sexual intercourse but, unfortunately, are also associated with reduced use of condoms and contraception. So by implication, some of this sex is unsafe and there is evidence that poor psychological health is linked to cis women having unwanted pregnancies. As women get older, stress and depression do to you what you'd expect – namely reduce sexual activity and satisfaction. Physical health also matters. The fitter you are, the more sex you are likely to have and the happier you are likely to feel about it. Trouble is that there are a lot of other factors that go along with this. In order to become fit, you generally need discretionary time and income and a positive mood, so untangling being better off and more in control of your life from the physical fitness itself is hard to do. Cis male and trans female partners who are physically fit and don't smoke are also more likely to be potent. That helps too.

Is it true that antidepressants can affect your sex life?

Yes, but it's not consistent which ones affect you more or less and then you have to take account of the sexual effects of your depression. You need to talk to your GP about choosing the medication with the least sexual side effects and be prepared to ask for a change if you don't like the one you're on. A big caveat though is how severe your depression is because changing medication has its own risks. Don't freelance with coming off an antidepressant 'cold'. There can be complications as your brain and body adjust. So do it in partnership with your doctor.

Do Viagra-like medications affect women's sexual desire and enjoyment? And if not, what does?

Quick take: There's not much evidence for Viagra or Cialis for women. Testosterone supplements may help postmenopausal cis women with female sexual interest/arousal disorder (FSIAD), if indeed you believe this is actually a disorder or rather part of a normal spectrum of sexual desire. They may also help younger women with antidepressant-induced sexual dysfunction. Some researchers are touting a combination of testosterone and either sildenafil (Viagra) or an anti-anxiety medication called buspirone but the evidence isn't great. Physical fitness, good general health, and expert psychological and relationship assistance may well get you further than meds. Psychotherapy in the form of sex-focused cognitive behavioural therapy, which teaches good sexual techniques and tries to reduce anxiety, can help. Mindfulness techniques and couples therapy may well work, too, but they haven't had many high-quality studies either. One thing which stands out is that gay and straight couples who are attentive to the other's needs and care about meeting their needs mutually do have higher levels of sexual desire and satisfaction.

Before I start on this, researchers have historically been much more interested in fixing up cis men's sexual problems than women's, partly through bias and partly because there's a very obvious and easy way to measure outcome in men: the erection. Few drug researchers have spent a lot of time on men's libido/desire for sex, which is ironic since drugs like Viagra and Cialis don't work very well unless there is sexual desire. But with cis women, where there are few outward manifestations, desire is mostly what researchers have to go on. Many doctors and all drug companies love labels and the current medical label for this problem is female sexual interest/arousal disorder (FSIAD). FSIAD requires that a woman is actually distressed by her low sexual desire and/or arousal. If it doesn't bother you, there's nothing wrong with that and you can be reassured you don't have a disorder. Call me a cynic, but creating a name for a problem is a prerequisite for the pharmaceutical industry to find a treatment. Anyway, before I get to Viagra-like drugs, let's start with a medication that was approved in the United States for hypoactive sexual desire disorder or HSDD (FSIAD's predecessor) – amid huge controversy: flibanserin. Flibanserin improved sexual desire a little and increased the number of sexual events a little, but at the expense of side effects such as sleepiness and interactions with drugs like alcohol, blood pressure lowering medications and antibiotics, causing in some women a fall in blood pressure which could lead to collapse.

There's a lot of interest and indeed prescribing of testosterone for FSIAD. An Australian study in nearly 7000 premenopausal women found that while higher levels of testosterone and related hormones were linked to sexual desire, orgasms and sexual self-image, the hormones only contributed about 1 per cent of the overall levels of these measures. What mattered more were the number of babies you'd had, whether you were with a partner and if you were on a medication like an antidepressant. And no hormone level predicted a woman's ability to be aroused or sexually responsive.

Having said that, the same research group has reviewed the published evidence for the safety and effectiveness of testosterone supplementation in postmenopausal women. They found 36 randomised trials involving more than

8000 women and when the results were brought together, testosterone supplements did significantly improve sexual functioning across a number of variables including orgasm, arousal and responsiveness, while lowering levels of concerns and distress. There were bad effects on blood fats when testosterone was taken by mouth but not when used as a patch. Testosterone did increase hair growth and the likelihood of developing acne.

In premenopausal women with loss of libido due to antidepressants, there is some evidence that testosterone patches can increase the number of sexually satisfying events a little. In premenopausal women with low testosterone levels, supplements can increase the number of sexually satisfying events by just under one a month. So it's not dramatic and a review of all the trials in the area showed little effect. There is also pretty good evidence to counter the idea that testosterone affects libido in premenopausal women. For example, those with polycystic ovarian syndrome (PCOS), who have trouble with fertility and weight among many other problems, can have relatively high levels of male hormones, causing problems with male pattern hair growth and hair loss, for example. When women with PCOS are given medications such as the oral contraceptive, which lower testosterone levels, they actually can have increases in libido. There's also a condition called androgen insensitivity syndrome (AIS) where those with AIS don't respond to testosterone and become feminised. Reduced libido or orgasms are in fact not prominent features of AIS. Having said that, testosterone does have complex effects on the brain.

Which brings us to sildenafil (Viagra). The evidence is thin that it helps women with FSIAD. There have been MRI studies of sildenafil and clitoral engorgement (trying to replicate what happens in penises) showing no significant effect, nor indeed that lack of clitoral engorgement is part of FSIAD.

There have been some poor quality trials of testosterone combined with either sildenafil or the anti-anxiety drug buspirone showing an increase in the number of satisfactory sexual events. Theoretically, testosterone may not work by itself because it only deals with the sex hormone side whereas serotonin in the brain may also play a role, which is where medications like buspirone may have a rationale.

May.

It could in future be possible to personalise the treatment of FSIAD. A study in 2018 suggested that genetic patterns (genotypes) in women with FSIAD could predict which drug combination would help them most: testosterone with sildenafil (Viagra) or testosterone with buspirone, compared to placebo. The gene score is called the phenotype prediction score and looks for genetic variation known to be linked to sexual behaviour.

Pregnancy and sex?

The answer is yes and it's safe unless you've been advised against it by your doctor. Best to avoid positions that put pressure on the baby.

Contraception

This is far better discussed at your family planning clinic because the choice is so individualised. The combined oral contraceptive pill is much safer than many people realise with reduced risks of cancer especially uterine, ovarian and bowel cancer. There is a small increased risk of liver cancer, but that is already very rare, and of cervical cancer, which should disappear as more women are immunised against HPV. Whether the Pill increases breast cancer risk is still controversial but if it does it's a small effect and disappears after stopping.

What's probably underutilised are the various forms of set and forget contraception usually associated with medicated intra-uterine devices or implants (also called long-acting reversible contraceptives).

I'm thinking of having cosmetic genital surgery but it's hard to get independent information

It's very easy for people to become judgemental about cosmetic surgery and even more sanctimonious when it comes to vulval surgery. Most of the information on the internet comes from clinics and doctors who do the procedure. First, the basics about choosing the surgeon:

1. Have they been trained in this procedure? If so, where and by whom? You wouldn't want anyone other than a gynaecologist or plastic surgeon to do this but they do need to show you where and when they were trained in this procedure. It's not necessarily part of their regular specialist training.
2. How many have they done and how many do they perform each year?
3. Where do they operate? If you've never heard of the hospital, or it's not part of one of the major chains which have a reputation for safety and quality, or it's in their own hospital or back office, abandon ship

and see someone else. A surgeon's results are closely linked to the quality of their team and the hospital they work in.

4. What's their infection rate?
5. What's their rate of post-operative problems with the clitoral hood? Sometimes surgery on the labia minora can make the clitoral hood appear more prominent than it used to.
6. How does the doctor define 'normal' vulvar anatomy? This goes to what should be done at operation. Labiaplasty focused on the labia minora is probably safer, less disruptive and associated with the highest satisfaction, but you need to ask about the implications for the surrounding anatomy. You don't want to be coming back for revision surgery or new procedures. If that happens, you're unlikely ever to achieve your concept of perfection.
7. What satisfaction measures do they collect from their patients and for how long after the procedure and can you see their data? No operation has amazing satisfaction levels, so if the number you're given feels too high, it probably is. The fact that in some countries there's a market for repairing botched genital surgery tells you a lot about being careful up front and limiting your expectations.
8. Can you speak to some of their patients who've had the procedure you're intending to have?
9. If the doctor is defensive or bridles at the questions, then move on to someone else.

For yourself, you need to keep front of mind that once a

surgeon – no matter how good she is (by the way, there is some evidence that female surgeons get better results) – operates on a part of your body, it can never return to normal. There's no going back. If you really need the operation, then that's an easier decision than whether to have a procedure which is cosmetic.

With genital surgery, the drive can come from pornography which usually features abnormal bodies masquerading as normal. The men have large penises, no body hair and six-packs (so I'm told), and the women have shapely breasts, not a trace of cellulite and vulvae that look like perfect flowers (so I'm told). There is emotional distress around this issue. In a study in Norway, one in three women contemplating and then undergoing cosmetic genital surgery had had negative comments from a sexual partner and more than one in three were influenced by what they'd seen in pornographic media. This caused lower self-esteem and feelings of sexual unattractiveness. Of the women who underwent surgery, 70 per cent were satisfied with the cosmetic result (which gives you a benchmark for the answers you get from your surgeon).

Coming out

Despite gender fluidity and more ease around sexual identity, we still live in a world that's dominated by heterosexuality and, sadly, 'coming out' to parents, friends and workmates can still be a challenge for many people.

It's a bit easier if you've found a group you're happy to identify with because it will usually be supportive. However, some people still find telling others hard especially if they identify as trans or queer about which there's even less understanding in the community than of gay culture.

Clinical psychologist Dr Catherine Boland, who regularly deals with the issues around coming out, says the degree of difficulty depends on a variety of personal and social factors including whether you have a confident, outgoing personality or are shy and introverted and fear being asked about the mechanics of gay sex. Whether you live in an area that accepts LGBTIQ people also matters. Very religious and conservative families or those from non-Anglo cultures may react more strongly. Again, there's no easy script but there is support available and examples – usually of good stories on coming out – on YouTube, Instagram and even TikTok.

Dr Boland says that although it can be hard, it is ultimately healthy to be authentic and true to who you are and stop worrying about being found out. Her advice for coming out includes:

- There's no one right way to do it – some do it in person, some do it in letter/ written format or on social media.
- It's not necessarily a 'one off' event. In fact many LGBTIQ people will continue to 'come out' for their entire lives.
- Take your time.
- Practise first with a trusted/ supportive friend.
- When telling your family, take your time to think about how you'll do it. It's not a great idea to do it in the middle of an argument; you might want to tell a more supportive family member first. Remember, their initial reactions are unlikely to last, so give them

time to absorb the information.
- Get support.

Sex and being trans

The evidence is that during adolescence and prior to hormone treatment or gender affirmative surgery, a significant percentage of transboys and trans girls have sexual experiences but at a lower rate than the age group as a whole. After surgery (for those who seek it, many don't), all forms of sexual activity increase but again at a level which is still lower than the average for the general population.

Sexual distress is part of the challenge that transpeople feel and it's related to discrimination and the psychological effects of social anxiety and of feeling uneasy with one's body, especially if features like hair growth don't match a person's gender identity. Hormone treatment helps relieve this sexual distress and improves desire and sexual function. Surgery can improve this further, but there are still challenges to be overcome such as post-operative pain and the psychological, social and physical adjustment. The message is that needing help with getting the most out of sex doesn't stop with surgery. Longer term follow-up has found that finding sexual partners and achieving orgasms were the main sexual difficulties. Surgery may not solve these problems, so specialised sexual counselling may have to continue for some time. So I suppose the message is, don't think that any of these options are easy. All require a significant pause for thought and talking them out with people you trust.

From one of the larger and better quality studies, it looks as though hormone treatment produces mainly short-term changes in sexual desire, although transwomen on hormone treatment aimed at feminisation do experience improved desire over the longer term, predominantly related to feeling and being affirmed as the women they have always been.

Transmen having hormone therapy aimed at masculinisation don't appear to experience a long-term change in desire from what it was at the start of treatment, even though they might feel a rise early on. There's also good news for transmen in that testosterone therapy does not appear to induce increased levels of anger when followed out to three years after commencing hormone treatment. Anger problems are more likely to arise from mental health issues associated with the stigma and discrimination which can be felt by transgender people as well as residual physical issues from incomplete masculinisation. It's yet another reason for long-term psychological support to help people through what can be difficult times especially if reality doesn't match expectations.

Having a partner and feeling positive make a big difference but finding the right person for you isn't easy if you're transgender. There are stigma and ignorance to deal with, as well as the labour of working out whether a potential partner is truly open to a mutual intimate sexual relationship. However, many transpeople report having no trouble finding a loving, intimate relationship.

PART 7

What about the kids?

Families ... I hear some of you groan while some will be very comfortable with the idea of family. For some of us it's traditional family: partners, kids, siblings, parents and more distant relatives. Others have had bad experiences of family and rely on friendships and community for the love and support that families might provide. I had a mixed experience. My brothers and I didn't grow up in a happy household. As a child I looked enviously at families which sat at the dinner table and had conversations; where there were books on the shelves and where they didn't seem to tiptoe around fearful that something innocently said would become a cause for warfare. I was determined that wouldn't happen when I became a father and I tried hard to avoid the verbally abusive pattern I grew up with. In my own family, I love those now-rare times when we all get together loudly around the table. Food and a warm hearth become the glue as time goes by. Whatever our definition of family, we need what it has to offer: love, support, giving and taking and participating in the cycle of life. What follows is less slushy but covers some of the issues that can stretch families.

Child development and tennis

Short version: After the nine months of pregnancy, there's no more important time in a person's life than early childhood, usually defined as birth to eight years old but with particular emphasis on the preschool years. It's when parents learn that setting boundaries doesn't detract from their love of their child. It's when the billions of connections in the brain are transformed into what are called networks for memory, learning, self-control and adaptation to stress. There are around a million new brain connections made every second, and these networks last a lifetime even though they continue to have capacity to change and adapt (plasticity). And you can think of it like a game of tennis.

*

I love babies and toddlers, even the Terrible Twos. Some people say, meh, that they prefer when the child can speak and interact because that's when they're fun, rather than the eating, sleeping and poo-ing machines of the first few months.

Any parent knows how wrong that is.

When I was training in paediatrics, there was a charismatic American paediatrician called T. Berry Brazelton who believed that you could tell a lot about mothers' wellbeing from their babies. Brazelton lived to just short of his 100th birthday, which might be partly credited to his sunny, optimistic disposition. He reckoned you could tell from the way an infant behaved whether the mother was depressed. Up until then, when a paediatrician assessed a newborn, they checked the hips, in case they were loose, felt the abdomen, looked for rudimentary signs that the baby's nervous system was intact, the tummy felt normal and there were no heart murmurs. But Brazelton transformed that assessment – at least for me – by developing a process to look at a baby's behaviour. You'd lift the baby and play with them in a semi-structured way, talking to them, seeing how they responded. It was actually fun and babies seemed to love it.

Serves: It was a bit like a game of tennis. You served something to the baby – like talking to them – and they returned serve with a reaction, a look or a sound. The baby might serve to you first with a look or a sound, and you had to be open to that signal and give the ball right back to them. A baby of a depressed mother wasn't very good at this behavioural tennis but improved immensely when the mother was helped because she was now able to join more fully in the delicious game of child development.

The baby was like a remote thermometer of mood.

As kids enter toddlerhood, the tennis rules change a bit. They're wary of strangers and take time to warm up. If you're a new person to them, you learn to wait for them to serve to you, rather than the gently boisterous Brazelton approach to the newborn. And when you return serve to a toddler, it's slower and further from the net so they can feel more in control.

The point is that parenting and child development work on this serve-and-return principle. Serve up talking and book reading from the get-go and the baby will return with engagement and interest and the acquisition of vocabulary, understanding, the ability to concentrate and focus, and the capacity for productive social and emotional interactions. Serve up consistent, firm and loving parenting and the baby will return with a lot of the above plus a palpable sense of security and the foundation for good mental health later in life. Serve up breast milk then fresh unprocessed food and vegetables then the baby will return (eventually) with better than average eating habits and food preferences.

Not everything is about parenting. The more general environment matters too, such as housing and air pollution, relationship stress and levels of domestic violence, drug and alcohol use in the vicinity of the growing child, child abuse and access to high-quality preschool education. Then when the child starts school it's critical there be zero tolerance for bullying and the school provides an engaging environment, models the firm but loving boundary-setting of good parenting, and facilitates strong peer connections in their children. The good news is that even when there is poverty and disadvantage, having one stable relationship with a parent or other caregiver can help to protect against the damage of what's been called the toxic stress of early childhood.

And not everything is set in stone in our genes.

The environment in which we grow up, how we interact with our parents and caregivers, and even the food that we eat as kids can cause chemical reactions in our genes which can switch them on or off or up or down like a volume control. These are the epigenetic effects I talked about earlier and can counter or modify the genetic hand of cards we were dealt at conception.

The tennis metaphor means that it's not enough to provide a nice place to live and material security. You've got to play the game with the baby and child, interacting with them reciprocally. The technical term is being prosocial – giving and being sensitive to a child's wellbeing.

It's easy to write this stuff and much harder to do at home. A child who is easygoing can have better emotional regulation and comply more readily than a child who is a bit cantankerous and difficult. This is where genes do matter. Research in Melbourne following large numbers of kids from birth found that children tend to be born with these temperaments and they last at least through to adolescence. So you've got to tailor parenting and teaching to these variations. The bottom line is to provide safe and stimulating environments, as one review of protective factors in childhood concluded.

Are we wrecking our kids by letting them use screens?

No, we're not. But we're right to be worried about it and need to be careful and strong.

Looking back to when I trained in paediatrics, parental worries were pretty basic: breast feeding, when to introduce solids (sooner rather than later to prevent allergies), sleep–wake cycles and tantrums. But these days, as soon as toddlerhood is reached, screens can become a major issue.

Researchers at the Telethon Kids Institute in Perth, Australia, have reviewed the evidence and provided some practical solutions for millennial parents.

The Telethon review notes that children are being exposed to digital technologies at increasingly earlier ages than their parents. We're referring here to smartphones, tablets, video game consoles and computers. They conclude there are risks from this early consumption.

The report finds that when used effectively, technology can promote children's active engagement and creativity, with new ways of learning and problem-solving skills.

Australian guidelines recommend a limit of one hour of screen time per day for children aged two and over. The American Academy of Pediatrics lowers the age boundary to 18 months. There are no definitive guidelines in the UK although it is recommended that no children of any age should have more than two hours a day. However, it's not just how much time children spend on technology, but the way it's used.

And remember, recreational sedentary screen use is linked to overweight, obesity and unhealthy diets, which is a less than ideal foundation for your kids' health and longevity.

How are children using technology?

We now have a generation of children who have had access to technology since birth and have no memory of life before the internet. More than half of Australian children aged between two and four use tablets for an average of 20 minutes per day. In the UK an estimated four in ten children have their own tablet by the age of six.

The touchscreen has implications for very young children. They learn to point their forefinger between the ages of ten and 14 months and can start interacting with the screen. You've probably seen toddlers navigate their way around a tablet screen with staggering competence, sometimes leaving their grandparents aghast. The touchscreen therefore gives very young children a huge level of autonomy far beyond their developmental capacity. A tablet (or smartphone) isn't a babysitter where you can set and forget, deluding yourself that you're nurturing a genius. The onus is on caregivers (and technology companies) to impose restrictions and think hard about what you're exposing your child to.

The pros of technology for kids

Technology has given us a new way of talking to one another. If you look at devices as a way to interact, think about all the new conversations that children and adults can have via the digital world.

Devices are often a substitute for busy parents and life with children is all about juggling. However, the research clearly shows that the best way for children to digest technology is with the aid of an adult who can provide encouragement and help to learn. Adults can also help their child to link digital material with real life.

The American Academy of Pediatrics has historically discouraged exposure to screens and other media for children under the age of two because of the potential for negative side effects. But they changed that recently, noting that video chats were an important way of connecting children who are geographically separated from family members. That argument resonates strongly now as the world emerges from the global COVID-19 pandemic.

Content is queen

There are arguments that when judiciously used, new technologies and devices enhance children's opportunities for learning, particularly when it comes to collaboration and problem-solving. The International Literacy Association brought together the evidence in 2019 and emphasised that it's not so much the screen as what's on it. They say the common elements of advice are:

- Selection of high-quality digital media conveying content that supports curricular and learning goals and includes minimal distractors (e.g. ads or links that take users away from a site)
- Integration of digital technologies in ways that complement and enhance learning with other essential materials and activities
- Use of technology that supports development of creativity, exploration, collaboration, problem-solving, and knowledge development
- Use of technology to strengthen home–school connections
- Access to assistive technologies to support equitable opportunities for learning.

Inexorably, new technologies including coding are being brought into schools. In the home, there's research that shows that technology can help bridge the gap in literacy outcomes between children from high and low socio-economic backgrounds. The Australian Telethon Kids Institute notes that having access to a computer in the home is significantly associated with a better vocabulary by the age of eight and that devices can unlock creativity in children.

Kids watch adults and copy them

Have you ever tried to take a tablet device off an eight-year-old playing Minecraft?

Have you ever tried to take a mobile phone away from an adult?

Have you argued with a 13-year-old to get off the laptop when they tell you earnestly that they just have to respond to other players just one more time?

Have you ever tried to get an adult to ignore that ping of a message on their phone, or that last check of Instagram to see what their friends are up to? Or to not check emails at 3 a.m. (mea culpa, mea culpa, mea maxima culpa)?

It's like taking a bottle of wine away from a daily drinker. You can be met with a tirade of abuse at best, sometimes violence at worst. And that's just from the adults.

Little kids watch what we do and because they adore us, they think that what we do is the right thing and want to emulate it. If you're worried about your kids' screen use – and you should be concerned enough to control it and choose carefully what they watch – we need first to look at whether our own screen use is getting in the way of good parenting.

So, in that context, we don't have to dig too deep to cite

some of the downsides of children using screens.

Excessive screen time during the early years of development has been linked to a number of psychological difficulties, associated with increased loneliness, depression, anxiety and attention problems. Children can resent and fail to understand why parents are taking away their electronic devices which make them feel good.

Technology can also affect physical development and has been associated with a higher body mass index. In this instance, children are using digital technologies instead of engaging in physical play, face-to-face interactions and adequate sleep. If your child is hunched over a tablet, or contorting their body with gaming consoles, it's almost impossible to achieve good posture, putting stress on muscles and joints.

Children risk accessing inappropriate content online. Research shows simulated violence through technology appears to affect the brain in the same way as when children are exposed to violence in real life. Children aged seven or under don't readily distinguish between the real and virtual worlds.

Then there's the big screen. Having the television on in the background can have a negative effect on children's language and cognitive development. Researchers recommend that background TV should be turned off, and for children under three, careful supervision is recommended when the TV is on. During the pandemic, parents noted that the only way to get home-schooling done with older children was to park young children in front of the TV. Sometimes you have no choice. But if the TV is on, parents should actively participate and watch with their children, and make sure that the media isn't fast-paced. High speed intercutting, especially in baby brain-boosting videos, can affect their development.

Screen guidelines for toddlers

Guidelines for the under threes from an evidence-based review by American child development specialists Dr Claire Lerner and Dr Rachel Barr include:

- Limit screen time so your child can explore the real world, preferably with you.
- Participate in screen activities in the same way you'd do with a book, constantly relating what they're seeing to the real world. In other words, talk a lot with your child, and don't let the screen content take over from you as their mum or dad. You're better than anything on a screen.
- Turn off background television – i.e. don't have the TV on when no-one's watching.
- Be super-careful about choosing screen content. Tips include making sure portrayals are positive, with good role models, are relatable in an everyday way, with strong stories and opportunities for interaction. Avoid like the plague content which is fast moving and changes scene every few seconds. High-paced video content can make you think it will stimulate the child's brain. Research has shown that it distorts brain development and can affect your child's ability to make decisions, plan ahead and control emotions. *Sesame Street* and other high-quality children's

programming rarely, if ever, uses short duration,
rapidly intercut shots.
- No violent content.
- Don't watch programming for grown-ups until the
kids are asleep.
- Don't get lost in the technological wonderment of the
screen. The content and story and how you use them
with the child are what count.
- No screens in the bedroom.
- No screen time just before bed.
- No eating in front of a screen (screen time is a strong
predictor of obesity throughout childhood and
probably in adulthood as well).
- No technology at the dining table.
- Put aside or limit your own technology when the kids
are around.

Apps for children

Spend some time searching for the best material and apps to fit
your child. Find content from reputable outlets that is fun and
playful and encourages children to engage and solve problems.
Remember, content matters.

While almost half of the top-selling apps are designed for
children between 0 and 12, three-quarters of them are full of
instructions, rather than allowing scope for open-ended play
and interaction with other children.

Most apps are marketed as 'educational' but research shows
that most haven't had input from developmental researchers or
been matched with specific school curricula.

Adolescents

Adolescents and screens are a slightly different story.

Teenagers increasingly use the internet for basic communication, education, and entertainment and socialising.

During adolescence, there's an increased risk of emotional crises, often accompanied by mood changes and periods of anxiety and depressive behaviour, which adolescents attempt to fight through withdrawal, avoidance of any extensive social contact, aggressive reactions, and potential addictive behaviour. Some researchers believe that this age group can become drawn to the internet as a form of release. The internet allows sociability and at the same time provides anonymity and belonging to a community.

One study of more than 1000 teenagers across Croatia, Poland and Finland showed what many parents already know, which is that they used the internet mostly for socialising and entertainment, closely followed by schoolwork. So when you challenge them, no doubt they use schoolwork as blackmail.

Social media play a big role in adolescents' lives. According to US researchers in 2018, 90 per cent of teens aged 13–17 have used social media – again, no shock for parents. Seventy-five per cent report having at least one active social media profile, and about half report visiting a social media site at least daily. Two-thirds of teens have their own mobile devices with internet capabilities. Teens can be online almost nine hours a day, not including time for homework.

It's a lot, and to say it's a very tricky path for parents to navigate is an understatement.

Setting screen rules for them, and us

Screens should be used with discretion which, of course, is the difficult bit. You might have to adapt your strategy to meet the specific needs of your child – for instance, do they tend to be a bit obsessive? Are they inclined to physical activity, or do they need to be shoehorned out of the house?

Blanket technology bans don't tend to work. Sometimes you hear frustrated parents declare, 'I'm taking away the iPad forever!'

I'm going to bet that the child will call your bluff. Or you'll realise soon enough that it's hard to ban a device that you rely on to read your morning newspaper. As I mentioned before, young children born in the 21st century are so tech-savvy that they're running rings around their parents. In the short term, it might feel good to 'ban' the internet, YouTube or Fortnite, but you'll need an iron will to hold firm on the ban and you might lose the opportunity to have a constructive conversation with your children about setting limits on their digital usage. Especially if you're not limiting yours.

Research suggests the best way through is to make a plan with your children governing healthy screen use. The Australian Telethon Kids Institute suggests that parents and caregivers communicate consistent and realistic messages about how much and what kind of screen time is allowed. As children grow older, prepare agreements that clearly describe how technology can be used by family members.

The UK council for internet safety suggests involving your child in creating a family plan for leisure and entertainment that balances time spent in front of the internet and TV with a variety of offline activities. Tie a physical activity to electronic time. Taking screens off children can lead to arguments and resentment. So gentle warnings like 'Ten minutes until we switch it off' can reduce conflict around switching off the screen.

The thing is that such rules should not just be for the kids in the house. It may be harder for us adults to comply than you'd imagine but all devices off at mealtimes is a start.

Try to avoid using your screens as an 'emotional pacifier' for yourself or your kids to keep them quiet. Children, like you and me, aren't robots and don't like being turned off for too long. No judgement, but try to keep a lid on it.

My child's health as an adult – what matters?

Researchers believe there are about six factors in childhood and adolescence which can make a big difference to their health and longevity as adults.

Alcohol: Try to delay the uptake of alcohol as long as possible (see Alcohol and Other Drugs).

Smoking: Ditto but the real aim is no tobacco at all since the first ten cigarettes a day have a disproportionate toxic effect.

Screen time: Minimise and reduce recreational, sedentary screen time – and that's all screens. It's associated with overweight, obesity and unhealthy diets. (See Dominated by Devices.)

Sleep: Try to increase sleep time in kids who don't get enough, and reduce it in kids who are sleeping too long.

Moderate to vigorous exercise: As much as you can get them to do! While bad habits set in during adolescence, so do good ones!

Sugar-sweetened drinks: Minimise or eliminate their consumption. That's about obesity, overweight and decayed teeth, which are a very bad foundation for good nutrition later in life.

Think ahead. Who said parenting was easy?

For parents of adolescents: delay is better

The older you are when you first have sex, in general the more likely you are to have safer sex. Gay men tend to start sexual experiences later and there is some evidence that their first experiences are less satisfying and more painful. This could be due to residual stigma in young people about being gay or sex education being more focused on heterosexual sex. There is not a lot of good research on the predictors or outcomes of early sex in cis women who have sex with women or transpeople of all genders.

There is evidence that for young people screen exposure to explicit sexual content predicts the risk of unsafe sex, teen pregnancy and early sexual initiation.

How do I prevent my child getting into drugs?

Quick answer: There is no quick answer.

*

Let's define 'getting into drugs' first because it depends. You really want to aim for first drug and alcohol use as late in adolescence as possible because that predicts safer use. Adolescence is a period where the huge brain development in childhood needs to be pruned and refined to set the teenager up for the rest of their life. So it's a highly sensitive time for brain development and if the pruning shears slip, long-term damage can be done to the young person's brain, cementing in behaviours and vulnerabilities. Toxic stress from disadvantage, abusive trauma, bullying and conflicts over sexual identity can adversely affect that pruning. But early drug use is the big one, across the spectrum from tobacco to alcohol to ice to cannabis and others. Early drug and alcohol use is more likely in kids who are depressed and anxious, find it hard to control their emotions, who go to a school which is not good at connecting with their students and tolerates bullying, who've seen drug use in their parents, who've lost a parent or loved one, who are poor, who are coming to terms with LGBTIQ identities and sexuality, whose peer group at school or elsewhere is into drugs, or who've had careless prescription of opioid pain relievers to treat pain.

A myth: That you can teach sensible drinking by letting your child have alcohol at the table. What that can do is prime them for alcohol abuse.

Another myth: That media campaigns are the solution. While they can work for smoking, safe sex, exercise and road safety, they don't seem to have an effect on consumption of alcohol and other non-tobacco drugs.

But ... What can work are school-based education programmes which have been designed with students and led by them. When young people have been involved in the design and it has been tailored to their needs, language and understanding, and sometimes with the use of cartoons and online media, you can see increased knowledge, reduced anxiety and lower alcohol use.

A big myth: That this is some kind of moral weakness and government regulation is just the nanny state in action and doesn't work. Price and availability are two important factors in young people taking up drugs. So taxation, advertising bans and restricted access to legal drugs like tobacco and alcohol make a huge difference. With tobacco, that includes restricting smoking in public places and in vehicles. In the UK, alcoholic drinks are taxed according to their alcohol by volume (abv) content. In addition, in Scotland any shop with a licence to sell alcohol must observe a minimum price per unit of alcohol – which at the time of writing is 50 pence.

An Australian review of the evidence on prevention quoted figures such as nearly eight out of ten people aged 14 and over had used alcohol recently, with nearly one in five drinking at dangerous levels. A survey by UK's Drinkaware observed that in England in 2018 more than 44 per cent of 11–15 year olds had consumed alcohol, and in Scotland, in 2015, 14 per cent of 11 year olds and 66 per cent of 15 year olds had had an alcoholic drink – these were the lowest figures since their surveys began in 1990. Alcohol use has dropped rapidly in young people in recent years with many young people choosing not to drink at all, which is great because that's where problem drinking usually begins. Up to the age of 44, alcohol and other drug use are the top two risk factors for death and illness.

Factors that are lowering the chances of drug and alcohol use include: bringing up a child to have good emotional regulation; going to a school which is well connected to its students and doesn't tolerate bullying; parents who maintain firm but loving parenting styles with clear and explicit rules, set an example about drug use, and minimise hostility between each other; and dealing with mental health and sexual identity issues early and sensitively. But the reality is that a young person's peer group has an enormous influence, as does the drug and alcohol use behaviour of their role models.

This all seems a little overwhelming, but the good news for teenagers is that they are learning machines and the Australian research out of the University of Sydney led by Professor Maree Teesson in co-design with young people has shown that by using digital technology, the old art of cartoon story-telling and psychological theory, we can give adolescents the skills they need to reduce the risks of harms from alcohol and other drugs.

After thought

You've probably thumbed through to this bit while standing in a bookshop wondering whether to buy the book. If you want to know what I really think about health, it's mostly above. I write this after thought nearly two years into the COVID-19 pandemic. My observation is that the general community now understands far more about molecular and cellular biology than they – or I – ever imagined they would. I've spent years translating complex science into terms that people will understand and take on board for their own decision making. But during all those years, I was never sure that listeners/readers/viewers really understood what a cell was, much less DNA, and even less than that, RNA. This new knowledge among so many people is a fantastic side effect of the pandemic but there is a risk, and that is the same one that medical researchers face: knowing more and more about less and less. It's the metaphor of the foxhole and the need to be brave enough to lift one's head and observe the world around to know what to do next. You know where I'm going with this.

Rejoice in your deeper understanding of how the human body works at a molecular level but never forget that what will get us through and keep us well is the health of the world around us, government for the people, the support of those we love and covering their back when they need it.

Norman Swan

Sydney, October 2021

Notes

There are references below that I have relied upon for several sections, usually because they are so wide ranging. One example is Tania Thodis's superb PhD and papers from the other members of this Melbourne nutrition group. Others include the Burden of Disease papers. So you might see an early section loaded up with references, and later ones which follow looking light-on. That's because we didn't want to repeat references endlessly and have this the size of the Five Books of Moses.

Introduction

Robinson H, 'Dualism', *The Stanford Encyclopedia of Philosophy*. Fall 2020 edition. Zalta EN (ed.), URL https://plato.stanford.edu/archives/fall2020/entries/dualism/

Descartes R (trans. J Cottingham), *Meditations on First Philosophy*. Cambridge

Part 1: What you put into yourself

Rise above nutrients

Deterre S, Leclair C, Bai J, Baldwin EA, Narciso JA, Plotto A. 'Chemical and Sensory Characterization of Orange (*Citrus sinensis*) Pulp, a by-Product of Orange Juice Processing Using Gas-Chromatography-Olfactometry', *Journal of Food Quality*. 2016; 39: 826–838. https://doi.org/10.1111/jfq.12226

Simons T, McNeil C, Pham VD, et al. 'Chemical and sensory analysis of commercial Navel oranges in California', *npj Sci Food* 3. 2019; 22. https://doi.org/10.1038/s41538-019-0055-7

https://www.morressier.com/article/role-roast-chemical-characteristics-cold-brew-coffee/5e736c70cd e2b641284abdff?

Calvo MM, de la Hoz L. 'Flavour of heated milks. A review', *International Dairy Journal*. 1992; volume 2, issue 2, pp. 69–81. ISSN 0958-6946. https://doi.org/10.1016/0958-6946(92)90001-3

Ryan L, Petit S. 'Addition of whole, semiskimmed, and skimmed bovine milk reduces the total antioxidant capacity of black tea', *Nutr Res*. 2010 Jan; 30(1): 14–20. doi: 10.1016/j. nutres.2009.11.005. PMID: 20116655

Kunnumakkara AB, Sailo BL, Banik K, et al. 'Chronic diseases, inflammation, and spices: how are they linked?', *J Transl Med*. 2018; 16: 14. https://doi.org/10.1186/s12967-018-1381-2

Chassot LN, Scolaro B, Roschel GG, Cogliati B, Cavalcanti MF, Abdalla DSP, Castro IA. 'Comparison between red wine and isolated trans-resveratrol on the prevention and regression of atherosclerosis in LDLr $^{(-/-)}$ mice', *J Nutr Biochem*. 2018 Nov; 61: 48–55. doi: 10.1016/j. jnutbio.2018.07.014. Epub 2018 Aug 16. PMID: 30184518

Hansen AS, Marckmann P, Dragsted LO, Finné Nielsen IL, Nielsen SE, Grønbaek M. 'Effect of red wine and red grape extract on blood lipids, haemostatic factors, and other risk factors for cardiovascular disease', *Eur J Clin Nutr*. 2005 Mar; 59(3): 449–55. doi: 10.1038/sj.ejcn.1602107. PMID: 15674304

Chiva-Blanch G, Magraner E, Condines X, Valderas-Martínez P, Roth I, Arranz S, Casas R, Navarro M, Hervas A, Sisó A, Martínez-Huélamo M, Vallverdú-Queralt A, Quifer-Rada P, Lamuela-Raventos RM, Estruch R. 'Effects of alcohol and polyphenols from beer on atherosclerotic biomarkers in high cardiovascular risk men: a randomized feeding trial', *Nutr Metab Cardiovasc Dis*. 2015 Jan; 25(1): 36–45. doi: 10.1016/j.numecd.2014.07.008. Epub 2014 Aug 2. PMID: 25183453

Arranz S, Chiva-Blanch G, Valderas-Martínez P, Medina-Remón A, Lamuela-Raventós RM, Estruch R. 'Wine, beer, alcohol and polyphenols on cardiovascular disease and cancer', *Nutrients*. 2012 Jul; 4(7): 759–81. doi: 10.3390/nu4070759. Epub 2012 Jul 10. PMID: 22852062; PMCID: PMC3407993
https://www.sourdough.co.uk/the-history-of-sourdough-bread/
https://www.mediterraneanliving.com/eat-real-mediterranean-diet/

Is it fat or *Game of Thrones*? There's always a trade-off
Sumithran P, et al. 'Long-term persistence of hormonal adaptations to weight loss' *N Engl J Med*. 2011 Oct 27; 365(17): 1597–1604. doi: 10.1056/NEJMoa1105816
Scientific Advisory Committee on Nutrition (SACN) *Saturated Fats and Health: SACN Report*. Public Health England 2019
Hu FB. 'Are refined carbohydrates worse than saturated fat?' *Am J Clin Nutr*. 2010 Jun; 91(6):1541–2. doi: 10.3945/ajcn.2010.29622. Epub 2010 Apr 21. PMID: 20410095; PMCID: PMC2869506
Siri-Tarino PW, Sun Q, Hu FB, Krauss RM. 'Meta-analysis of prospective cohort studies evaluating the association of saturated fat with cardiovascular disease' *Am J Clin Nutr*. 2010 Mar; 91(3):535–46. doi: 10.3945/ajcn.2009.27725. Epub 2010 Jan 13. PMID: 20071648; PMCID: PMC2824152
Siri-Tarino PW, Sun Q, Hu FB, Krauss RM. 'Saturated fat, carbohydrate, and cardiovascular disease' *Am J Clin Nutr*. 2010 Mar; 91(3):502–9. doi: 10.3945/ajcn.2008.26285. Epub 2010 Jan 20. PMID: 20089734; PMCID: PMC2824150
Briggs MA, Petersen KS, Kris-Etherton PM. 'Saturated fatty acids and cardiovascular disease: replacements for saturated fat to reduce cardiovascular risk' *Healthcare*. 2017; 5(2), 29. https://doi.org/10.3390/healthcare5020029
Astrup A, Geiker NRW, Magkos F. 'Effects of full-fat and fermented dairy products on cardiometabolic disease: food is more than the sum of its parts' *Adv Nutr*. 2019 Sep 1; 10(5):924S–930S. doi: 10.1093/advances/nmz069. PMID: 31518411; PMCID: PMC6743821
Mozaffarian D, Micha R, Wallace S. 'Effects on coronary heart disease of increasing polyunsaturated fat in place of saturated fat: a systematic review and meta-analysis of randomized controlled trials' *PLoS Med*. 2010 Mar 23; doi:10.1371/journal.pmed.1000252
Mozaffarian D, Ludwig DS. 'Dietary guidelines in the 21st century – a time for food' *JAMA*. 2010; 304(6):681–682. doi:10.1001/jama.2010.1116

Cuisine counts – but not by itself
Hairston KG, Ducharme JL, Treuth MS, Hsueh WC, Jastreboff AM, Ryan KA, Shi X, Mitchell BD, Shuldiner AR, Snitker S. 'Comparison of BMI and physical activity between old order Amish children and non-Amish children', *Diabetes Care*. 2013 Apr; 36(4): 873–8. doi: 10.2337/dc12-0934. Epub 2012 Oct 23. PMID: 23093661; PMCID: PMC3609522
Radd S, Kouris-Blazos A, Singh MF, Flood V. 'Evolution of Mediterranean diets and cuisine: Concepts and definitions', *Asia Pacific Journal of Clinical Nutrition*. 2017; 26: 749–763. doi: 10.6133/apjcn.082016.0
Thodis A. 'MEDiterranean ISlands – Australia Study: Greek Mediterranean Diet Pattern Adherence, Successful Aging and Associations in Greek Australian Island-Born Long-Term Migrants [Short title: MEDIS-Australia Study]'. PhD thesis, La Trobe University, June 2019
Goff LM, 'Ethnicity and Type 2 Diabetes in the UK', *Diabetic Medicine*. 2019; 36 (8):927–38. doi.org/10.1111/dme.13895
https://www.diabetes.org.uk/resources-s3/2017-11/south_asian_report.pdf

Maybe culture counts more
https://geriatrics.stanford.edu/wp-content/uploads/downloads/ethnomed/japanese/downloads/japanese_american.pdf
Hastings KG, Eggleston K, Boothroyd D, et al. 'Mortality outcomes for Chinese and Japanese immigrants in the USA and countries of origin (Hong Kong, Japan): a comparative analysis using national mortality records from 2003 to 2011', *BMJ Open*. 2016; 6: e012201. doi:10.1136/
Harriss LR, English DR, Powles J, Giles GG, Tonkin AM, Hodge AM, Brazionis L, O'Dea K. 'Dietary patterns and cardiovascular mortality in the Melbourne Collaborative Cohort Study', *Am J Clin*

Nutr. 2007 Jul; 86(1): 221–9. doi: 10.1093/ajcn/86.1.221. PMID: 17616784

Micha R, Shulkin ML, Peñalvo JL, Khatibzadeh S, Singh GM, Rao M, Fahimi S, Powles J, Mozaffarian D. 'Etiologic effects and optimal intakes of foods and nutrients for risk of cardiovascular diseases and diabetes: Systematic reviews and meta-analyses from the Nutrition and Chronic Diseases Expert Group (NutriCoDE)', *PLoS One.* 2017 Apr 27; 12(4): e0175149. doi: 10.1371/journal.pone.0175149. PMID: 28448503; PMCID: PMC5407851

Micha R, Khatibzadeh S, Shi P, Fahimi S, Lim S, Andrews KG, et al. 'Global, regional, and national consumption levels of dietary fats and oils in 1990 and 2010: a systematic analysis including 266 country-specific nutrition surveys', *BMJ.* 2014; 348: g2272 doi:10.1136/bmj.g2272

Singh GM, Micha R, Khatibzadeh S, Lim S, Ezzati M, Mozaffarian D; Global Burden of Diseases Nutrition and Chronic Diseases Expert Group (NutriCoDE). 'Estimated Global, Regional, and National Disease Burdens Related to Sugar-Sweetened Beverage Consumption in 2010', *Circulation.* 2015 Aug 25; 132(8): 639–66. doi: 10.1161/CIRCULATIONAHA.114.010636. Epub 2015 Jun 29. PMID: 26124185; PMCID: PMC4550496

Imamura F, Micha R, Khatibzadeh S, Fahimi S, Shi P, Powles J, Mozaffarian Dr PH. 'Dietary quality among men and women in 187 countries in 1990 and 2010: A systematic assessment', *The Lancet Global Health.* 2015; 3: e132–42. doi: 10.1016/S2214-109X(14)70381-X

Micha R, Khatibzadeh S, Shi P, Andrews KG, Engell RE, Mozaffarian D; Global Burden of Diseases Nutrition and Chronic Diseases Expert Group (NutriCoDE). 'Global, regional and national consumption of major food groups in 1990 and 2010: a systematic analysis including 266 country-specific nutrition surveys worldwide', *BMJ Open.* 2015 Sep 24; 5(9): e008705. doi: 10.1136/bmjopen-2015-008705. PMID: 26408285; PMCID: PMC4593162

Wang Q, Afshin A, Yakoob MY, Singh GM, Rehm CD, Khatibzadeh S, Micha R, Shi P, Mozaffarian D; Global Burden of Diseases Nutrition and Chronic Diseases Expert Group (NutriCoDE). 'Impact of Nonoptimal Intakes of Saturated, Polyunsaturated, and Trans Fat on Global Burdens of Coronary Heart Disease', *J Am Heart Assoc.* 2016 Jan 20; 5(1): e002891. doi: 10.1161/JAHA.115.002891. Erratum in: *J Am Heart Assoc.* 2016 Jan; 5(1). p. ii: e002076. doi: 10.1161/JAHA.115.002076. Erratum in: *J Am Heart Assoc.* 2017 Nov 8; 6(11): PMID: 26790695; PMCID: PMC4859401

Yakoob MY, Micha R, Khatibzadeh S, Singh GM, Shi P, Ahsan H, Balakrishna N, Brahmam GN, Chen Y, Afshin A, Fahimi S, Danaei G, Powles JW, Ezzati M, Mozaffarian D; Global Burden of Diseases, Injuries, and Risk Factors: Nutrition and Chronic Diseases Expert Group; Metabolic Risk Factors of Chronic Diseases Collaborating Group. 'Impact of Dietary and Metabolic Risk Factors on Cardiovascular and Diabetes Mortality in South Asia: Analysis from the 2010 Global Burden of Disease Study', *Am J Public Health.* 2016 Dec; 106(12): 2113–2125. doi: 10.2105/AJPH.2016.303368. Epub 2016 Oct 13. PMID: 27736219; PMCID: PMC5104988

Afshin A, Micha R, Khatibzadeh S; On behalf of the 2010 Global Burden of Diseases, Injuries, and Risk Factors Study: Nutrition and Chronic Diseases Expert Group (NutriCoDE), and Metabolic Risk Factors of Chronic Diseases Collaborating Group, et al. 'The impact of dietary habits and metabolic risk factors on cardiovascular and diabetes mortality in countries of the Middle East and North Africa in 2010: a comparative risk assessment analysis', *BMJ Open.* 2015; 5: e006385. doi: 10.1136/bmjopen-2014-006385

Nicastro HL, Ross SA, Milner JA. 'Garlic and onions: their cancer prevention properties', *Cancer Prev Res (Phila).* 2015 Mar; 8(3): 181–9. doi: 10.1158/1940-6207.CAPR-14-0172. Epub 2015 Jan 13. PMID: 25586902; PMCID: PMC4366009

Lim SS, et al. 'A comparative risk assessment of burden of disease and injury attributable to 67 risk factors and risk factor clusters in 21 regions, 1990–2010: a systematic analysis for the Global Burden of Disease Study 2010', *Lancet.* 2012 Dec 15; 380(9859): 2224–60. doi: 10.1016/S0140-6736(12)61766-8. Erratum in: *Lancet.* 2013 Apr 13; 381(9874): 1276. Erratum in: *Lancet.* 2013 Feb 23; 381(9867): 628. Al Mazroa MA [added]; Memish ZA [added]. PMID: 23245609; PMCID: PMC4156511

Forget the French … the paradox is Greek

Kouris-Blazos A, Itsiopoulos C. 'Low all-cause mortality despite high cardiovascular risk in elderly Greek-born Australians: attenuating potential of diet?', *Asia Pac J Clin Nutr.* 2014; 23(4): 532–44. doi: 10.6133/apjcn.2014.23.4.16. PMID: 25516310

Kouris-Blazos A, Itsiopoulos C. 'Longevity in elderly Greek migrants to Australia may be explained by adherence to a traditional Greek Mediterranean diet?', in: Tsianikas M, Couvalis G, Palaktsoglou M (eds), 'Reading, interpreting, experiencing: an inter-cultural journey into Greek letters', *Modern Greek Studies Association of New Zealand*. 2015; 217–38. Published version of the paper reproduced here with permission from the publisher

Pillen H, Tsourtos G, Coveney J, Thodis A, Itsiopoulos C, Kouris-Blazos A. 'Retaining Traditional Dietary Practices among Greek Immigrants to Australia: The Role of Ethnic Identity', *Ecol Food Nutr*. 2017 Jul–Aug; 56(4): 312–328. doi: 10.1080/03670244.2017.1333000. Epub 2017 Jun 28. PMID: 28657346

Bruce MA, Martins D, Duru K, Beech BM, Sims M, Harawa N, et al. 'Church attendance, allostatic load and mortality in middle aged adults', *PLoS ONE*. 2017; 12(5): e0177618. https://doi.org/10.1371/journal.pone.0177618

Chliaoutakis JE, Drakou I, Gnardellis C, Galariotou S, Carra H, Chliaoutaki M. 'Greek Christian Orthodox ecclesiastical lifestyle: could it become a pattern of health-related behaviour?', *Prev Med*. 2002; 34: 428–435

Rate your diet

Chiuve SE, Fung TT, Rimm EB, Hu FB, MMcCullough ML, Wang M, Stampfer MJ, Willett WC. 'Alternative Dietary Indices Both Strongly Predict Risk of Chronic Disease', *The Journal of Nutrition*. June 2012; volume 142, issue 6, pp. 1009–1018. https://doi.org/10.3945/jn.111.157222

What is the Mediterranean dietary pattern anyway?

Mayr HL, Tierney AC, Kucianski T, Thomas CJ, Itsiopoulos C. 'Australian patients with coronary heart disease achieve high adherence to 6-month Mediterranean diet intervention: preliminary results of the AUSMED Heart Trial', *Nutrition*. 2019; volume 61, pp. 21–31. ISSN 0899-9007. https://doi.org/10.1016/j.nut.2018.10.02.

George ES, Kucianski T, Mayr HL, Moschonis G, Tierney AC, Itsiopoulos CA. 'Mediterranean Diet Model in Australia: Strategies for Translating the Traditional Mediterranean Diet into a Multicultural Setting', *Nutrients*. 2018 Apr 9; 10(4): 465. doi: 10.3390/nu10040465. PMID: 29642557; PMCID: PMC5946250

Lakshminarayana R, Raju M, Krishnakantha TP, Baskaran V. 'Lutein and zeaxanthin in leafy greens and their bioavailability: olive oil influences the absorption of dietary lutein and its accumulation in adult rats', *J Agric Food Chem*. 2007 Jul 25; 55(15): 6395–400. doi: 10.1021/jf070482z. Epub 2007 Jun 30. PMID: 17602649

La J, Roberts NH, Yafi FA. 'Diet and Men's Sexual Health', *Sex Med Rev*. 2018 Jan; 6(1): 54–68. doi: 10.1016/j.sxmr.2017.07.004. Epub 2017 Aug 1. PMID: 28778698

Kouidrat Y, Pizzol D, Cosco T, Thompson T, Carnaghi M, Bertoldo A, Solmi M, Stubbs B, Veronese N. 'High prevalence of erectile dysfunction in diabetes: a systematic review and meta-analysis of 145 studies', *Diabet Med*. 2017 Sep; 34(9): 1185–1192. doi: 10.1111/dme.13403. Epub 2017 Jul 18. PMID: 28722225

Ashworth A, Mitchell K, Blackwell J, Vanhatalo A, Jones A. 'High-nitrate vegetable diet increases plasma nitrate and nitrite concentrations and reduces blood pressure in healthy women', *Public Health Nutrition*. 2015; 18(14): 2669–2678. doi: 10.1017/S1368980015000038

Van der Avoort CMT, Van Loon LJC, Hopman MTE, Verdijk LB. 'Increasing vegetable intake to obtain the health promoting and ergogenic effects of dietary nitrate', *Eur J Clin Nutr*. 2018 Nov; 72(11): 1485–1489. doi: 10.1038/s41430-018-0140-z. Epub 2018 Mar 20. PMID: 29559721

Santos HO, de Moraes WMAM, da Silva GAR, Prestes J, Schoenfeld BJ. 'Vinegar (acetic acid) intake on glucose metabolism: A narrative review', *Clin Nutr ESPEN*. 2019 Aug; 32: 1–7. doi: 10.1016/j.clnesp.2019.05.008. Epub 2019 May 31. PMID: 31221273

Budak NH, Aykin E, Seydim AC, Greene AK, Guzel-Seydim ZB. 'Functional properties of vinegar', *J Food Sci*. 2014 May; 79(5): R757–64. doi: 10.1111/1750-3841.12434. PMID: 24811350

Sarri KO, Linardakis MK, Bervanaki FN, Tzanakis NE, Kafatos AG. 'Greek Orthodox fasting rituals: a hidden characteristic of the Mediterranean diet of Crete', *Br J Nutr*. 2004 Aug; 92(2): 277–84. doi: 10.1079/BJN20041197. PMID: 15333159

Kromhout D, Keys A, Aravanis C, Buzina R, Fidanza F, Giampaoli S, Jansen A, Menotti A, Nedeljkovic S, Pekkarinen M, et al. 'Food consumption patterns in the 1960s in seven countries', *Am J Clin*

Nutr. 1989 May; 49(5): 889–94. doi: 10.1093/ajcn/49.5.889. PMID: 2718924

Chliaoutakis JE, Drakou I, Gnardellis C, Galariotou S, Carra H, Chliaoutaki M. 'Greek Christian Orthodox ecclesiastical lifestyle: could it become a pattern of health-related behaviour?', *Prev Med.* 2002; 34: 428–435

The paleo myth

Johnson AR. 'The paleo diet and the American weight loss utopia, 1975–2014' *Utopian Studies* 2015 26 (1): 101–124, Special issue: Utopia and Food

Buckley HR, Buikstra JE. 'Stone agers in the fast lane? How bioarchaeologists can address the paleo diet myth' In: Buikstra J eds *Bioarchaeologists Speak Out. Bioarchaeology and Social Theory.* 2019. Springer, Cham. https://doi.org/10.1007/978-3-319-93012-1_7

Trinkaus E. 'Late Pleistocene adult mortality patterns and modern human establishment', *Proc Natl Acad Sci USA.* 2011 Jan 25; 108(4): 1267–71. doi: 10.1073/pnas.1018700108. Epub 2011 Jan 10. PMID: 21220336; PMCID: PMC3029716

16/8 and 5:2 ... when hunger is a luxury

Harvie MN, Pegington M, Mattson MP, Frystyk J, Dillon B, Evans G, Cuzick J, Jebb SA, Martin B, Cutler RG, et al. 'The effects of intermittent or continuous energy restriction on weight loss and metabolic disease risk markers: A randomized trial in young overweight women', *Int J Obes (Lond).* 2011; 35: 714–727

Varady KA, Bhutani S, Klempel MC, Kroeger CM, Trepanowski JF, Haus JM, Hoddy KK, Calvo YL. 'Alternate day fasting for weight loss in normal weight and overweight subjects: A randomized controlled trial', *Nutr J.* 2013: 12: 146

Eshghinia S, Mohammadzadeh F. 'The effects of modified alternate-day fasting diet on weight loss and CAD risk factors in overweight and obese women', *J Diabetes Metab Disord.* 2013; 12: 4

Teng NIMF, Shahar S, Rajab NF, Manaf ZA, Ngah WZ. 'Improvement of metabolic parameters in healthy older adult men following a fasting calorie restriction intervention', *Aging Male.* 2013; 16: 177–183

Harvie MN, Wright C, Pegington M, McMullan D, Mitchell E, Martin B, Cutler RG, Evans G, Whiteside S, Maudsley S, et al. 'The effect of intermittent energy and carbohydrate restriction v. daily energy restriction on weight loss and metabolic disease risk markers in overweight women', *Br J Nutr.* 2013; 110: 1534–1547

Kerndt PR, Naughton JL, Driscoll CE, Loxterkamp DA. 'Fasting: the history, pathophysiology and complications', *West J Med.* 1982 Nov; 137(5): 379–99. PMID: 6758355; PMCID: PMC1274154

Heyman SN, Bursztyn M, Szalat A, Muszkat M, Abassi Z. 'Fasting-Induced Natriuresis and SGLT: A New Hypothesis for an Old Enigma', *Front Endocrinol (Lausanne).* 2020 May 7; 11: 217. doi: 10.3389/fendo.2020.00217. PMID: 32457696; PMCID: PMC7221140

Choi IY, Lee C, Longo VD. 'Nutrition and fasting mimicking diets in the prevention and treatment of autoimmune diseases and immunosenescence', *Mol Cell Endocrinol.* 2017 Nov 5; 455: 4–12. doi: 10.1016/j.mce.2017.01.042. Epub 2017 Jan 28. PMID: 28137612; PMCID: PMC5862044

Cheng CW, Villani V, Buono R, Wei M, Kumar S, Yilmaz OH, Cohen P, Sneddon JB, Perin L, Longo VD. 'Fasting-Mimicking Diet Promotes Ngn3-Driven β-Cell Regeneration to Reverse Diabetes', *Cell.* 2017 Feb 23; 168(5): 775–788. e12. doi: 10.1016/j.cell.2017.01.040. PMID: 28235195; PMCID: PMC5357144

Longo VD, Panda S. 'Fasting, Circadian Rhythms, and Time-Restricted Feeding in Healthy Lifespan', *Cell Metab.* 2016 Jun 14; 23(6): 1048–1059. doi: 10.1016/j.cmet.2016.06.001. PMID: 27304506; PMCID: PMC5388543

Vallianou N, Stratigou T, Christodoulatos GS, Dalamaga M. 'Understanding the Role of the Gut Microbiome and Microbial Metabolites in Obesity and Obesity-Associated Metabolic Disorders: Current Evidence and Perspectives', *Curr Obes Rep.* 2019 Sep; 8(3): 317–332. doi: 10.1007/s13679-019-00352-2. PMID: 31175629

Lee CJ, Sears CL, Maruthur N. 'Gut microbiome and its role in obesity and insulin resistance', *Ann NY Acad Sci.* 2020 Feb; 1461(1): 37–52. doi: 10.1111/nyas.14107. Epub 2019 May 14. PMID: 31087391

Pavlik Z. 'Population and development', *Acta Univ Carol Geogr.* 1995; 30(1–2): 43–51. PMID: 12292830

Caspari R, Lee S-H. 'Is human longevity a consequence of cultural change or modern biology?', *Am J Phys Anthropol.* 2006, 129: 512–517. https://doi.org/10.1002/ajpa.20360

Lowe DA, Wu N, Rohdin-Bibby L, Moore AH, Kelly N, Liu YE, Philip E, Vittinghoff E, Heymsfield SB, Olgin JE, Shepherd JA, Weiss EJ. 'Effects of Time-Restricted Eating on Weight Loss and Other Metabolic Parameters in Women and Men With Overweight and Obesity: The TREAT Randomized Clinical Trial', *JAMA Intern Med*. 2020 Nov 1; 180(11): 1491–1499. doi: 10.1001/jamainternmed.2020.4153. PMID: 32986097; PMCID: PMC7522780

Campbell BI, Aguilar D, Colenso-Semple LM, Hartke K, Fleming AR, Fox CD, Longstrom JM, Rogers GE, Mathas DB, Wong V, Ford S, Gorman J. 'Intermittent Energy Restriction Attenuates the Loss of Fat Free Mass in Resistance Trained Individuals. A Randomized Controlled Trial', *J Funct Morphol Kinesiol*. 2020 Mar 8; 5(1): 19. doi: 10.3390/jfmk5010019. PMID: 33467235; PMCID: PMC7739314

Kim C, Pinto AM, Bordoli C, Buckner LP, Kaplan PC, Del Arenal IM, Jeffcock EJ, Hall WL, Thuret S. 'Energy Restriction Enhances Adult Hippocampal Neurogenesis-Associated Memory after Four Weeks in an Adult Human Population with Central Obesity; a Randomized Controlled Trial', *Nutrients*. 2020 Feb 28; 12(3): 638. doi: 10.3390/nu12030638. PMID: 32121111; PMCID: PMC7146388

Rynders CA, Thomas EA, Zaman A, Pan Z, Catenacci VA, Melanson EL. 'Effectiveness of Intermittent Fasting and Time-Restricted Feeding Compared to Continuous Energy Restriction for Weight Loss', *Nutrients*. 2019 Oct 14; 11(10): 2442. doi: 10.3390/nu11102442. PMID: 31614992; PMCID: PMC6836017

Malinowski B, Zalewska K, Węsierska A, Sokołowska MM, Socha M, Liczner G, Pawlak-Osińska K, Wiciński M. 'Intermittent Fasting in Cardiovascular Disorders – An Overview', *Nutrients*. 2019 Mar 20; 11(3): 673. doi: 10.3390/nu11030673. PMID: 30897855; PMCID: PMC6471315

Grajower MM, Horne BD. 'Clinical Management of Intermittent Fasting in Patients with Diabetes Mellitus', *Nutrients*. 2019 Apr 18; 11(4): 873. doi: 10.3390/nu11040873. PMID: 31003482; PMCID: PMC6521152

Mager DE, Wan R, Brown M, Cheng A, Wareski P, Abernethy DR, et al. 'Caloric restriction and intermittent fasting alter spectral measures of heart rate and blood pressure variability in rats', *FASEB*. 2006; 20(6): 631–7

Mattson MP, Longo VD, Harvie M. 'Impact of intermittent fasting on health and disease processes', *Ageing Research Reviews*. 2017; volume 39, pp. 46–58. ISSN 1568-1637. https://doi.org/10.1016/j.arr.2016.10.005

Jane L, Atkinson G, Jaime V, Hamilton S, Waller G, Harrison S. 'Intermittent fasting interventions for the treatment of overweight and obesity in adults aged 18 years and over. A systematic review protocol', *JBI Database Syst Rev Implement Rep*. 2015; 13: 60–68

Harvie M, Howell A. 'Potential benefits and harms of intermittent energy restriction and intermittent fasting amongst obese, overweight, and normal weight subjects – A narrative review of human and animal evidence', *Behav Sci*. 2017; 7: E4

Carter S, Clifton PM, Keogh JB. 'The effects of intermittent compared to continuous energy restriction on glycaemic control in type 2 diabetes; a pragmatic pilot trial', *Diabetes Res Clin Pract*. 2016; 122: 106–112

Patterson RE, Sears DD. 'Metabolic Effects of Intermittent Fasting', *Annu Rev Nutr*. 2017; 37: 371–393

Heilbronn LK, Smith SR, Martin CK, Anton SD, Ravussin E. 'Alternate-day fasting in nonobese subjects: Effects on body weight, body composition, and energy metabolism', *Am J Clin Nutr*. 2005; 81: 69–73

Moro T, Tinsley G, Bianco A, Marcolin G, Pacelli QF, Battaglia G, Palma A, Gentil P, Neri M, Paoli A. 'Effects of eight weeks of time-restricted feeding (16/8) on basal metabolism, maximal strength, body composition, inflammation, and cardiovascular risk factors in resistance-trained males', *J Transl Med*. 2016; 14: 290

Harvie MN, Pegington M, Mattson MP, Frystyk J, Dillon B, Evans G, Cuzick J, Jebb SA, Martin B, Cutler RG, et al. 'The effects of intermittent or continuous energy restriction on weight loss and metabolic disease risk markers: A randomized trial in young overweight women', *Int J Obes (Lond)*. 2011; 35: 714–727

Varady KA, Bhutani S, Klempel MC, Kroeger CM, Trepanowski JF, Haus JM, Hoddy KK, Calvo YL. 'Alternate day fasting for weight loss in normal weight and overweight subjects: A randomized controlled trial', *Nutr J*. 2013; 12: 146

Eshghinia S, Mohammadzadeh F. 'The effects of modified alternate-day fasting diet on weight loss and

CAD risk factors in overweight and obese women', *J Diabetes Metab Disord*. 2013; 12: 4

Teng NIMF, Shahar S, Rajab NF, Manaf ZA, Ngah WZ. 'Improvement of metabolic parameters in healthy older adult men following a fasting calorie restriction intervention', *Aging Male*. 2013; 16: 177–183

Harvie MN, Wright C, Pegington M, McMullan D, Mitchell E, Martin B, Cutler RG, Evans G, Whiteside S, Maudsley S, et al. 'The effect of intermittent energy and carbohydrate restriction v. daily energy restriction on weight loss and metabolic disease risk markers in overweight women', *Br J Nutr*. 2013; 110: 1534–1547

How important is breakfast, really?

Chowdhury EA, Richardson JD, Holman GD, Tsintzas K, Thompson D, Betts JA. 'The causal role of breakfast in energy balance and health: A randomized controlled trial in obese adults', *Am J Clin Nutr*. 2016; 103: 747–756

Monzani A, Ricotti R, Caputo M, Solito A, Archero F, Bellone S, Prodam F. 'A Systematic Review of the Association of Skipping Breakfast with Weight and Cardiometabolic Risk Factors in Children and Adolescents. What Should We Better Investigate in the Future?' *Nutrients*. 2019 Feb 13; 11(2): 387. doi: 10.3390/nu11020387. PMID: 30781797; PMCID: PMC6412508

Edefonti V, Rosato V, Parpinel M, Nebbia G, Fiorica L, Fossali E, Ferraroni M, Decarli A, Agostoni C. 'The effect of breakfast composition and energy contribution on cognitive and academic performance: a systematic review', *Am J Clin Nutr*. 2014 Aug; 100(2): 626–56. doi: 10.3945/ajcn.114.083683. Epub 2014 May 7. PMID: 24808492

Hoyland A, Dye L, Lawton CL. 'A systematic review of the effect of breakfast on the cognitive performance of children and adolescents', *Nutr Res Rev*. 2009 Dec; 22(2): 220–43. doi: 10.1017/S0954422409990175. PMID: 19930787

Mahoney CR, Taylor HA, Kanarek RB, Samuel P. 'Effect of breakfast composition on cognitive processes in elementary school children', *Physiol Behav*. 2005 Aug 7; 85(5): 635–45. doi: 10.1016/j.physbeh.2005.06.023. PMID: 16085130

Widenhorn-Müller K, Hille K, Klenk J, Weiland U. 'Influence of having breakfast on cognitive performance and mood in 13- to 20-year-old high school students: results of a crossover trial', *Pediatrics*. 2008 Aug; 122(2): 279–84. doi: 10.1542/peds.2007-0944. PMID: 18676544

Edefonti V, Bravi F, Ferraroni M. 'Breakfast and behavior in morning tasks: Facts or fads?', *J Affect Disord*. 2017 Dec 15; 224: 16–26. doi: 10.1016/j.jad.2016.12.028. Epub 2016 Dec 24. PMID: 28062077

Adolphus K, Lawton CL, Dye L. 'Associations Between Habitual School-Day Breakfast Consumption Frequency and Academic Performance in British Adolescents', *Front Public Health*. 2019 Nov 20; 7: 283. doi: 10.3389/fpubh.2019.00283. PMID: 31824903; PMCID: PMC6879673

Sievert K, Hussain SM, Page MJ, Wang Y, Hughes HJ, Malek M, Cicuttini FM. 'Effect of breakfast on weight and energy intake: systematic review and meta-analysis of randomised controlled trials', *BMJ*. 2019 Jan 30; 364: l42. doi: 10.1136/bmj.l42. PMID: 30700403; PMCID: PMC6352874.

Chowdhury EA, Richardson JD, Holman GD, Tsintzas K, Thompson D, Betts JA. 'The causal role of breakfast in energy balance and health: A randomized controlled trial in obese adults', *Am J Clin Nutr*. 2016; 103: 747–756

Quatela A, Patterson A, Callister R, et al. 'Breakfast consumption habits of Australian men participating in the "Typical Aussie Bloke" study', *BMC Nutr*. 2020; 6: 1. https://doi.org/10.1186/s40795-019-0317-4

O'Neil CE, Nicklas TA, Fulgoni VL 3rd. 'Nutrient intake, diet quality, and weight/adiposity parameters in breakfast patterns compared with no breakfast in adults: National Health and Nutrition Examination Survey 2001–2008', *J Acad Nutr Diet*. 2014 Dec; 114(12 Suppl): S27–43. doi: 10.1016/j.jand.2014.08.021. Epub 2014 Nov 24. PMID: 25458992

Hoyland A, Lawton C, Dye L. 'Influence of breakfast on cognitive performance, appetite and mood in healthy young adults', *Appetite*. 2008; volume 50, issues 2–3, p. 560. ISSN 0195-6663. https://doi.org/10.1016/j.appet.2007.09.036

González-Garrido AA, Brofman-Epelbaum JJ, Gómez-Velázquez FR, Balart-Sánchez SA, Ramos-Loyo J. 'Skipping breakfast affects the early steps of cognitive processing: An event-related brain potentials study', *Journal of Psychophysiology*. 2019; 33(2): 109–118. https://doi.org/10.1027/0269-8803/a000214

Komiyama T, Sudo M, Okuda N, Yasuno T, Kiyonaga A, Tanaka H, Higaki Y, Ando S. 'Cognitive function at rest and during exercise following breakfast omission', *Physiol Behav*. 2016 Apr 1;

157: 178–84. doi: 10.1016/j.physbeh.2016.02.013. Epub 2016 Feb 11. PMID: 26876456

Keto … or low carb … or is it that you want to be ripped?
https://opentextbc.ca/anatomyandphysiology/chapter/24-4-protein-metabolism/
https://opentextbc.ca/anatomyandphysiology/chapter/24-4-lipid-metabolism/
https://biologydictionary.net/ketone-bodies/
Gibson AA, Seimon RV, Lee CM, Ayre J, Franklin J, Markovic TP, Caterson ID, Sainsbury A. 'Do ketogenic diets really suppress appetite? A systematic review and meta-analysis', *Obes Rev*. 2015 Jan; 16(1): 64–76. doi: 10.1111/obr.12230. Epub 2014 Nov 17. PMID: 25402637
Nymo S, Coutinho SR, Jørgensen J, Rehfeld JF, Truby H, Kulseng B, Martins C. 'Timeline of changes in appetite during weight loss with a ketogenic diet', *Int J Obes (Lond)*. 2017 Aug; 41(8): 1224–1231. doi: 10.1038/ijo.2017.96. Epub 2017 Apr 25. PMID: 28439092; PMCID: PMC5550564
Barry D, Ellul S, Watters L, Lee D, Haluska R Jr, White R. 'The ketogenic diet in disease and development', *International Journal of Developmental Neuroscience*. 2018; 68: 53–58. doi: 10.1016/j.ijdevneu.2018.04.005
Rusek M, Pluta R, Ułamek-Kozioł M, Czuczwar SJ. 'Ketogenic Diet in Alzheimer's Disease', *Int J Mol Sci*. 2019 Aug 9; 20(16): 3892. doi: 10.3390/ijms20163892. PMID: 31405021; PMCID: PMC6720297
Seidelmann SB, Claggett B, Cheng S, Henglin M, Shah A, Steffen LM, Folsom AR, Rimm EB, Willett WC, Solomon SD. 'Dietary carbohydrate intake and mortality: a prospective cohort study and meta-analysis', *Lancet Public Health*. 2018 Sep; 3(9): e419–e428. doi: 10.1016/S2468-2667(18)30135-X. Epub 2018 Aug 17. PMID: 30122560; PMCID: PMC6339822

Green is a good colour
Huang J, Liao LM, Weinstein SJ, Sinha R, Graubard BI, Albanes D. 'Association Between Plant and Animal Protein Intake and Overall and Cause-Specific Mortality', *JAMA Intern Med*. 2020 Sep 1; 180(9): 1173–1184. doi: 10.1001/jamainternmed.2020.2790. PMID: 32658243; PMCID: PMC7358979
Kwok CS, Umar S, Myint PK, Mamas MA, Loke YK. 'Vegetarian diet, Seventh Day Adventists and risk of cardiovascular mortality: a systematic review and meta-analysis', *Int J Cardiol*. 2014 Oct 20; 176(3): 680–6. doi: 10.1016/j.ijcard.2014.07.080. Epub 2014 Aug 4. PMID: 25149402
Rosell M, Appleby P, Spencer E, Key T. 'Weight gain over 5 years in 21,966 meat-eating, fish-eating, vegetarian, and vegan men and women in EPIC-Oxford', *Int J Obes (Lond)*. 2006 Sep; 30(9): 1389–96. doi: 10.1038/sj.ijo.0803305. Epub 2006 Mar 14. PMID: 16534521
Sebastiani G, Herranz Barbero A, Borrás-Novell C, Alsina Casanova M, Aldecoa-Bilbao V, Andreu-Fernández V, Pascual Tutusaus M, Ferrero Martínez S, Gómez Roig MD, García-Algar O. 'The Effects of Vegetarian and Vegan Diet during Pregnancy on the Health of Mothers and Offspring', *Nutrients*. 2019 Mar 6; 11(3): 557. doi: 10.3390/nu11030557. PMID: 30845641; PMCID: PMC6470702
Tuso PJ, Ismail MH, Ha BP, Bartolotto C. 'Nutritional update for physicians: plant-based diets', *Perm J*. 2013 Spring; 17(2): 61–6. doi: 10.7812/TPP/12-085. PMID: 23704846; PMCID: PMC3662288
Medawar E, Huhn S, Villringer A, Veronica Witte A. 'The effects of plant-based diets on the body and the brain: a systematic review', *Transl Psychiatry*. 2019 Sep 12; 9(1): 226. doi: 10.1038/s41398-019-0552-0. PMID: 31515473; PMCID: PMC6742661
Mahase E. 'Vegetarian and pescatarian diets are linked to lower risk of ischaemic heart disease, study finds', *BMJ*. 2019 Sep 4; 366: l5397. doi: 10.1136/bmj.l5397. PMID: 31488424

Is there a gene for garlic?
Menni C, Zhai G, Macgregor A, Prehn C, Römisch-Margl W, Suhre K, Adamski J, Cassidy A, Illig T, Spector TD, Valdes AM. 'Targeted metabolomics profiles are strongly correlated with nutritional patterns in women', *Metabolomics*. 2013 Apr; 9(2): 506–514. doi: 10.1007/s11306-012-0469-6. Epub 2012 Oct 6. PMID: 23543136; PMCID: PMC3608890
Makrecka-Kuka M, Sevostjanovs E, Vilks K, Volska K, Antone U, Kuka J, Makarova E, Pugovics O, Dambrova M, Liepinsh E. 'Plasma acylcarnitine concentrations reflect the acylcarnitine profile in cardiac tissues', *Sci Rep*. 2017 Dec 13; 7(1): 17528. doi: 10.1038/s41598-017-17797-x. PMID: 29235526; PMCID: PMC5727517

Strand E, Pedersen ER, Svingen GF, Olsen T, Bjørndal B, Karlsson T, Dierkes J, Njølstad PR, Mellgren G, Tell GS, Berge RK, Svardal A, Nygård O. 'Serum Acylcarnitines and Risk of Cardiovascular Death and Acute Myocardial Infarction in Patients With Stable Angina Pectoris', *J Am Heart Assoc.* 2017 Feb 3; 6(2): e003620. doi: 10.1161/JAHA.116.003620. PMID: 28159823; PMCID: PMC5523736

Pallister T, Sharafi M, Lachance G, Pirastu N, Mohney RP, MacGregor A, Feskens EJ, Duffy V, Spector TD, Menni C. 'Food Preference Patterns in a UK Twin Cohort', *Twin Res Hum Genet.* 2015 Dec; 18(6): 793–805. doi: 10.1017/thg.2015.69. Epub 2015 Sep 28. PMID: 26412323

Martins N, Petropoulos S, Ferreira IC. 'Chemical composition and bioactive compounds of garlic (*Allium sativum L.*) as affected by pre- and post-harvest conditions: A review', *Food Chem.* 2016 Nov 15; 211: 41–50. doi: 10.1016/j.foodchem.2016.05.029. Epub 2016 May 6. PMID: 27283605

Nicastro HL, Ross SA, Milner JA. 'Garlic and onions: their cancer prevention properties', *Cancer Prev Res (Phila).* 2015 Mar; 8(3): 181–9. doi: 10.1158/1940-6207.CAPR-14-0172. Epub 2015 Jan 13. PMID: 25586902; PMCID: PMC4366009

Bahadoran Z, Mirmiran P, Momenan AA, Azizi F. 'Allium vegetable intakes and the incidence of cardiovascular disease, hypertension, chronic kidney disease, and type 2 diabetes in adults: a longitudinal follow-up study', *J Hypertens.* 2017 Sep; 35(9): 1909–1916. doi: 10.1097/HJH.0000000000001356. PMID: 28319598

Platel K, Srinivasan K. 'Bioavailability of Micronutrients from Plant Foods: An Update', *Crit Rev Food Sci Nutr.* 2016 Jul 26; 56(10): 1608–19. doi: 10.1080/10408398.2013.781011. PMID: 25748063

Rinaldi de Alvarenga JF, Quifer-Rada P, Francetto Juliano F, Hurtado-Barroso S, Illan M, Torrado-Prat X, Lamuela-Raventós RM. 'Using Extra Virgin Olive Oil to Cook Vegetables Enhances Polyphenol and Carotenoid Extractability: A Study Applying the *sofrito* Technique', *Molecules.* 2019 Apr 19; 24(8): 1555. doi: 10.3390/molecules24081555. PMID: 31010212; PMCID: PMC6514867

Galeone C, Tavani A, Pelucchi C, Negri E, La Vecchia C. 'Allium vegetable intake and risk of acute myocardial infarction in Italy', *Eur J Nutr.* 2009 Mar; 48(2): 120–3. doi: 10.1007/s00394-008-0771-2. Epub 2009 Jan 13. PMID: 19142565

Red is a very good colour

Fielding JM, Rowley KG, Cooper P, O'Dea K. 'Increases in plasma lycopene concentration after consumption of tomatoes cooked with olive oil', *Asia Pac J Clin Nutr.* 2005; 14(2): 131–6. PMID: 15927929

Rock CL, Lovalvo JL, Emenhiser C, Ruffin MT, Flatt SW, Schwartz SJ. 'Bioavailability of beta-carotene is lower in raw than in processed carrots and spinach in women', *J Nutr* 1998; 128: 913–6

Johnson EJ, Qin J, Krinsky NI, Russell RM. 'Ingestion by men of a combined dose of beta-carotene and lycopene does not affect the absorption of beta-carotene but improves that of lycopene', *J Nutr.* 1997; 127: 1833–7

Lee A, Thurnham DI, Chopra M. 'Consumption of tomato products with olive oil but not sunflower oil increases the antioxidant activity of plasma', *Free Radic Biol Med* 2000; 29: 1051–5

Clifford T, Howatson G, West DJ, Stevenson EJ. 'The potential benefits of red beetroot supplementation in health and disease', *Nutrients.* 2015 Apr 14; 7(4): 2801–22. doi: 10.3390/nu7042801. PMID: 25875121; PMCID: PMC4425174

Grabowska M, Wawrzyniak D, Rolle K, Chomczyński P, Oziewicz S, Jurga S, Barciszewski J. 'Let food be your medicine: nutraceutical properties of lycopene', *Food Funct.* 2019 Jun 19; 10(6): 3090–3102. doi: 10.1039/c9fo00580c. PMID: 31120074

Costa-Rodrigues J, Pinho O, Monteiro PRR. 'Can lycopene be considered an effective protection against cardiovascular disease?', *Food Chem.* 2018 Apr 15; 245: 1148–1153. doi: 10.1016/j.foodchem.2017.11.055. Epub 2017 Nov 15. PMID: 29287334

Crowe-White KM, Phillips TA, Ellis AC. 'Lycopene and cognitive function', *J Nutr Sci.* 2019 May 29; 8: e20. doi: 10.1017/jns.2019.16. PMID: 31217968; PMCID: PMC6558668

Akbaraly NT, Faure H, Gourlet V, et al. 'Plasma carotenoid levels and cognitive performance in an elderly population: results of the EVA study', *J Gerontol A Biol Sci Med Sci.* 2007; 62: 308–316. 23

Polidori MC, Praticóc D, Mangialasche F, et al. 'High fruit and vegetable intake is positively correlated with antioxidant status and cognitive performance in healthy subjects', *J Alzheimers Dis.* 2009; 17: 921–927

Lauretani F, Semba RD, Dayhoff-Brannigan M, et al. 'Low total plasma carotenoids are independent predictors of mortality among older persons: the InCHIANTI Study', *Eur J Nutr.* 2008; 47: 335–340

Shardell MD, Alley DE, Hicks GE, et al. 'Low-serum carotenoid concentrations and carotenoid interactions predict mortality in US adults: the Third National Health and Nutrition Examination Survey', *Nutr Res.* 2011; 31: 178–189

Rinaldi de Alvarenga JF, Quifer-Rada P, Westrin V, Hurtado-Barroso S, Torrado-Prat X, Lamuela-Raventós RM. 'Mediterranean sofrito home-cooking technique enhances polyphenol content in tomato sauce', *J Sci Food Agric.* 2019 Nov; 99(14): 6535–6545. doi: 10.1002/jsfa.9934. Epub 2019 Aug 13. PMID: 31321777

Olas B. 'Anti-Aggregatory Potential of Selected Vegetables-Promising Dietary Components for the Prevention and Treatment of Cardiovascular Disease', *Adv Nutr.* 2019 Mar 1; 10(2): 280–290. doi: 10.1093/advances/nmy085. PMID: 30759176; PMCID: PMC6416036

Frond AD, Iuhas CI, Stirbu I, Leopold L, Socaci S, Andreea S, Ayvaz H, Andreea S, Mihai S, Diaconeasa Z, Carmen S. 'Phytochemical Characterization of Five Edible Purple-Reddish Vegetables: Anthocyanins, Flavonoids, and Phenolic Acid Derivatives', *Molecules.* 2019 Apr 18; 24(8): 1536. doi: 10.3390/molecules24081536. PMID: 31003505; PMCID: PMC6514853

Be bioactive: on antioxidants and tubas
Biesalski HK, Grune T, Tinz J, Zöllner I, Blumberg JB. 'Reexamination of a meta-analysis of the effect of antioxidant supplementation on mortality and health in randomized trials', *Nutrients.* 2010 Sep; 2(9): 929–49. doi: 10.3390/nu2090929. Epub 2010 Aug 30. PMID: 22254063; PMCID: PMC3257709

Yang CS, Ho CT, Zhang J, Wan X, Zhang K, Lim J. 'Antioxidants: Differing Meanings in Food Science and Health Science', *J Agric Food Chem.* 2018 Mar 28; 66(12): 3063–3068. doi: 10.1021/acs.jafc.7b05830. Epub 2018 Mar 14. PMID: 29526101

Smith RE. 'The Effects of Dietary Supplements that Overactivate the Nrf2/ARE System', *Curr Med Chem.* 2020; 27(13): 2077–2094. doi: 10.2174/0929867326666190517113533. PMID: 31099320

Vasconcelos AR, Dos Santos NB, Scavone C, Munhoz CD. 'Nrf2/ARE Pathway Modulation by Dietary Energy Regulation in Neurological Disorders', *Front Pharmacol.* 2019 Feb 4; 10: 33. doi: 10.3389/fphar.2019.00033. PMID: 30778297; PMCID: PMC6369171

Anderson G, Maes M. 'How immune-inflammatory processes link CNS and psychiatric disorders: classification and treatment implications', *CNS Neurol Disord Drug Targets.* 2017; 16: 266–278. doi: 10.2174/1871527315666161122144659

Anderson G, Seo M, Berk M, Carvalho AF, Maes M. 'Gut permeability and microbiota in Parkinson's disease: role of depression, tryptophan catabolites, oxidative and nitrosative stress and melatonergic pathways', *Curr Pharm Des.* 2016; 22: 6142–6151. doi: 10.2174/1381612822666160 906161513

Sporn MB, Liby KT. 'NRF2 and cancer: the good, the bad and the importance of context', *Nat Rev Cancer.* 2012; 12: 564–571. doi: 10.1038/nrc3278

Buendia I, Michalska P, Navarro E, Gameiro I, Egea J, León R. 'Nrf2-ARE pathway: An emerging target against oxidative stress and neuroinflammation in neurodegenerative diseases', *Pharmacol Ther.* 2016 Jan; 157: 84–104. doi: 10.1016/j.pharmthera.2015.11.003. Epub 2015 Nov 23. PMID: 26617217

Childs A, Jacobs C, Kaminski T, Halliwell B, Leeuwenburgh C. 'Supplementation with vitamin C and V-acetyl-cysteine increases oxidative stress in humans after an acute muscle injury induced by eccentric exercise', *Free Radic Biol Med.* 2001; 31: 745–53. doi: 10.1016/S0891-5849(01)00640-2

Bast A, Haenen GR. 'Ten misconceptions about antioxidants', *Trends Pharmacol Sci.* 2013 Aug; 34(8): 430–6. doi: 10.1016/j.tips.2013.05.010. Epub 2013 Jun 24. PMID: 23806765

Park S-J, Myung S-K, Lee Y, Lee Y-J. 'Effects of Vitamin and Antioxidant Supplements in Prevention of Bladder Cancer: a Meta-Analysis of Randomized Controlled Trials', *Journal of Korean Medical Science.* 2017; 32: 628. doi: 10.3346/jkms.2017.32.4.628

Krinsky NI, Johnson EJ. 'Carotenoid actions and their relation to health and disease', *Mol Aspects Med.* 2005; 26: 459–516 [PubMed: 16309738]

El-Agamey A, Lowe GM, McGarvey DJ, et al. 'Carotenoid radical chemistry and antioxidant/prooxidant properties', *Arch Biochem Biophys.* 2004; 430: 37–48 [PubMed: 15325910]

Bach Knudsen KE, Lærke HN, Hedemann MS, Nielsen TS, Ingerslev AK, Gundelund Nielsen DS, Theil PK, Purup S, Hald S, Schioldan AG, Marco ML, Gregersen S, Hermansen K. 'Impact of Diet-Modulated Butyrate Production on Intestinal Barrier Function and Inflammation', *Nutrients.* 2018 Oct 13; 10(10): 1499. doi: 10.3390/nu10101499. PMID: 30322146; PMCID: PMC6213552

Brown isn't such a good colour
Uribarri J, Woodruff S, Goodman S, Cai W, Chen X, Pyzik R, Yong A, Striker GE, Vlassara H. 'Advanced glycation end products in foods and a practical guide to their reduction in the diet', *J Am Diet Assoc.* 2010 Jun; 110(6): 911–16. e12. doi: 10.1016/j.jada.2010.03.018. PMID: 20497781; PMCID: PMC3704564
Kim NY, Goddard TN, Sohn S, Spiegel DA, Crawford JM. 'Biocatalytic Reversal of Advanced Glycation End Product Modification', *Chembiochem.* 2019 Sep 16; 20(18): 2402–2410. doi: 10.1002/cbic.201900158. Epub 2019 Aug 9. PMID: 31013547; PMCID: PMC6768434
Wautier MP, Guillausseau PJ, Wautier JL. 'Activation of the receptor for advanced glycation end products and consequences on health', *Diabetes Metab Syndr.* 2017 Oct–Dec; 11(4): 305–309. doi: 10.1016/j.dsx.2016.09.009. Epub 2016 Sep 4. PMID: 27612394
Ruiz HH, Ramasamy R, Schmidt AM. 'Advanced Glycation End Products: Building on the Concept of the "Common Soil" in Metabolic Disease', *Endocrinology.* 2020 Jan 1; 161(1): bqz006. doi: 10.1210/endocr/bqz006. PMID: 31638645; PMCID: PMC7188081
Spauwen PJ, van Eupen MG, Köhler S, Stehouwer CD, Verhey FR, van der Kallen CJ, Sep SJ, Koster A, Schaper NC, Dagnelie PC, Schalkwijk CG, Schram MT, van Boxtel MP. 'Associations of advanced glycation end-products with cognitive functions in individuals with and without type 2 diabetes: the maastricht study', *J Clin Endocrinol Metab.* 2015 Mar; 100(3): 951–60. doi: 10.1210/jc.2014-2754. Epub 2014 Dec 2. PMID: 25459912
Hanssen NM, Beulens JW, van Dieren S, Scheijen JL, van der A DL, Spijkerman AM, van der Schouw YT, Stehouwer CD, Schalkwijk CG. 'Plasma advanced glycation end products are associated with incident cardiovascular events in individuals with type 2 diabetes: a case-cohort study with a median follow-up of 10 years (EPIC-NL)', *Diabetes.* 2015 Jan; 64(1): 257–65. doi: 10.2337/db13-1864. Epub 2014 May 21. PMID: 24848072

Immune boosters, *Pulp Fiction* and *The Sopranos*
Cohen J. 'Waning immunity', *Science.* 2019 Apr 19; 364(6437): 224–227. doi: 10.1126/science.364.6437.224. Epub 2019 Apr 18. PMID: 31000646
Campbell JP, Turner JE. 'Debunking the Myth of Exercise-Induced Immune Suppression: Redefining the Impact of Exercise on Immunological Health Across the Lifespan', *Front Immunol.* 2018 Apr 16; 9: 648. doi: 10.3389/fimmu.2018.00648. PMID: 29713319; PMCID: PMC5911985
Miller LE, Lehtoranta L, Lehtinen MJ. 'Short-term probiotic supplementation enhances cellular immune function in healthy elderly: systematic review and meta-analysis of controlled studies', *Nutr Res.* 2019 Apr; 64: 1–8. doi: 10.1016/j.nutres.2018.12.011. Epub 2018 Dec 28. PMID: 30802719
Gui Q, Wang A, Zhao X, et al. 'Effects of probiotic supplementation on natural killer cell function in healthy elderly individuals: a meta-analysis of randomized controlled trials', *Eur J Clin Nutr.* 2020; 74: 1630–1637. https://doi.org/10.1038/s41430-020-0670-z
Jasiulionis MG. 'Abnormal Epigenetic Regulation of Immune System during Aging', *Front Immunol.* 2018 Feb 12; 9: 197. doi: 10.3389/fimmu.2018.00197. PMID: 29483913; PMCID: PMC5816044
Dhabhar FS. 'Effects of stress on immune function: the good, the bad, and the beautiful', *Immunol Res.* 2014 May; 58(2-3): 193–210. doi: 10.1007/s12026-014-8517-0. PMID: 24798553
Soldati L, Di Renzo L, Jirillo E, Ascierto PA, Marincola FM, De Lorenzo A. 'The influence of diet on anti-cancer immune responsiveness', *J Transl Med.* 2018 Mar 20; 16(1): 75. doi: 10.1186/s12967-018-1448-0. PMID: 29558945; PMCID: PMC5859494
Mayr HL, Itsiopoulos C, Tierney AC, Ruiz-Canela M, Hebert JR, Shivappa N, Thomas CJ. 'Improvement in dietary inflammatory index score after 6-month dietary intervention is associated with reduction in interleukin-6 in patients with coronary heart disease: The AUSMED heart trial', *Nutr Res.* 2018 Jul; 55: 108–121. doi: 10.1016/j.nutres.2018.04.007. Epub 2018 Apr 25. PMID: 29807669
Mayr HL, Thomas CJ, Tierney AC, Kucianski T, George ES, Ruiz-Canela M, Hebert JR, Shivappa

N, Itsiopoulos C. 'Randomization to 6-month Mediterranean diet compared with a low-fat diet leads to improvement in Dietary Inflammatory Index scores in patients with coronary heart disease: the AUSMED Heart Trial', *Nutr Res.* 2018 Jul; 55: 94–107. doi: 10.1016/j. nutres.2018.04.006. Epub 2018 Apr 14. PMID: 29754829

García-Calzón S, Zalba G, Ruiz-Canela M, Shivappa N, Hébert JR, Martínez JA, Fitó M, Gómez-Gracia E, Martínez-González MA, Marti A. 'Dietary inflammatory index and telomere length in subjects with a high cardiovascular disease risk from the PREDIMED-NAVARRA study: cross-sectional and longitudinal analyses over 5 y', *Am J Clin Nutr.* 2015 Oct; 102(4): 897–904. doi: 10.3945/ajcn.115.116863. Epub 2015 Sep 9. PMID: 26354530; PMCID: PMC4588745

Bodén S, Wennberg M, Van Guelpen B, Johansson I, Lindahl B, Andersson J, Shivappa N, Hebert JR, Nilsson LM. 'Dietary inflammatory index and risk of first myocardial infarction; a prospective population-based study', *Nutr J.* 2017 Apr 4; 16(1): 21. doi: 10.1186/s12937-017-0243-8. PMID: 28376792; PMCID: PMC5379659

Is butter that bad? The dairy paradox

Forouhi NG, Krauss RM, Taubes G, Willett W. 'Dietary fat and cardiometabolic health: evidence, controversies, and consensus for guidance', *BMJ.* 2018; 316: k2139. doi:10.1136/bmj.k2139

Appel LJ, Van Horn L. 'Did the PREDIMED trial test a Mediterranean diet?' *N Engl J Med.* 2013 Apr 4; 368(14): 1353–4. doi: 10.1056/NEJMe1301582. PMID: 23550674

Pimpin L, Wu JHY, Haskelberg H, Del Gobbo L, Mozaffarian D. 'Is Butter Back? A Systematic Review and Meta-Analysis of Butter Consumption and Risk of Cardiovascular Disease, Diabetes, and Total Mortality', *PLoS ONE.* 2016; 11(6): e0158118. https://doi.org/10.1371/journal.pone.0158118

Qin L-Q, Xu J-Y, Han S-F, Zhang Z-L, Zhao Y-Y, Szeto IM. 'Dairy consumption and risk of cardiovascular disease: An updated meta-analysis of prospective cohort studies', *Asia Pacific Journal of Clinical Nutrition.* 2015; 24(1): 90–100

O'Sullivan TA, Hafekost K, Mitrou F, Lawrence D. 'Food sources of saturated fat and the association with mortality: a meta-analysis', *Am J Public Health.* 2013 Sep; 103(9): e31–42. doi: 10.2105/AJPH.2013.301492. Epub 2013 Jul 18. PMID: 23865702; PMCID: PMC3966685

Teng M, Zhao YJ, Khoo AL, Yeo TC, Yong QW, Lim BP. 'Impact of coconut oil consumption on cardiovascular health: a systematic review and meta-analysis', *Nutr Rev.* 2020 Mar 1; 78(3): 249–259. doi: 10.1093/nutrit/nuz074. PMID: 31769848

Khaw KT, Sharp SJ, Finikarides L, Afzal I, Lentjes M, Luben R, Forouhi NG. 'Randomised trial of coconut oil, olive oil or butter on blood lipids and other cardiovascular risk factors in healthy men and women', *BMJ Open.* 2018 Mar 6; 8(3): e020167. doi: 10.1136/bmjopen-2017-020167. PMID: 29511019; PMCID: PMC5855206

https://fingertips.phe.org.uk/profile/tobacco-control

www.nhs.uk/conditions/nhs-health-check/your-nhs-health-check-results-and-action-plan – QRISK

Which milk? (This is the farting bit)

Vanga SK, Raghavan V. 'How well do plant based alternatives fare nutritionally compared to cow's milk?', *J Food Sci Technol.* 2018 Jan; 55(1): 10–20. doi: 10.1007/s13197-017-2915-y. Epub 2017 Nov 2. PMID: 29358791; PMCID: PMC5756203

Rivas M, Garay RP, Escanero JF, Cia P Jr, Cia P, Alda JO. 'Soya Milk Lowers Blood Pressure in Men and Women with Mild to Moderate Essential Hypertension', *The Journal of Nutrition.* July 2002; volume 132, issue 7, pp. 1900–1902. https://doi.org/10.1093/jn/132.7.1900

Zhao Y, Martin BR, Weaver CM. 'Calcium Bioavailability of Calcium Carbonate Fortified Soyamilk Is Equivalent to Cow's Milk in Young Women', *The Journal of Nutrition.* October 2005; volume 135, issue 10, pp. 2379–2382. https://doi.org/10.1093/jn/135.10.2379

https://theconversation.com/soya-versus-dairy-which-milk-is-better-for-you-9379

Önning G, Åkesson B, Öste R, Lundquist I. 'Effects of Consumption of Oat Milk, Soya Milk, or Cow's Milk on Plasma Lipids and Antioxidative Capacity in Healthy Subjects', *Ann Nutr Metab.* 1998; 42: 211–220. doi: 10.1159/000012736

https://www.health.harvard.edu/staying-healthy/plant-milk-or-cows-milk-which-is-better-for-you

https://theconversation.com/soya-versus-dairy-whats-the-footprint-of-milk-8498

Singhal S, Baker RD, Baker SS. 'A Comparison of the Nutritional Value of Cow's Milk and Nondairy

Beverages', *Journal of Pediatric Gastroenterology and Nutrition*. May 2017; volume 64, issue 5, pp. 799–805. doi: 10.1097/MPG.0000000000001380

Swagerty DL Jr, Walling AD, Klein RM. 'Lactose intolerance', *Am Fam Physician*. 2002 May 1; 65(9): 1845–50. Erratum in: *Am Fam Physician*. 2003 Mar 15; 67(6): 1195. PMID: 12018807

Our salt addiction (well, mine at least)

https://www.heartfoundation.org.au/health-professional-tools/sodium-and-salt-converter?gclid=Cj0K CQjwzbv7BRDIARIsAM-A6-0wmul9XZDWXj6faimxu3QLrRYbpCfqiz2rhQGVUMGmSorFiU ElPSUaAuy3EALw_wcB

www.nhs.uk/Livewell/Goodfood/Documents/having-too-much-salt-survival-guide

Land MA, Neal BC, Johnson C, Nowson CA, Margerison C, Petersen KS. 'Salt consumption by Australian adults: a systematic review and meta-analysis', *Med J Aust*. 2018 Feb 5; 208(2): 75–81. doi: 10.5694/mja17.00394. PMID: 29385968

Fang X, Wei J, He X, An P, Wang H, Jiang L, Shao D, Liang H, Li Y, Wang F, Min J. 'Landscape of dietary factors associated with risk of gastric cancer: A systematic review and dose-response meta-analysis of prospective cohort studies', *Eur J Cancer*. 2015 Dec; 51(18): 2820–32. doi: 10.1016/j. ejca.2015.09.010. Epub 2015 Nov 14. PMID: 26589974

Scrivo R, Perricone C, Altobelli A, Castellani C, Tinti L, Conti F, Valesini G. 'Dietary Habits Bursting into the Complex Pathogenesis of Autoimmune Diseases: The Emerging Role of Salt from Experimental and Clinical Studies', *Nutrients*. 2019 May 5; 11(5): 1013. doi: 10.3390/nu11051013. PMID: 31060286; PMCID: PMC6566149

Sharif K, Amital H, Shoenfeld Y. 'The role of dietary sodium in autoimmune diseases: The salty truth', *Autoimmun Rev*. 2018 Nov; 17(11): 1069–1073. doi: 10.1016/j.autrev.2018.05.007. Epub 2018 Sep 11. Erratum in: *Autoimmun Rev*. 2019 Feb; 18(2): 214. PMID: 30213699

Wang XQ, Terry PD, Yan H. 'Review of salt consumption and stomach cancer risk: epidemiological and biological evidence', *World J Gastroenterol*. 2009 May 14; 15(18): 2204–13. doi: 10.3748/ wjg.15.2204. PMID: 19437559; PMCID: PMC2682234

Grillo A, Salvi L, Coruzzi P, Salvi P, Parati G. 'Sodium Intake and Hypertension', *Nutrients*. 2019 Aug 21; 11(9): 1970. doi: 10.3390/nu11091970. PMID: 31438636; PMCID: PMC6770596

D'Elia L, Rossi G, Ippolito R, Cappuccio FP, Strazzullo P. 'Habitual salt intake and risk of gastric cancer: a meta-analysis of prospective studies', *Clin Nutr*. 2012 Aug; 31(4): 489–98. doi: 10.1016/j. clnu.2012.01.003. Epub 2012 Jan 31. PMID: 22296873

Brook RD, Appel LJ, Rubenfire M, Ogedegbe G, Bisognano JD, Elliott WJ, Fuchs FD, Hughes JW, Lackland DT, Staffileno BA, Townsend RR, Rajagopalan S; American Heart Association Professional Education Committee of the Council for High Blood Pressure Research, Council on Cardiovascular and Stroke Nursing, Council on Epidemiology and Prevention, and Council on Nutrition, Physical Activity. 'Beyond medications and diet: alternative approaches to lowering blood pressure: a scientific statement from the American Heart Association', *Hypertension*. 2013 Jun; 61(6): 1360–83. doi: 10.1161/HYP.0b013e318293645f. Epub 2013 Apr 22. PMID: 23608661

Mozaffarian D, Fahimi S, Singh GM, Micha R, Khatibzadeh S, Engell RE, Lim S, Danaei G, Ezzati M, Powles J; Global Burden of Diseases Nutrition and Chronic Diseases Expert Group. 'Global sodium consumption and death from cardiovascular causes', *N Engl J Med*. 2014 Aug 14; 371(7): 624–34. doi: 10.1056/NEJMoa1304127. PMID: 25119608

Powles J, Fahimi S, Micha R, Khatibzadeh S, Shi P, Ezzati M, Engell RE, Lim SS, Danaei G, Mozaffarian D; Global Burden of Diseases Nutrition and Chronic Diseases Expert Group (NutriCoDE). 'Global, regional and national sodium intakes in 1990 and 2010: a systematic analysis of 24 h urinary sodium excretion and dietary surveys worldwide', *BMJ Open*. 2013 Dec 23; 3(12): e003733. doi: 10.1136/bmjopen-2013-003733. PMID: 24366578; PMCID: PMC3884590

Kendig MD, Morris MJ. 'Reviewing the effects of dietary salt on cognition: mechanisms and future directions', *Asia Pac J Clin Nutr*. 2019; 28(1): 6–14. doi: 10.6133/apjcn.201903_28(1).0002. PMID: 30896408

Faraco G, Hochrainer K, Segarra SG, Schaeffer S, Santisteban MM, Menon A, Jiang H, Holtzman DM, Anrather J, Iadecola C. 'Dietary salt promotes cognitive impairment through tau phosphorylation', *Nature*. 2019 Oct; 574(7780): 686–690. doi: 10.1038/s41586-019-1688-z. Epub 2019 Oct 23. Erratum in: *Nature*. 2020 Feb; 578(7793): E9. PMID: 31645758; PMCID: PMC7380655

Mariutti LR, Bragagnolo N. 'Influence of salt on lipid oxidation in meat and seafood products: A review', *Food Res Int.* 2017 Apr; 94: 90–100. doi: 10.1016/j.foodres.2017.02.003. Epub 2017 Feb 8. PMID: 28290372

Emorine M, Septier C, Andriot I, Martin C, Salles C, Thomas-Danguin T. 'Combined heterogeneous distribution of salt and aroma in food enhances salt perception', *Food Funct.* 2015 May; 6(5): 1449–59. doi: 10.1039/c4fo01067a. PMID: 25856503

Our sugar addiction (yours and mine)
Prinz P. 'The role of dietary sugars in health: molecular composition or just calories?', *Eur J Clin Nutr.* 2019; 73: 1216–1223. https://doi.org/10.1038/s41430-019-0407-z

Hu FB. 'Resolved: there is sufficient scientific evidence that decreasing sugar-sweetened beverage consumption will reduce the prevalence of obesity and obesity-related diseases', *Obes Rev.* 2013 Aug; 14(8): 606–19. doi: 10.1111/obr.12040. Epub 2013 Jun 13. PMID: 23763695; PMCID: PMC5325726

DiNicolantonio JJ, O'Keefe JH, Wilson WL. 'Sugar addiction: is it real? A narrative review', *Br J Sports Med.* 2018 Jul; 52(14): 910–913. doi: 10.1136/bjsports-2017-097971. Epub 2017 Aug 23. PMID: 28835408

Pearlman M, Obert J, Casey L. 'The Association Between Artificial Sweeteners and Obesity', *Curr Gastroenterol Rep.* 2017 Nov 21; 19(12): 64. doi: 10.1007/s11894-017-0602-9. PMID: 29159583

Bian X, Chi L, Gao B, Tu P, Ru H, Lu K. 'The artificial sweetener acesulfame potassium affects the gut microbiome and body weight gain in CD-1 mice', *PLoS ONE.* 2017; 12(6): e0178426. https://doi.org/10.1371/journal. pone.0178426

Suez J, Korem T, Zeevi D, et al. 'Artificial sweeteners induce glucose intolerance by altering the gut microbiota', *Nature.* 2014; 514: 181–186. https://doi.org/10.1038/nature13793

Blundell JE, Hill AJ. 'Paradoxical effects of an intense sweetener (aspartame) on appetite', *Lancet.* 1986; 1(8489): 1092–3 [PubMed: 2871354]

Fowler SP, Williams K, Resendez RG, et al. 'Fueling the obesity epidemic? Artificially sweetened beverage use and long-term weight gain', *Obesity.* 2008; 16(8): 1894–900 [PubMed: 18535548]

Stellman SD, Garfinkel L. 'Artificial sweetener use and one-year weight change among women', *Prev Med.* 1986; 15(2): 195–202 [PubMed: 3714671] 13

Colditz GA, Willett WC, Stampfer MJ, et al. 'Patterns of weight change and their relation to diet in a cohort of healthy women', *Am J Clin Nutr.* 1990; 51(6): 1100–5 [PubMed: 2349925]

Duffey KJ, Popkin BM. 'Adults with healthier dietary patterns have healthier beverage patterns', *J Nutr.* 2006; 136(11): 2901–7 [PubMed: 17056820]

Lutsey PL, Steffen LM, Stevens J. 'Dietary intake and the development of the metabolic syndrome: the Atherosclerosis Risk in Communities study', *Circulation.* 2008; 117(6): 754–61 [PubMed: 18212291]

Enhanced foods – be careful what you wish for
Wanyama R, Gödecke T, Jager M and Qaim M. 'Poor consumers' preferences for nutritionally enhanced foods' *British Food Journal.* 2019 121(3): 755–770. https://doi.org/10.1108/BFJ-09-2018-0622

Hasler CM, Brown AC, American Dietetic Association. 'Position of the American Dietetic Association: functional foods' *Journal of the American Dietetic Association.* 2009 Apr; 109(4):735–746. DOI: 10.1016/j.jada.2009.02.023

Marinangeli CP, Jones PJ. 'Gazing into the crystal ball: future considerations for ensuring sustained growth of the functional food and nutraceutical marketplace' *Nutr Res Rev.* 2013 Jun; 26(1):12–21. doi: 10.1017/S0954422412000236

Saing S, Haywood P, van der Linden N, Manipis K, Meshcheriakova E, Goodall S. 'Real-world cost effectiveness of mandatory folic acid fortification of bread-making flour in Australia' *Appl Health Econ Health Policy.* 2019 Apr; 17(2):243–254. doi: 10.1007/s40258-018-00454-3. PMID: 30617458

D'Antoine H, Bower C, 'Folate status and neural tube defects in Aboriginal Australians: the success of mandatory fortification in reducing a health disparity' *Current Developments in Nutrition,* 2019 Aug; 3(8). https://doi.org/10.1093/cdn/nzz071

www.gov.uk/government/consultations/adding-folic-acid-to-flour/proposal-to-add-folic-acid-to-flour-consultation-document

www.bda.uk.com/resource/vitamin-d

www.gov.uk/government/publications/health-matters-reproductive-health-and-pregnancy-planning/
health-matters-reproductive-health-and-pregnancy-planning

Okay, I've held off this long … time for the microbiome

Ong TG, Gordon M, Banks SS, Thomas MR, Akobeng AK. 'Probiotics to prevent infantile colic',
Cochrane Database Syst Rev. 2019 Mar 13; 3(3): CD012473. doi: 10.1002/14651858.CD012473.
pub2. PMID: 30865287; PMCID: PMC6415699

Liu H, Wang J, He T, Becker S, Zhang G, Li D, Ma X. 'Butyrate: A Double-Edged Sword for Health?'
Adv Nutr. 2018 Jan 1; 9(1): 21–29. doi: 10.1093/advances/nmx009. PMID: 29438462; PMCID:
PMC6333934

Parker EA, Roy T, D'Adamo CR, Wieland LS. 'Probiotics and gastrointestinal conditions: An overview
of evidence from the Cochrane Collaboration', *Nutrition.* 2018 Jan; 45: 125–134. e11. doi:
10.1016/j.nut.2017.06.024. Epub 2017 Jul 6. PMID: 28870406; PMCID: PMC5683921

Abid MB, Koh CJ. 'Probiotics in health and disease: fooling Mother Nature?', *Infection.* 2019; 47: 911–
917. https://doi.org/10.1007/s15010-019-01351-0

Bagga D, Reichert JL, Koschutnig K, Aigner CS, Holzer P, Koskinen K, Moissl-Eichinger C, Schöpf
V. 'Probiotics drive gut microbiome triggering emotional brain signatures', *Gut Microbes.*
2018; 9: 6, 486–496, doi: 10.1080/19490976.2018.1460015

Wilmes L, Collins JM, O'Riordan KJ, O'Mahony SM, Cryan JF, Clarke G. 'Of bowels, brain and
behavior: A role for the gut microbiota in psychiatric comorbidities in irritable bowel
syndrome', *Neurogastroenterology & Motility.* 2021; 33: e14095. https://doi.org/10.1111/
nmo.14095

Chahwan B, Kwan S, Isik A, van Hemert S, Burke C, Roberts L. 'Gut feelings: A randomised, triple-
blind, placebo-controlled trial of probiotics for depressive symptoms', *J Affect Disord.* 2019 Jun
15; 253: 317–326. doi: 10.1016/j.jad.2019.04.097. Epub 2019 May 9. PMID: 31078831

Forsythe P, Sudo N, Dinan T, Taylor VH, Bienenstock J. 'Mood and gut feelings', *Brain Behav
Immun.* 2010 Jan; 24(1): 9–16. doi: 10.1016/j.bbi.2009.05.058. Epub 2009 May 28. PMID:
19481599

Desbonnet L, Garrett L, Clarke G, Bienenstock J, Dinan TG. 'The probiotic *Bifidobacteria infantis*: An
assessment of potential antidepressant properties in the rat', *J Psychiatr Res.* 2008 Dec; 43(2):
164–74. Epub 2008 May 5

Bienenstock J, Kunze W, Forsythe P. 'Microbiota and the gut–brain axis', *Nutrition Reviews.* 1 August
2015; volume 73, issue suppl_1, pp. 28–31. https://doi.org/10.1093/nutrit/nuv019

Bravo JA, Forsythe P, Chew MV, Escaravage E, Savignac HM, Dinan TG, Bienenstock J, Cryan JF.
'Ingestion of *Lactobacillus* strain regulates emotional behavior and central GABA receptor
expression in a mouse via the vagus nerve', *Proc Natl Acad Sci USA.* 2011 Sep 20; 108(38):
16050–5. doi: 10.1073/pnas.1102999108. Epub 2011 Aug 29. PMID: 21876150; PMCID:
PMC3179073

Champagne-Jorgensen K, Kunze WA, Forsythe P, Bienenstock J, McVey Neufeld KA. 'Antibiotics and
the nervous system: More than just the microbes?', *Brain Behav Immun.* 2019 Mar; 77: 7–15.
doi: 10.1016/j.bbi.2018.12.014. Epub 2018 Dec 21. PMID: 30582961

Du X, Wang L, Wu S, Yuan L, Tang S, Xiang Y, Qu X, Liu H, Qin X, Liu C. 'Efficacy of probiotic
supplementary therapy for asthma, allergic rhinitis, and wheeze: a meta-analysis of
randomized controlled trials', *Allergy Asthma Proc.* 2019 Jul 1; 40(4): 250–260. doi: 10.2500/
aap.2019.40.4227. PMID: 31262380

Hagan T, et al. 'Antibiotics-Driven Gut Microbiome Perturbation Alters Immunity to Vaccines in
Humans', *Cell.* 2019; volume 178, issue 6, pp. 1313–1328, e13. ISSN 0092-8674. https://doi.
org/10.1016/j.cell.2019.08.010

Becattini S, Taur Y, Pamer EG. 'Antibiotic-Induced Changes in the Intestinal Microbiota and Disease',
Trends Mol Med. 2016 Jun; 22(6): 458–478. doi: 10.1016/j.molmed.2016.04.003. Epub 2016 May
10. PMID: 27178527; PMCID: PMC4885777

Dethlefsen L, Relman DA. 'Incomplete recovery and individualized responses of the human distal
gut microbiota to repeated antibiotic perturbation', *Proc Natl Acad Sci USA.* 2011 Mar 15; 108
Suppl 1(Suppl 1): 4554–61. doi: 10.1073/pnas.1000087107. Epub 2010 Sep 16. PMID: 20847294;
PMCID: PMC3063582

Modi SR, Collins JJ, Relman DA. 'Antibiotics and the gut microbiota', *J Clin Invest.* 2014 Oct; 124(10):

4212–8. doi: 10.1172/JCI72333. Epub 2014 Oct 1. PMID: 25271726; PMCID: PMC4191029

Patel RM, Underwood MA. 'Probiotics and necrotizing enterocolitis', *Semin Pediatr Surg.* 2018 Feb; 27(1): 39–46. doi: 10.1053/j.sempedsurg.2017.11.008. Epub 2017 Nov 6. PMID: 29275816; PMCID: PMC5844696

Cryan JF, O'Riordan KJ, Sandhu K, Peterson V, Dinan TG. 'The gut microbiome in neurological disorders', *Lancet Neurol.* 2020 Feb; 19(2): 179–194. doi: 10.1016/S1474-4422(19)30356-4. Epub 2019 Nov 18. PMID: 31753762

Dalton A, Mermier C, Zuhl M. 'Exercise influence on the microbiome–gut–brain axis', *Gut Microbes.* 2019; 10: 5, 555–568. doi: 10.1080/19490976.2018.1562268

Weingarden AR, Vaughn BP. 'Intestinal microbiota, fecal microbiota transplantation, and inflammatory bowel disease', *Gut Microbes.* 2017; 8: 3, 238–252. doi: 10.1080/19490976.2017.1290757

Crovesy L, Ostrowski M, Ferreira D, et al. 'Effect of *Lactobacillus* on body weight and body fat in overweight subjects: a systematic review of randomized controlled clinical trials', *Int J Obes.* 2017; 41: 1607–1614. https://doi.org/10.1038/ijo.2017.161

Adan RAH, van der Beek EM, Buitelaar JK, Cryan JF, Hebebrand J, Higgs S, Schellekens H, Dickson SL. 'Nutritional psychiatry: Towards improving mental health by what you eat', *Eur Neuropsychopharmacol.* 2019 Dec; 29(12): 1321–1332. doi: 10.1016/j.euroneuro.2019.10.011. Epub 2019 Nov 14. PMID: 31735529

Ford AC, Quigley EM, Lacy BE, Lembo AJ, Saito YA, Schiller LR, Soffer EE, Spiegel BM, Moayyedi P. 'Efficacy of prebiotics, probiotics, and synbiotics in irritable bowel syndrome and chronic idiopathic constipation: systematic review and meta-analysis', *Am J Gastroenterol.* 2014 Oct; 109(10): 1547–61; quiz 1546, 1562. doi: 10.1038/ajg.2014.202. Epub 2014 Jul 29. PMID: 25070051

Heintz-Buschart A, Wilmes P. 'Human Gut Microbiome: Function Matters', *Trends Microbiol.* 2018 Jul; 26(7): 563–574. doi: 10.1016/j.tim.2017.11.002. Epub 2017 Nov 22. PMID: 29173869

Temraz S, Nassar F, Nasr R, Charafeddine M, Mukherji D, Shamseddine A. 'Gut Microbiome: A Promising Biomarker for Immunotherapy in Colorectal Cancer', *Int J Mol Sci.* 2019 Aug 25; 20(17): 4155. doi: 10.3390/ijms20174155. PMID: 31450712; PMCID: PMC6747470

Winter G, Hart RA, Charlesworth RPG, Sharpley CF. 'Gut microbiome and depression: what we know and what we need to know', *Rev Neurosci.* 2018 Aug 28; 29(6): 629–643. doi: 10.1515/revneuro-2017-0072. PMID: 29397391

Li W, Deng Y, Chu Q, Zhang P. 'Gut microbiome and cancer immunotherapy', *Cancer Lett.* 2019 Apr 10; 447: 41–47. doi: 10.1016/j.canlet.2019.01.015. Epub 2019 Jan 23. PMID: 30684593

Chaput N, et al. 'Baseline gut microbiota predicts clinical response and colitis in metastatic melanoma patients treated with ipilimumab', *Ann Oncol.* 2017 Jun 1; 28(6): 1368–1379. doi: 10.1093/annonc/mdx108. Erratum in: *Ann Oncol.* 2019 Dec 1; 30(12): 2012. Erratum in: *Ann Oncol.* 2019 Dec; 30(12): 2012. PMID: 28368458

Vallianou N, Stratigou T, Christodoulatos GS, Dalamaga M. 'Understanding the Role of the Gut Microbiome and Microbial Metabolites in Obesity and Obesity-Associated Metabolic Disorders: Current Evidence and Perspectives', *Curr Obes Rep.* 2019 Sep; 8(3): 317–332. doi: 10.1007/s13679-019-00352-2. PMID: 31175629

Lee CJ, Sears CL, Maruthur N. 'Gut microbiome and its role in obesity and insulin resistance', *Ann NY Acad Sci.* 2020 Feb; 1461(1): 37–52. doi: 10.1111/nyas.14107. Epub 2019 May 14. PMID: 31087391

Lu QY, Summanen PH, Lee RP, Huang J, Henning SM, Heber D, Finegold SM, Li Z. 'Prebiotic Potential and Chemical Composition of Seven Culinary Spice Extracts', *J Food Sci.* 2017 Aug; 82(8): 1807–1813. doi: 10.1111/1750-3841.13792. Epub 2017 Jul 5. PMID: 28678344; PMCID: PMC5600121

Petrelli F, Ghidini M, Ghidini A, Perego G, Cabiddu M, Khakoo S, Oggionni E, Abeni C, Hahne JC, Tomasello G, Zaniboni A. 'Use of Antibiotics and Risk of Cancer: A Systematic Review and Meta-Analysis of Observational Studies', *Cancers (Basel).* 2019 Aug 14; 11(8): 1174. doi: 10.3390/cancers11081174. PMID: 31416208; PMCID: PMC6721461

Sánchez-Alcoholado L, Ramos-Molina B, Otero A, Laborda-Illanes A, Ordóñez R, Medina JA, Gómez-Millán J, Queipo-Ortuño MI. 'The Role of the Gut Microbiome in Colorectal Cancer Development and Therapy Response', *Cancers (Basel).* 2020 May 29; 12(6): 1406. doi: 10.3390/cancers12061406. PMID: 32486066; PMCID: PMC7352899

DR NORMAN SWAN

You get thirsty for a reason – and don't bottle it up

Hew-Butler T, Rosner MH, Fowkes-Godek S, Dugas JP, Hoffman MD, Lewis DP, Maughan RJ, Miller KC, Montain SJ, Rehrer NJ, Roberts WO, Rogers IR, Siegel AJ, Stuempfle KJ, Winger JM, Verbalis JG. 'Statement of the Third International Exercise-Associated Hyponatremia Consensus Development Conference, Carlsbad, California, 2015', *Clin J Sport Med.* 2015 Jul; 25(4): 303–20. doi: 10.1097/JSM.0000000000000221. PMID: 26102445

https://www.nutrition.org.uk/nutritionscience/life/dehydrationelderly.html

James LJ, Funnell MP, James RM, et al. 'Does Hypohydration Really Impair Endurance Performance? Methodological Considerations for Interpreting Hydration Research', *Sports Med.* 2019; 49: 103–114. https://doi.org/10.1007/s40279-019-01188-5

Beis LY, Willkomm L, Ross R, et al. 'Food and macronutrient intake of elite Ethiopian distance runners', *J Int Soc Sports Nutr.* 2011; 8: 7. https://doi.org/10.1186/1550-2783-8-7

Armstrong LE, Costill DL, Fink WJ. 'Influence of diuretic-induced dehydration on competitive running performance', *Med Sci Sports Exerc.* 1985 Aug; 17(4): 456–61. doi: 10.1249/00005768-198508000-00009. PMID: 4033401

Coyle EF. 'Fluid and fuel intake during exercise', *J Sports Sci.* 2004 Jan; 22(1): 39–55. doi: 10.1080/0264041031000140545. PMID: 14971432

Sui Z, Zheng M, Zhang M, Rangan A. 'Water and Beverage Consumption: Analysis of the Australian 2011–2012 National Nutrition and Physical Activity Survey', *Nutrients.* 2016 Oct 26; 8(11): 678. doi: 10.3390/nu8110678. PMID: 27792184; PMCID: PMC5133066

https://www.nytimes.com/2020/01/04/style/self-care/hydrate-hydrate-hydrate.html

https://www.health.harvard.edu/staying-healthy/how-much-water-should-you-drink

Is the sparkle worth it?

Eweis DS, Abed F, Stiban J. 'Carbon dioxide in carbonated beverages induces ghrelin release and increased food consumption in male rats: Implications on the onset of obesity', *Obes Res Clin Pract.* 2017 Sep-Oct; 11(5): 534–543. doi: 10.1016/j.orcp.2017.02.001. Epub 2017 Feb 20. PMID: 28228348

Sichert-Hellert W, Kersting M. 'Home-made carbonated water and the consumption of water and other beverages in children and adolescents: results of the DONALD study', *Acta Paediatr.* 2004 Dec; 93(12): 1583–7. doi: 10.1080/08035250410033925. PMID: 15841765

Wakisaka S, Nagai H, Mura E, Matsumoto T, Moritani T, Nagai N. 'The effects of carbonated water upon gastric and cardiac activities and fullness in healthy young women', *J Nutr Sci Vitaminol (Tokyo).* 2012; 58(5): 333–8. doi: 10.3177/jnsv.58.333. PMID: 23327968

Cuomo R, Grasso R, Sarnelli G, Capuano G, Nicolai E, Nardone G, Pomponi D, Budillon G, Ierardi E. 'Effects of carbonated water on functional dyspepsia and constipation', *Eur J Gastroenterol Hepatol.* 2002 Sep; 14(9): 991–9. doi: 10.1097/00042737-200209000-00010. PMID: 12352219

Nisell O. 'Does intake of sugarless carbonated water at physical activity cause type 2 diabetes? ', *Acta Physiol (Oxf).* 2013 May; 208(1): 6–8. doi: 10.1111/apha.12035. PMID: 23577668

Morishita M, Mori S, Yamagami S, Mizutani M. 'Effect of carbonated beverages on pharyngeal swallowing in young individuals and elderly inpatients', *Dysphagia.* 2014 Apr; 29(2): 213–22. doi: 10.1007/s00455-013-9493-6. Epub 2013 Oct 30. PMID: 24170038

Schoppen S, Pérez-Granados AM, Carbajal A, de la Piedra C, Pilar Vaquero M. 'Bone remodelling is not affected by consumption of a sodium-rich carbonated mineral water in healthy postmenopausal women', *Br J Nutr.* 2005 Mar; 93(3): 339–44. doi: 10.1079/bjn20041332. PMID: 15877873

Mun JH, Jun SS. 'Effects of carbonated water intake on constipation in elderly patients following a cerebrovascular accident', *J Korean Acad Nurs.* 2011 Apr; 41(2): 269–75. Korean. doi: 10.4040/jkan.2011.41.2.269. PMID: 21551998

Simons CT, Dessirier JM, Carstens MI, O'Mahony M, Carstens E. 'Neurobiological and psychophysical mechanisms underlying the oral sensation produced by carbonated water', *J Neurosci.* 1999 Sep 15; 19(18): 8134–44. doi: 10.1523/JNEUROSCI.19-18-08134.1999. Erratum in: *J Neurosci.* 1999 Nov 15; 19(22): 10191. PMID: 10479713; PMCID: PMC6782458

Koelkebeck KW, Harrison PC, Madindou T. 'Research note: effect of carbonated drinking water on production performance and bone characteristics of laying hens exposed to high environmental temperatures', *Poult Sci.* 1993 Sep; 72(9): 1800–3. doi: 10.3382/ps.0721800. PMID: 8234140

Santos A, Martins MJ, Guimarães JT, Severo M, Azevedo I. 'Sodium-rich carbonated natural mineral water ingestion and blood pressure', *Rev Port Cardiol.* 2010 Feb; 29(2): 159–72. English, Portuguese. PMID: 20545244

Costa-Vieira D, Monteiro R, Martins MJ. 'Metabolic Syndrome Features: Is There a Modulation Role by Mineral Water Consumption? A Review', *Nutrients.* 2019 May 22; 11(5): 1141. doi: 10.3390/nu11051141. PMID: 31121885; PMCID: PMC6566252

Schorr U, Distler A, Sharma AM. 'Effect of sodium chloride- and sodium bicarbonate-rich mineral water on blood pressure and metabolic parameters in elderly normotensive individuals: a randomized double-blind crossover trial', *J Hypertens.* 1996 Jan; 14(1): 131–5. PMID: 12013486

Toxqui L, Vaquero MP. 'Aldosterone changes after consumption of a sodium-bicarbonated mineral water in humans. A four-way randomized controlled trial', *J Physiol Biochem.* 2016 Dec; 72(4): 635–641. doi: 10.1007/s13105-016-0502-8. Epub 2016 Jun 29. PMID: 27356528

Ogoh S, Washio T, Suzuki K, Ikeda K, Hori T, Olesen ND, Muraoka Y. 'Effect of leg immersion in mild warm carbonated water on skin and muscle blood flow', *Physiol Rep.* 2018 Sep; 6(18): e13859. doi: 10.14814/phy2.13859. PMID: 30221833; PMCID: PMC6139710

Caffeine hits

Yang I, Mao Q-X, Xu H-X, Ma X, Zeng C-Y. 'Tea consumption and risk of type 2 diabetes mellitus: a systematic review and meta-analysis update', *BMJ Open.* Jul 2014; 4(7): e005632. doi: 10.1136/bmjopen-2014-005632

van den Brandt PA. 'Coffee or Tea? A prospective cohort study on the associations of coffee and tea intake with overall and cause-specific mortality in men versus women', *Eur J Epidemiol.* 2018; 33: 183–200. https://doi.org/10.1007/s10654-018-0359-y

Leurs LJ, Schouten LJ, Goldbohm RA, van den Brandt PA. 'Total fluid and specific beverage intake and mortality due to IHD and stroke in the Netherlands Cohort Study', *Br J Nutr.* 2010 Oct; 104(8): 1212–21. doi: 10.1017/S0007114510001923. Epub 2010 May 11. PMID: 20456812

Zhang C, Linforth R, Fisk ID. 'Cafestol extraction yield from different coffee brew mechanisms', *Food Research International.* 2012; volume 49, issue 1, pp. 27–31. ISSN 0963-9969. https://doi.org/10.1016/j.foodres.2012.06.032

Urgert R, Schulz AG, Katan MB. 'Effects of cafestol and kahweol from coffee grounds on serum lipids and serum liver enzymes in humans', *The American Journal of Clinical Nutrition.* January 1995; volume 61, issue 1, pp. 149–154. https://doi.org/10.1093/ajcn/61.1.149

White JR Jr, Padowski JM, Zhong Y, Chen G, Luo S, Lazarus P, Layton ME, McPherson S. 'Pharmacokinetic analysis and comparison of caffeine administered rapidly or slowly in coffee chilled or hot versus chilled energy drink in healthy young adults', *Clinical Toxicology.* 2016; 54(4): 308–312. doi: 10.3109/15563650.2016.1146740

Franklin KM, Hauser SR, Bell RL, Engleman EA. 'Caffeinated Alcoholic Beverages – An Emerging Trend in Alcohol Abuse', *J Addict Res Ther.* 2013 Aug 20; Suppl 4: S4–012. doi: 10.4172/2155-6105.S4-012. PMID: 25419478; PMCID: PMC4238293

Bagwath PL. 'Energy Drinks and the Neurophysiological Impact of Caffeine', *Frontiers in Neuroscience.* 2011; volume 5, p. 116. https://www.frontiersin.org/article/10.3389/fnins.2011.00116 doi=10.3389/fnins.2011.00116

Forester SC, Lambert JD. 'The role of antioxidant versus pro-oxidant effects of green tea polyphenols in cancer prevention', *Mol Nutr Food Res.* 2011; 55: 844–854. https://doi.org/10.1002/mnfr.201000641

Fujiki H, Suganuma M, Imai K, Nakachi K. 'Green tea: cancer preventive beverage and/or drug', *Cancer Letters.* 2002; volume 188, issues 1–2, pp. 9–13. ISSN 0304-3835

Jung Y, Kim M, Shin B, et al. 'EGCG, a major component of green tea, inhibits tumour growth by inhibiting VEGF induction in human colon carcinoma cells', *Br J Cancer.* 2001; 84: 844–850. https://doi.org/10.1054/bjoc.2000.1691

Sharangi AB. 'Medicinal and therapeutic potentialities of tea (*Camellia sinensis L.*) – A review', *Food Research International.* 2009; volume 42, issues 5–6, pp. 529–535. ISSN 0963-9969

Luciano M, Kirk KM, Heath AC, Martin NG. 'The genetics of tea and coffee drinking and preference for source of caffeine in a large community sample of Australian twins', *Addiction.* 2005 Oct; 100(10): 1510–7. doi: 10.1111/j.1360-0443.2005.01223.x. PMID: 16185212

Loftfield E, Gunter MJ, Sinha R. 'Coffee and Colorectal Cancer: Is Improved Survival a "Perk" of Coffee

Drinking?', *JAMA Oncol.* 2020; 6(11): 1721–1722. doi: 10.1001/jamaoncol.2020.3313

Mackintosh C, Yuan C, Ou F, et al. 'Association of Coffee Intake With Survival in Patients With Advanced or Metastatic Colorectal Cancer', *JAMA Oncol.* 2020; 6(11): 1713–1721. doi: 10.1001/jamaoncol.2020.3938

van Dam RM, Hu FB, Willett WC. 'Coffee, Caffeine, and Health', *N Engl J Med.* 2020 Jul 23; 383(4): 369–378. doi: 10.1056/NEJMra1816604. PMID: 32706535

Ding M, Satija A, Bhupathiraju SN, Hu Y, Sun Q, Han J, Lopez-Garcia E, Willett W, van Dam RM, Hu FB. 'Association of Coffee Consumption With Total and Cause-Specific Mortality in 3 Large Prospective Cohorts', *Circulation.* 2015 Dec 15; 132(24): 2305–15. doi: 10.1161/CIRCULATIONAHA.115.017341. Epub 2015 Nov 16. PMID: 26572796; PMCID: PMC4679527

Chen ZM, Lin Z. 'Tea and human health: biomedical functions of tea active components and current issues', *J Zhejiang Univ Sci B.* 2015 Feb; 16(2): 87–102. doi: 10.1631/jzus.B1500001. PMID: 25644464; PMCID: PMC4322420

Nurk E, Refsum H, Drevon CA, Tell GS, Nygaard HA, Engedal K, Smith AD. 'Intake of flavonoid-rich wine, tea, and chocolate by elderly men and women is associated with better cognitive test performance', *J Nutr.* 2009 Jan; 139(1): 120–7. doi: 10.3945/jn.108.095182. Epub 2008 Dec 3. PMID: 19056649

Khan N, Mukhtar H. 'Tea and health: studies in humans', *Curr Pharm Des.* 2013; 19(34): 6141–7. doi: 10.2174/1381612811319340008. PMID: 23448443; PMCID: PMC4055352

Khan N, Afaq F, Mukhtar H. 'Cancer chemoprevention through dietary antioxidants: progress and promise', *Antioxid Redox Signal.* 2008 Mar; 10(3): 475–510. doi: 10.1089/ars.2007.1740. PMID: 18154485

Bøhn SK, Ward NC, Hodgson JM, Croft KD. 'Effects of tea and coffee on cardiovascular disease risk', *Food Funct.* 2012 Jun; 3(6): 575–91. doi: 10.1039/c2fo10288a. PMID: 22456725

Goldfarb DS, Fischer ME, Keich Y, Goldberg J. 'A twin study of genetic and dietary influences on nephrolithiasis: a report from the Vietnam Era Twin (VET) Registry', *Kidney Int.* 2005 Mar; 67(3): 1053–61. doi: 10.1111/j.1523-1755.2005.00170.x. PMID: 15698445

Treur JL, Taylor AE, Ware JJ, Nivard MG, Neale MC, McMahon G, Hottenga JJ, Baselmans BML, Boomsma DI, Munafò MR, Vink JM. 'Smoking and caffeine consumption: a genetic analysis of their association', *Addict Biol.* 2017 Jul; 22(4): 1090–1102. doi: 10.1111/adb.12391. Epub 2016 Mar 30. PMID: 27027469; PMCID: PMC5045318

Cornelis MC. 'Genetic determinants of beverage consumption: Implications for nutrition and health', *Adv Food Nutr Res.* 2019; 89: 1–52. doi: 10.1016/bs.afnr.2019.03.001. Epub 2019 Apr 19. PMID: 31351524; PMCID: PMC7047661

Negronis and other alcoholic drinks

Rohsenow DJ, Howland J. 'The role of beverage congeners in hangover and other residual effects of alcohol intoxication: a review', *Curr Drug Abuse Rev.* 2010 Jun; 3(2): 76–9. doi: 10.2174/1874473711003020076. PMID: 20712591

Di Castelnuovo A, Costanzo S, Bagnardi V, Donati MB, Iacoviello L, de Gaetano G. 'Alcohol dosing and total mortality in men and women: an updated meta-analysis of 34 prospective studies', *Arch Intern Med.* 2006 Dec 11–25; 166(22): 2437–45. doi: 10.1001/archinte.166.22.2437. PMID: 17159008

https://www.aihw.gov.au/getmedia/65567981-9e45-48e0-b829-f73a36ee6ff0/aihw-phe-221-AODTSInfographic-YP.pdf.aspx

The Alcohol & Drug Foundation – adf.org.au. https://adf.org.au/insights/harm-reduction-pides/

Slade T, Chapman C, Swift W, Keyes K, Tonks Z, Teesson M. 'Birth cohort trends in the global epidemiology of alcohol use and alcohol-related harms in men and women: systematic review and meta-regression', *BMJ Open.* 2016; 6(10): e011827

Clare PJ, Dobbins T, Bruno R, et al. 'The overall effect of parental supply of alcohol across adolescence on alcohol-related harms in early adulthood—a prospective cohort study', *Addiction.* 2020; 115: 1833–1843

Mewton L, Lees B, Rao Rahul T. 'Lifetime perspective on alcohol and brain health', *BMJ.* 2020; 371: m4691

www.alcoholchange.org.uk/alcohol-facts/fact-sheets/alcohol-statistics

SO YOU THINK YOU KNOW WHAT'S GOOD FOR YOU?

Alcohol and other drugs

Caldwell TM, Rodgers B, Jorm AF, Christensen H, Jacomb PA, Korten AE, Lynskey MT. 'Patterns of association between alcohol consumption and symptoms of depression and anxiety in young adults', *Addiction*. 2002; 97: 583–594

Lees B, Mewton L, Jacobus J, Valadez E, Stapinski L, Teesson M, Tapert S, Squeglia LM. 'Association of Prenatal Alcohol Exposure With Psychological, Behavioral, and Neurodevelopmental Outcomes in Children From the Adolescent Brain Cognitive Development Study', *The American Journal of Psychiatry*. 2020 Nov 1; 177(11):1060–1072

Lees B, Mewton L, Stapinski LA, Teesson M, Squeglia LM. 'Association of prenatal alcohol exposure with preadolescent alcohol sipping in the ABCD Study', *Drug and Alcohol Dependence*. 2020 Sep 1; 214:108–187

Center for Behavioral Health Statistics and Quality. 'Key substance use and mental health indicators in the United States: Results from the 2015 National Survey on Drug Use and Health'. 2016. (HHS Publication No. SMA 16-4984, NSDUH Series H-51)

Di Castelnuovo A, Costanzo S, Bagnardi V, Donati MB, Iacoviello L, de Gaetano G. 'Alcohol dosing and total mortality in men and women: an updated meta-analysis of 34 prospective studies', *Arch Intern Med*. 2006 Dec 11–25; 166(22): 2437–45. doi: 10.1001/archinte.166.22.2437. PMID: 17159008

https://www.aihw.gov.au/getmedia/65567981-9e45-48e0-b829-f73a36ee6ff0/aihw-phe-221-AODTSInfographic-YP.pdf.aspx

https://cracksintheice.org.au/pdf/download/how-many-people-use-ice-summary.pdf

https://cracksintheice.org.au/why-do-people-use-ice

https://cracksintheice.org.au/community-toolkit/webinars/current-and-promising-treatment-options-for-crystal-methamphetamine-dependence

https://ndarc.med.unsw.edu.au/resource/cannabis-related-death-australia

https://ndarc.med.unsw.edu.au/resource/cocaine-0

https://www.ons.gov.uk/peoplepopulationandcommunity/crimeandjustice/articles/drugmisuseinenglandandwales/yearendingmarch2020

www.who.int/news-room/fact-sheets/detail/opioid-overdose

https://www.bmj.com/content/362/bmj.k3208

Supplements for big muscles

http://www.perseus.tufts.edu/Olympics/running.html

Shimko KM, O'Brien JW, Barron L, et al. 'A pilot wastewater-based epidemiology assessment of anabolic steroid use in Queensland, Australia', *Drug Test Anal*. 2019; 11: 937–949. https://doi.org/10.1002/dta.2591

Van de Ven K, Maher L, W and H, Memedovic S, Jackson E, Iversen J. 'Health risk and health seeking behaviours among people who inject performance and image enhancing drugs who access needle syringe programs in Australia', *Drug Alcohol Rev*. 2018 Nov; 37(7): 837–846. doi: 10.1111/dar.12831. Epub 2018 Jul 2. PMID: 29968372

Smit DL, Buijs MM, de Hon O, den Heijer M, de Ronde W. 'Positive and negative side effects of androgen abuse. The HAARLEM study: A one-year prospective cohort study in 100 men' *Scand J Med Sci Sports*. 2021 Feb; 31(2):427–438. doi: 10.1111/sms.13843. Epub 2020 Nov 4. PMID: 33038020

https://www1.racgp.org.au/newsgp/clinical/push-to-measure-steroid-use-in-general-practice

Is testosterone worth taking?

Sartorius G, Spasevska S, Idan A, Turner L, Forbes E, Zamojska A, Allan CA, Ly LP, Conway AJ, McLachlan RI, Handelsman DJ. 'Serum testosterone, dihydrotestosterone and estradiol concentrations in older men self-reporting very good health: the healthy man study', *Clin Endocrinol (Oxf)*. 2012 Nov; 77(5): 755–63. doi: 10.1111/j.1365-2265.2012.04432.x. PMID: 22563890

Yeap BB, Wu FCW. 'Clinical practice update on testosterone therapy for male hypogonadism: Contrasting perspectives to optimize care', *Clin Endocrinol (Oxf)*. 2019 Jan; 90(1): 56–65. doi: 10.1111/cen.13888. Epub 2018 Dec 3. PMID: 30358898

Ford AH, Yeap BB, Flicker L, Hankey GJ, Chubb SAP, Golledge J, Almeida OP. 'Sex hormones and incident dementia in older men: The health in men study', *Psychoneuroendocrinology*. 2018 Dec;

98: 139–147. doi: 10.1016/j.psyneuen.2018.08.013. Epub 2018 Aug 9. PMID: 30144781

Yeap B, Grossmann M, McLachlan R, Handelsman D, Wittert G, Conway A, Stuckey B, Lording D, Allan C, Zajac J, Burger H. 'Endocrine Society of Australia position statement on male hypogonadism (part 2): treatment and therapeutic considerations', *The Medical Journal of Australia*. 2016; 205: 228–231. doi: 10.5694/mja16.00448

Handelsman DJ. 'Testosterone and Male Aging: Faltering Hope for Rejuvenation', *JAMA*. 2017 Feb 21; 317(7): 699–701. doi: 10.1001/jama.2017.0129. PMID: 28241336

Hsu B, Cumming RG, Naganathan V, Blyth FM, Le Couteur DG, Hirani V, Waite LM, Seibel MJ, Handelsman DJ. 'Temporal Changes in Androgens and Estrogens Are Associated With All-Cause and Cause-Specific Mortality in Older Men', *J Clin Endocrinol Metab*. 2016 May; 101(5): 2201–10. doi: 10.1210/jc.2016-1025. Epub 2016 Mar 10. PMID: 26963953

Hirschberg AL, Elings Knutsson J, Helge T, Godhe M, Ekblom M, Bermon S, Ekblom B. 'Effects of moderately increased testosterone concentration on physical performance in young women: a double blind, randomised, placebo controlled study', *Br J Sports Med*. 2020 May; 54(10): 599–604. doi: 10.1136/bjsports-2018-100525. Epub 2019 Oct 15. PMID: 31615775

Zheng J, Islam RM, Skiba MA, Bell RJ, Davis SR. 'Associations between androgens and sexual function in premenopausal women: a cross-sectional study', *Lancet Diabetes Endocrinol*. 2020 Aug; 8(8): 693–702. doi: 10.1016/S2213-8587(20)30239-4. PMID: 32707117

Rowen TS, Davis SR, Parish S, Simon J, Vignozzi L. (2020). 'Methodological Challenges in Studying Testosterone Therapies for Hypoactive Sexual Desire Disorder in Women', *Journal of Sexual Medicine*. 2020; 17(4): 585–594. https://doi.org/10.1016/j.jsxm.2019.12.013

Parish SJ, Hahn SR. 'Hypoactive Sexual Desire Disorder: A Review of Epidemiology, Biopsychology, Diagnosis, and Treatment', *Sex Med Rev*. 2016 Apr; 4(2): 103–120. doi: 10.1016/j.sxmr.2015.11.009. Epub 2016 Feb 6. PMID: 27872021

Chan YX, Knuiman MW, Divitini ML, Handelsman DJ, Beilby JP, Yeap BB. 'Lower Circulating Androgens Are Associated with Overall Cancer Risk and Prostate Cancer Risk in Men Aged 25-84 Years from the Busselton Health Study', *Horm Cancer*. 2018 Dec; 9(6): 391–398. doi: 10.1007/s12672-018-0346-5. Epub 2018 Aug 10. PMID: 30097782

Yeap BB, Knuiman MW, Divitini ML, Handelsman DJ, Beilby JP, Beilin J, McQuillan B, Hung J. 'Differential associations of testosterone, dihydrotestosterone and oestradiol with physical, metabolic and health-related factors in community-dwelling men aged 17–97 years from the Busselton Health Survey', *Clin Endocrinol*. 2014; 81: 100–108. http://dx.doi.org/10.1111/cen.12407

Yeap B. 'Are declining testosterone levels a major risk factor for ill-health in aging men?', *Int J Impot Res*. 2009; 21: 24–36. https://doi.org/10.1038/ijir.2008.60

Sartorius G, Spasevska S, Idan A, Turner L, Forbes E, Zamojska A, Allan C, Ly L, Conway A, McLachlan R, Handelsman DJ. 'Serum Testosterone, Dihydrotestosterone and Estradiol Concentrations in Older Men Self-Reporting Very Good Health: The Healthy Man Study', *Journal of Clinical Endocrinology (Oxf)*. 2012. 1365-2265.2012.04432.x.

Vitamins and mineral supplements

http://www.roymorgan.com/findings/8456-australian-vitamin-market-march-2020-202006290736

https://www.csiro.au/en/News/News-releases/2018/Diets-lacking-in-essential-vitamins-and-minerals

https://foodfoundation.org.uk/wp-content/uploads/2018/10/Affordability-of-the-Eatwell-Guide_Final.pdf

Pilz S, Zittermann A, Trummer C, et al. 'Vitamin D testing and treatment: a narrative review of current evidence', *Endocrine Connections*. 2019 Feb; 8(2): R27–R43. doi: 10.1530/ec-18-0432

https://www.cancercouncil.com.au/wp-content/uploads/2013/04/CAN6647_Viatmin_D.pdf

Miles LM, Allen E, Clarke R, Mills K, Uauy R, Dangour AD. 'Impact of baseline vitamin B12 status on the effect of vitamin B12 supplementation on neurologic function in older people: secondary analysis of data from the OPEN randomised controlled trial', *Eur J Clin Nutr*. 2017 Oct; 71(10): 1166–1172. doi: 10.1038/ejcn.2017.7. Epub 2017 Feb 22. PMID: 28225050

https://www.abc.net.au/radionational/programs/healthreport/vitamin-b12-supplementation/3823160

Kibirige D, Mwebaze R. 'Vitamin B12 deficiency among patients with diabetes mellitus: is routine screening and supplementation justified?', *J Diabetes Metab Disord*. 2013 May 7; 12(1): 17. doi: 10.1186/2251-6581-12-17. PMID: 23651730; PMCID: PMC3649932

Spence JD, Stampfer MJ. 'Understanding the Complexity of Homocysteine Lowering With Vitamins', (Commentary) *JAMA*. December 21, 2011; 306; 23: 2610–2611

House AA, et al. 'Effect of B-Vitamin Therapy on Progression of Diabetic Nephropathy. A Randomized Controlled Trial', *JAMA*. April 28, 2010; 303; 16: 1603–1609

Spence JD. 'Atrial fibrillation, stroke prevention therapy and aging. News & Views', *Nature*. July 2009; 6: 1–2

Spence JD. 'Homocysteine-lowering therapy: a role in stroke prevention?' *Lancet Neurology*. 2007; 7: 830–8

Spence JD, et al. 'Vitamin Intervention for Stroke Prevention Trial: an efficacy analysis', *Stroke*. 2005; 36: 2404–9

Lonn E, Yusuf S, Arnold MJ, Sheridan P, Pogue J, Micks M, McQueen MJ, Probstfield J, Fodor G, Held C, Genest J Jr; Heart Outcomes Prevention Evaluation (HOPE) 2 Investigators. 'Homocysteine lowering with folic acid and B vitamins in vascular disease', *N Engl J Med*. 2006 Apr 13; 354(15): 1567–77. doi: 10.1056/NEJMoa060900. Epub 2006 Mar 12. Erratum in: *N Engl J Med*. 2006 Aug 17; 355(7): 746. PMID: 16531613

Spence JD, et al. 'Vitamin Intervention for Stroke Prevention (VISP) trial: rationale and design', *Neuroepidemiology*. 2001 Feb; 20(1): 16–25

Tummala R, Ghosh RK, Jain V, Devanabanda AR, Bandyopadhyay D, Deedwania P, Aronow WS. 'Fish Oil and Cardiometabolic Diseases: Recent Updates and Controversies', *Am J Med*. 2019 Oct; 132(10): 1153–1159. doi: 10.1016/j.amjmed.2019.04.027. Epub 2019 May 8. PMID: 31077653

Danthiir V, Hosking DE, Nettelbeck T, Vincent AD, Wilson C, O'Callaghan N, Calvaresi E, Clifton P, Wittert GA. 'An 18-mo randomized, double-blind, placebo-controlled trial of DHA-rich fish oil to prevent age-related cognitive decline in cognitively normal older adults', *Am J Clin Nutr*. 2018 May 1; 107(5): 754–762. doi: 10.1093/ajcn/nqx077. PMID: 29722833

Abdelhamid AS, Brown TJ, Brainard JS, Biswas P, Thorpe GC, Moore HJ, Deane KHO, Al Abdulghafoor FK, Summerbell CD, Worthington HV, Song F, Hooper L. 'Omega 3 fatty acids for the primary and secondary prevention of cardiovascular disease', *Cochrane Database of Systematic Reviews*. 2018; issue 7. Art. No.: CD003177. doi: 10.1002/14651858.CD003177.pub3

Part 2: What you take out of yourself – making sure it's not too much

The control factor (this is the stress bit)

D'Souza RM, Stradzins L, Lim L, Broom D, Rodgers B. 'Work and health in a contemporary society: Demands, control and insecurity', *Journal of Epidemiology and Community Health*. 2003; 57: 849–854

Strazdins L, D'Souza RM, Lim LL-Y, Broom DH, Rodgers B. 'Job strain, job insecurity and health: rethinking the relationship', *Journal of Occupational and Health Psychology*. 2004; 9(4): 296–305

D'Souza RM, Strazdins L, Broom DH, Rogders B, Berry H. 'Work demands, job insecurity and sickness absence from work. How productive is the new, flexible labour force?', *Australian and New Zealand Journal of Public Health*. 2006; 30, 3: 205–212

Leach LS, Christensen H, Mackinnon AJ, Windsor TD, Butterworth P. 'Gender differences in depression and anxiety across the adult lifespan: The role of psychosocial mediators', *Social Psychiatry and Psychiatric Epidemiology*. 2008; 43: 983–998

Tsey K. 'The control factor: a neglected social determinant of health', *Lancet*. 2008 Nov 8; 372(9650): 1629. doi: 10.1016/S0140-6736(08)61678-5. PMID: 18994654

https://www.abc.net.au/radionational/programs/healthreport/mastering-the-control-factor-part-one/3566112

https://www.abc.net.au/radionational/programs/healthreport/mastering-the-control-factor-part-two/3554360

https://www.abc.net.au/radionational/programs/healthreport/mastering-the-control-factor-part-three/3554354

https://www.abc.net.au/radionational/programs/healthreport/mastering-the-control-factor-part-four/3554368

https://www.abc.net.au/radionational/programs/healthreport/effects-of-stress-on-the-immune-system/3564390

Health isn't evenly spread

Marmot M. 'Health equity in England: the Marmot review 10 years on', *BMJ*. 2020 Feb 24; 368: m693. doi: 10.1136/bmj.m693. PMID: 32094110

Marmot M. *The Health Gap*. 2015. Bloomsbury: London

Yen IH. 'Historical perspective: S. Leonard Syme's influence on the development of social epidemiology and where we go from there', *Epidemiol Perspect Innov*. 2005 May 25; 2: 3. doi: 10.1186/1742-5573-2-3. PMID: 15916710; PMCID: PMC1175097

Seligman ME, Maier SF, Geer JH. 'Alleviation of learned helplessness in the dog' In: Keehn JD ed. *Origins of Madness*. 1979. Pergamon, pp. 401–409

Adler NE, Boyce WT, Chesney MA, Folkman S, Syme SL. 'Socioeconomic inequalities in health. No easy solution', *JAMA*. 1993 Jun 23–30; 269(24): 3140–5. PMID: 8505817

North FM, Syme SL, Feeney A, Shipley M, Marmot M. 'Psychosocial work environment and sickness absence among British civil servants: the Whitehall II study', *Am J Public Health*. 1996 Mar; 86(3): 332–40. doi: 10.2105/ajph.86.3.332. Erratum in: *Am J Public Health*. 1996 Aug; 86(8 Pt 1): 1093. PMID: 8604757; PMCID: PMC1380513

Kagan A, Harris BR, Winkelstein W Jr, Johnson KG, Kato H, Syme SL, Rhoads GG, Gay ML, Nichaman MZ, Hamilton HB, Tillotson J. 'Epidemiologic studies of coronary heart disease and stroke in Japanese men living in Japan, Hawaii and California: demographic, physical, dietary and biochemical characteristics', *J Chronic Dis*. 1974 Sep; 27(7–8): 345–64. doi: 10.1016/0021-9681(74)90014-9. PMID: 4436426

Pantell M, Rehkopf D, Jutte D, Syme SL, Balmes J, Adler N. 'Social isolation: a predictor of mortality comparable to traditional clinical risk factors', *Am J Public Health*. 2013 Nov; 103(11): 2056–62. doi: 10.2105/AJPH.2013.301261. Epub 2013 Sep 12. PMID: 24028260; PMCID: PMC3871270

Stansfeld SA, Marmot MG *Stress and the heart: Psychosocial pathways to coronary heart disease*. BMJ Books, 2002

Syme SL. 'Control and health: A personal perspective', *Advances*. 1991; 7(2): 16–27

Chetty R, Stepner M, Abraham S, Lin S, Scuderi B, Turner N, Bergeron A, Cutler D. 'The Association Between Income and Life Expectancy in the United States, 2001–2014', *JAMA*. 2016 Apr 26; 315(16): 1750–66. doi: 10.1001/jama.2016.4226. Erratum in: *JAMA*. 2017 Jan 3; 317(1): 90. PMID: 27063997; PMCID: PMC4866586

Preston SH. 'The changing relation between mortality and level of economic development' *International Journal of Epidemiology*. 2007; 36 (3): 484–90. doi: 10.1093/ije/dym075. PMC: 257236

https://www.oecd.org/berlin/47570194.pdf

http://www.oecd.org/els/health-systems/health-data.htm

Iacobucci G. 'Life expectancy gap between rich and poor in England widens', *BMJ*. 2019 Mar 28; 364: l1492. doi: 10.1136/bmj.l1492. PMID: 30923046

ABS Oct 2020: Australia's Leading Causes of Death 2019. https://www.abs.gov.au/statistics/health/causes-death

Overload and the brain

Cassell JC. 'Life stress and mental health: the midtown Manhattan study', *Am J Public Health Nations Health*. 1964 Sep; 54(9): 1624–5. PMCID: PMC1255021

Adler NE, Marmot M, McEwen BS, Stewart J. (eds) 'Socioeconomic Status and Health in Industrial Nations: Social, Psychological, and Biological Pathways', *Annals of the New York Academy of Sciences: New York*. 1999

McEwen BS, Wingfield JC. 'The concept of allostasis in biology and biomedicine', *Horm. & Behav*. 2003; 43: 2–15

McEwen BS. 'Protective and damaging effects of stress mediators', *New England J Med*. 1998; 338: 171–179

Shonkoff JP, Boyce WT, McEwen BS. 'Neuroscience, molecular biology, and the childhood roots of health disparities', *JAMA*. 2009; 301: 2252–2259

Seeman T, Epel E, Gruenewald T, Karlamangla A, McEwen BS. 'Socio-economic differentials in peripheral biology: Cumulative allostatic load', *Ann NY Acad Sci*. 2010; 1186: 223–239

Reknes I, Visockaite G, Liefooghe A, Lovakov A, Einarsen SV. 'Locus of Control Moderates the Relationship Between Exposure to Bullying Behaviors and Psychological Strain', *Front Psychol*. 2019 Jun 6; 10: 1323. doi: 10.3389/fpsyg.2019.01323. PMID: 31244725; PMCID: PMC6563764

Wang L, Lv M. 'Internal-External Locus of Control Scale', in: Zeigler-Hill V, Shackelford T. (eds) *Encyclopedia of Personality and Individual Differences.* 2017; Springer, Cham. https://doi. org/10.1007/978-3-319-28099-8_41-1

Di Pentima L, Toni A, Schneider BH, Tomás JM, Oliver A, Attili G. 'Locus of control as a mediator of the association between attachment and children's mental health', *J Genet Psychol.* 2019 Nov–Dec; 180(6): 251–265. doi: 10.1080/00221325.2019.1652557. Epub 2019 Sep 9. PMID: 31496445

Johnson RE, Rosen CC, Chang CH, Lin SH. 'Getting to the core of locus of control: Is it an evaluation of the self or the environment?', *J Appl Psychol.* 2015 Sep; 100(5): 1568–78. doi: 10.1037/apl0000011. Epub 2015 Feb 9. PMID: 25664470

Wallston BD, Wallston KA. 'Locus of control and health: a review of the literature', *Health Educ Monogr.* 1978 Spring; 6(2): 107–17. doi: 10.1177/109019817800600102. PMID: 357347

Tang K. 'A reciprocal interplay between psychosocial job stressors and worker well-being? A systematic review of the "reversed" effect', *Scand J Work Environ Health.* 2014 Sep; 40(5): 441–56. doi: 10.5271/sjweh.3431. Epub 2014 Apr 22. PMID: 24756578

Stress and shoelaces

Ornish D, Lin J, Chan JM, Epel E, Kemp C, Weidner G, Marlin R, Frenda SJ, Magbanua MJM, Daubenmier J, Estay I, Hills NK, Chainani-Wu N, Carroll PR, Blackburn EH. 'Effect of comprehensive lifestyle changes on telomerase activity and telomere length in men with biopsy-proven low-risk prostate cancer: 5-year follow-up of a descriptive pilot study', *Lancet Oncol.* 2013 Oct; 14(11): 1112–1120. doi: 10.1016/S1470-2045(13)70366-8. Epub 2013 Sep 17. PMID: 24051140

Epel ES, Blackburn EH, Lin J, Dhabhar FS, Adler NE, Morrow JD, Cawthon RM. 'Accelerated telomere shortening in response to life stress', *Proc Natl Acad Sci USA.* 2004 Dec 7; 101(49): 17312–5. doi: 10.1073/pnas.0407162101. Epub 2004 Dec 1. PMID: 15574496; PMCID: PMC534658

Blackburn EH, Epel ES, Lin J. 'Human telomere biology: A contributory and interactive factor in aging, disease risks, and protection', *Science.* 2015 Dec 4; 350(6265): 1193–8. doi: 10.1126/science. aab3389. PMID: 26785477

Epel ES, Lin J, Dhabhar FS, Wolkowitz OM, Puterman E, Karan L, Blackburn EH. 'Dynamics of telomerase activity in response to acute psychological stress', *Brain, Behavior, and Immunity.* 2010; 24(4): 531–539. doi: 10.1016/j.bbi.2009.11.018. PMC: 2856774; PMID: 20018236

Jacobs TL, Epel ES, Lin J, Blackburn EH, Wolkowitz OM, Bridwell DA, Zanesco AP, Aichele SR, Sahdra BK, Maclean KA, King BG, Shaver PR, Rosenberg EL, Ferrer E, Wallace BA, Saron CD. 'Intensive meditation training, immune cell telomerase activity, and psychological mediators', *Psychoneuroendocrinology.* 2010; 36 (5): 664–681. doi: 10.1016/j. psyneuen.2010.09.010. PMID: 21035949

Epel E, Daubenmier J, Tedlie Moskowitz J, Folkman S, Blackburn E. 'Can meditation slow rate of cellular aging? cognitive stress, mindfulness, and telomeres', *Annals of the New York Academy of Sciences.* 2009; 1172(1): 34–53. Bibcode: 2009NYASA1172...34E. doi: 10.1111/j.1749-6632.2009.04414.x. PMC: 3057175; PMID: 19735238

Humphreys J, Epel ES, Cooper BA, Lin J, Blackburn EH, Lee KA. 'Telomere Shortening in Formerly Abused and Never Abused Women', *Biological Research for Nursing.* 2012; 14 (2): 115–123. doi: 10.1177/1099800411398479. PMC: 3207021; PMID: 21385798

What to do about it and where anxiety fits in

https://www.blackdoginstitute.org.au/resources-support/anxiety/treatment/

Thibaut F. 'Anxiety disorders: a review of current literature' *Dialogues Clin Neurosci.* 2017 Jun; 19(2): 87–88. doi: 10.31887/DCNS.2017.19.2/fthibaut. PMID: 28867933; PMCID: PMC5573565

Jorm AF, Patten SB, Brugha TS, Mojtabai R. 'Has increased provision of treatment reduced the prevalence of common mental disorders? Review of the evidence from four countries' *World Psychiatry.* 2017 Feb; 16(1): 90–99. doi: 10.1002/wps.20388. PMID: 28127925; PMCID: PMC5269479

Creswell C, Waite P, Hudson J. 'Practitioner review: anxiety disorders in children and young people – assessment and treatment' *J Child Psychol Psychiatry.* 2020 Jun; 61(6): 628–643. doi: 10.1111/jcpp.13186. Epub 2020 Jan 21. PMID: 31960440

Zimmermann M, Chong AK, Vechiu C, Papa A. 'Modifiable risk and protective factors for anxiety disorders among adults: a systematic review' *Psychiatry Res*. 2020 Mar; 285: 112705. doi: 10.1016/j.psychres.2019.112705. Epub 2019 Dec 4. PMID: 31839417

The bigger picture and what it means for living younger longer
World Bank. 'World Development Report 1993: Investing in Health'. 1993; New York: Oxford University Press. © World Bank. https://openknowledge.worldbank.org/handle/10986/5976 License: CC BY 3.0 IGO.
https://www.worldometers.info/demographics/life-expectancy/
Commission on the Social Determinants of Health. 'Closing the gap in a generation: health equity through action on the social determinants of health. Final report of the Commission on Social Determinants of Health'. 2008; Geneva: World Health Organization.
Marmot M, Bell R. 'Fair society, healthy lives', *Public Health*. 2012 Sep; 126 Suppl 1: S4–S10. doi: 10.1016/j.puhe.2012.05.014. Epub 2012 Jul 10. PMID: 22784581

History and your health (this is the pandemic bit)
https://www.unaids.org/en/resources/fact-sheet
Caldwell J, Caldwell P, Quiggin P. 'The Social Context of AIDS in sub-Saharan Africa', *Population and Development Review*. 1989; 15(2): 185–234. doi: 10.2307/1973703
Worobey M, et al. 'Island biogeography reveals the deep history of SIV', *Science*. 2010; 329(5998): 1487
Sharp PM, Hahn BH. 'Origins of HIV and the AIDS pandemic', *Cold Spring Harbour Perspectives in Medicine*. 2011; 1(1): a006841
Gao F, et al. 'Origin of HIV-1 in the chimpanzee Pan troglodytes troglodytes', *Nature*. 1999; 397(6718): 436–441
Bailes E, et al. 'Hybrid Origin of SIV in Chimpanzees', *Science*. 2003; 300(5626): 1713
Reddy BL, Saier MHJ. 'The Causal Relationship between Eating Animals and Viral Epidemics', *Microb Physiol*. 2020; 30(1-6): 2–8. doi: 10.1159/000511192. Epub 2020 Sep 21. PMID: 32957108; PMCID: PMC7573891
Pickrell JK, Reich D. 'Toward a new history and geography of human genes informed by ancient DNA', *Trends Genet*. 2014 Sep; 30(9): 377–89. doi: 10.1016/j.tig.2014.07.007. Epub 2014 Aug 26. PMID: 25168683; PMCID: PMC4163019
Harper KN, Zuckerman MK, Harper ML, Kingston JD, Armelagos GJ. 'The origin and antiquity of syphilis revisited: an appraisal of Old World pre-Columbian evidence for treponemal infection', *Am J Phys Anthropol*. 2011; 146 Suppl 53: 99–133. doi: 10.1002/ajpa.21613. PMID: 22101689
Tampa M, Sarbu I, Matei C, Benea V, Georgescu SR. 'Brief history of syphilis', *J Med Life*. 2014 Mar 15; 7(1): 4–10. Epub 2014 Mar 25. PMID: 24653750; PMCID: PMC3956094
Chimaobi Kalu M. 'Birth of the Black Plague: The Mongol Siege on Caffa', *War History Online*. July 2018.
CBC. Oct 2019. https://www.cbc.ca/news/canada/manitoba/national-microbiology-lab-scientist-investigation-china-1.5307424
https://nationalpost.com/news/canadian-lab-immersed-in-rcmp-probe-sent-ebola-and-another-deadly-virus-to-china-health-agency
https://nationalpost.com/news/covid-19-pandemic-wuhan-institute-of-virology-ebola-national-microbiology-laboratory
https://besacenter.org/perspectives-papers/china-biological-warfare/
https://www.nbcboston.com/news/local/top-harvard-professor-indicted-in-china-case/2139972/

Your genes as history in the making – but they're not destiny
Schultz M. 'Rudolf Virchow', *Emerg Infect Dis*. 2008; 14 (9): 1480–1481. doi: 10.3201/eid1409.086672. PMC: 2603088
Virchow RC. 'Report on the typhus epidemic in Upper Silesia, 1848', *Am J Public Health*. 2006 Dec; 96(12): 2102–5. doi: 10.2105/ajph.96.12.2102. PMID: 17123938; PMCID: PMC1698167
https://www.nobelprize.org/prizes/medicine/1905/koch/biographical/
Barlow FK. 'Nature vs. nurture is nonsense: on the necessity of an integrated genetic, social, developmental, and personality psychology' *Australian Journal of Psychology*. 2019; 71(1): 68–79. doi: 10.1111/ajpy.12240

Heine SJ, Dar-Nimrod I, Cheung BY, Proulx T, 'Chapter Three – Essentially biased: why people are fatalistic about genes' in Olson JM, *Advances in Experimental Social Psychology*. Academic Press, 55, 2017: 137–192. ISSN 0065-2601, ISBN 9780128121153, https://doi.org/10.1016/bs.aesp.2016.10.003

Gericke, N., Carver, R., Castéra, J. et al. Exploring Relationships Among Belief in Genetic Determinism, Genetics Knowledge, and Social Factors. *Sci & Educ* 26, 1223–1259 (2017). https://doi.org/10.1007/s11191-017-9950-y

Your destiny can affect your genes

Notterman DA, Mitchell C. 'Epigenetics and Understanding the Impact of Social Determinants of Health', *Pediatr Clin North Am*. 2015 Oct; 62(5): 1227–40. doi: 10.1016/j.pcl.2015.05.012. PMID: 26318949; PMCID: PMC4555996

Ward-Caviness C, Pu S, Martin C, Galea S, Uddin M, Wildman D, Koenen K, Aiello A. 'Epigenetic predictors of all-cause mortality are associated with objective measures of neighborhood disadvantage in an urban population', *Clinical Epigenetics. 2020;* 12. 10.1186/s13148-020-00830-8

Simmons D. 'Epigenetic influence and disease', *Nature Education*. 2008; 1(1): 6

Scorza P, Duarte CS, Hipwell AE, Posner J, Ortin A, Canino G, Monk C; Program Collaborators for Environmental influences on Child Health Outcomes. 'Research Review: Intergenerational transmission of disadvantage: epigenetics and parents' childhoods as the first exposure', *J Child Psychol Psychiatry*. 2019 Feb; 60(2): 119–132. doi: 10.1111/jcpp.12877. Epub 2018 Feb 23. PMID: 29473646; PMCID: PMC6107434

Merrill SM, Gladish N, Kobor MS. 'Social Environment and Epigenetics', *Curr Top Behav Neurosci*. 2019; 42: 83–126. doi: 10.1007/7854_2019_114. PMID: 31485989

Heinbockel T, Csoka AB. 'Epigenetic Effects of Drugs of Abuse', *Int J Environ Res Public Health*. 2018 Sep 25; 15(10): 2098. doi: 10.3390/ijerph15102098. PMID: 30257440; PMCID: PMC6210395

Ganesan A, Arimondo PB, Rots MG, Jeronimo C, Berdasco M. 'The timeline of epigenetic drug discovery: from reality to dreams', *Clin Epigenetics*. 2019 Dec 2; 11(1): 174. doi: 10.1186/s13148-019-0776-0. PMID: 31791394; PMCID: PMC6888921

Ashapkin VV, Kutueva LI, Vanyushin BF. 'Epigenetic Clock: Just a Convenient Marker or an Active Driver of Aging?', *Adv Exp Med Biol*. 2019; 1178: 175–206. doi: 10.1007/978-3-030-25650-0_10. PMID: 31493228

Unnikrishnan A, Freeman WM, Jackson J, Wren JD, Porter H, Richardson A. 'The role of DNA methylation in epigenetics of aging', *Pharmacol Ther*. 2019 Mar; 195: 172–185. doi: 10.1016/j.pharmthera.2018.11.001. Epub 2018 Nov 9. PMID: 30419258; PMCID: PMC6397707

Gobsmacked: gene testing your spit

https://www.hgsa.org.au/resources/genetic-testing-and-life-insurance

Savard J, Terrill B, Dunlop K, Samanek A, Metcalfe S. (2020). 'Human Genetics Society of Australasia Position Statement: Online DNA Testing', *Twin Research and Human Genetics*. 2020; 23(4): 256–258. doi: 10.1017/thg.2020.67

Long S, Goldblatt J. 'MTHFR genetic testing: Controversy and clinical implications', *Aust Fam Physician*. 2016 Apr; 45(4): 237–40. PMID: 27052143

Horne J, Gilliland J, Madill J, Shelley J. 'A critical examination of legal and ethical considerations for nutrigenetic testing with recommendations for improving regulation in Canada: from science to consumer', *Journal of Law and the Biosciences*. 2020; lsaa003, https://doi.org/10.1093/jlb/lsaa003

Browne K. 'Are home DNA kits reliable? ', *CHOICE*. 2018; https://www.choice.com.au/health-and-body/health-practitioners/prevention/articles/dna-tests?gclid=CjwKCAiAkan9BRAqEiwAP9X6UQpx4G1qfTgNHJGC4M6n6dHJCWRVrdazxdxGsPa9ITyg4v2R0N_9qBoCZtwQAvD_BwE

'DNA dilemmas – What do ancestry DNA test results mean?' *Know Pathology*. https://knowpathology.com.au/2018/04/27/dna-tests/?gclid=CjwKCAiAkan9BRAqEiwAP9X6UcYKRh4IgVe03HHeVfx_1G2Xn0AIYJyDJ6lgXa7-6Jf3CzW8rRBWuRoCnfsQAvD_BwE

Shelton JF, Shastri AJ, Ye C, Weldon CH, Filshtein-Somnez T, Coker D, Symons A, Esparza-Gordillo J, The 23andMe Team, Aslibekyan S, Auton A. 'Trans-ethnic analysis reveals genetic and non-genetic associations with COVID-19 susceptibility and severity', medRxiv 2020.09.04.20188318; doi: https://doi.org/10.1101/2020.09.04.20188318

https://www.wired.com/story/theres-no-such-thing-as-family-secrets-in-the-age-of-23andme/

Johnson EC, et al. 'A large-scale genome-wide association study meta-analysis of cannabis use disorder', *Lancet Psychiatry*. 2020 Dec; 7(12): 1032–1045. doi: 10.1016/S2215-0366(20)30339-4. Epub 2020 Oct 20. PMID: 33096046; PMCID: PMC7674631

Coleman JRI, et al. 'Genome-wide gene-environment analyses of major depressive disorder and reported lifetime traumatic experiences in UK Biobank', *Mol Psychiatry*. 2020 Jul; 25(7): 1430–1446. doi: 10.1038/s41380-019-0546-6. Epub 2020 Jan 23. Erratum in: *Mol Psychiatry*. 2020 May 18. PMID: 31969693; PMCID: PMC7305950

Part 3: Living younger longer

Staying young as old as possible

Stallard E. 'Compression of Morbidity and Mortality: New Perspectives', *N Am Actuar J*. 2016; 20(4): 341–354. doi: 10.1080/10920277.2016.1227269. Epub 2016 Oct 4. PMID: 28740358; PMCID: PMC5520809

Rizzuto D, Orsini N, Qiu C, Wang H-X, Fratiglioni L. 'Lifestyle, social factors, and survival after age 75: Population based study', *BMJ*. 2012; 345: e5568. doi: 10.1136/bmj.e5568

Foreman KJ, Marquez N, Dolgert A, et al. 'Forecasting life expectancy, years of life lost, and all-cause and cause-specific mortality for 250 causes of death: reference and alternative scenarios for 2016–40 for 195 countries and territories', *Lancet*. 2018; 392: 2052–2090

Anstey KJ, Low L-F, Christensen H, Sachdev P. 'Level of cognitive performance as a correlate and predictor of health behaviors that protect against cognitive decline in late life: The PATH Through Life Study', *Intelligence*. 2009; 37: 600–606

http://cmhr.anu.edu.au/path/pdf/PATH_papers_published.pdf

Kumar R, Anstey KJ, Wen W, Sachdev PS. 'Association of Type 2 Diabetes With Depression, Brain Atrophy, and Reduced Fine Motor Speed in a 60–64-Year-Old Community Sample', *American Journal of Geriatric Psychiatry*. 2008; 16: 989–998

Lawrence D, Hancock KJ, Kisely S. 'The gap in life expectancy from preventable physical illness in psychiatric patients in Western Australia: retrospective analysis of population based registers', *BMJ*. 2013 May 21; 346: f2539. doi: 10.1136/bmj.f2539. PMID: 23694688; PMCID: PMC3660620

Hatton T. 'How Have Europeans Grown so Tall?', *Oxford Economic Papers*. 2011; 2. doi: 10.1093/oep/gpt030

Bonner C, Raffoul N, Battaglia T, Mitchell JA, Batcup C, Stavreski B. 'Experiences of a National Web-Based Heart Age Calculator for Cardiovascular Disease Prevention: User Characteristics, Heart Age Results, and Behavior Change Survey', *J Med Internet Res*. 2020; 22(8): e19028. doi: 10.2196/19028 PMID: 32763875; PMCID: 7442940

Bruce ML, Leaf PJ, Rozal GPM, et al. 'Psychiatric status and 9-year mortality in the New Haven Epidemiologic Catchment Area study', *American Journal of Psychiatry*. 1994; 151: 716–721

Lallo C, Raitano M. 'Life expectancy inequalities in the elderly by socioeconomic status: evidence from Italy', *Popul Health Metr*. 2018 Apr 12; 16(1): 7. doi: 10.1186/s12963-018-0163-7. PMID: 29650013; PMCID: PMC5898057

Berr C, Balard F, Blain H, Robine JM. 'Vieillissement, l'émergence d'une nouvelle population [How to define old age: successful aging and/or longevity]', *Med Sci (Paris)*. 2012 Mar; 28(3): 281–7. French. doi: 10.1051/medsci/2012283016. Epub 2012 Apr 6. PMID: 22480652

Labat-Robert J, Robert L. 'Longevity and aging. Mechanisms and perspectives', *Pathol Biol (Paris)*. 2015 Dec; 63(6): 272–6. doi: 10.1016/j.patbio.2015.08.001. Epub 2015 Sep 26. PMID: 26416405

Foreman KJ, et al. 'Forecasting life expectancy, years of life lost, and all-cause and cause-specific mortality for 250 causes of death: reference and alternative scenarios for 2016-40 for 195 countries and territories', *Lancet*. 2018 Nov 10; 392(10159): 2052–2090. doi: 10.1016/S0140-6736(18)31694-5. Epub 2018 Oct 16. PMID: 30340847; PMCID: PMC6227505

Huang Y, Filshtein T, Gentleman R, Aslibekyan S. 'An Environment-Wide Study of Adult Cognitive Performance in the 23andMe Cohort'. 2019. doi: 10.1101/19009076

Don't know your limits

https://www.ons.gov.uk/peoplepopulationandcommunity/birthsdeathsandmarriages/lifeexpectancies/

articles/ethnicdifferencesinlifeexpectancyandmortalityfromselectedcausesinenglandandwale
s/2011to2014

Bending your genes

Guillot M, Gavrilova N, Pudrovska T. 'Understanding the "Russian mortality paradox" in Central Asia: evidence from Kyrgyzstan' *Demography*. 2011 Aug; 48(3): 1081–104. doi: 10.1007/s13524-011-0036-1. PMID: 21618068; PMCID: PMC3315848

Trovato F, Lalu NM. 'Narrowing sex differentials in life expectancy in the industrialized world: early 1970s to early 1990s' *Social Biology*. 1996; 43: 1-2, 20-37. doi: 10.1080/19485565.1996.9988911

Sebastiani P, Perls TT. 'The genetics of extreme longevity: lessons from the New England centenarian study' *Front Genet*. 2012 Nov 30; 3: 277. doi: 10.3389/fgene.2012.00277. PMID: 23226160; PMCID: PMC3510428

Govindaraju D, Atzmon G, Barzilai N. 'Genetics, lifestyle and longevity: lessons from centenarians' *Appl Transl Genom*. 2015 Feb 4; 4: 23–32. doi: 10.1016/j.atg.2015.01.001. PMID: 26937346; PMCID: PMC4745363

Galioto A, Dominguez LJ, Pineo A, Ferlisi A, Putignano E, Belvedere M, Costanza G, Barbagallo M. 'Cardiovascular risk factors in centenarians' *Exp Gerontol*. 2008 Feb; 43(2): 106–13. doi: 10.1016/j.exger.2007.06.009. Epub 2007 Jul 4. PMID: 17689040

Life-shorteners hunt in packs

Taylor R, Dobson A, Mirzaei M. 'Contribution of changes in risk factors to the decline of coronary heart disease mortality in Australia over three decades', *Eur J Cardiovasc Prev Rehabil*. 2006; 13: 760–768

Life-shortening factors aren't equal

http://healthyweight.health.gov.au/wps/portal/Home/get-started/are-you-a-healthy-weight/waist-circumference

GBD 2016 Alcohol Collaborators. 'Alcohol use and burden for 195 countries and territories, 1990-2016: a systematic analysis for the Global Burden of Disease Study 2016', *Lancet*. 2018 Sep 22; 392(10152): 1015–1035. doi: 10.1016/S0140-6736(18)31310-2. Epub 2018 Aug 23. Erratum in: *Lancet*. 2018 Sep 29; 392(10153): 1116. Erratum in: *Lancet*. 2019 Jun 22; 393(10190): e44. PMID: 30146330; PMCID: PMC6148333

GBD Mortality Collaborators. 'Global, regional, and national under-5 mortality, adult mortality, age-specific mortality, and life expectancy, 1970–2016: a systematic analysis for the Global Burden of Disease Study 2016', *Lancet*. 2017; 390: 1084–1150

Pirie K, Peto R, Reeves GK, et al; Million Women Study Collaborators. 'The 21st century hazards of smoking and benefits of stopping: a prospective study of one million women in the UK', *Lancet*. 2013; 381: 133–141

Ezzati M, Obermeyer Z, Tzoulaki I, Mayosi BM, Elliott P, Leon DA. 'Contributions of risk factors and medical care to cardiovascular mortality trends', *Nat Rev Cardiol*. 2015 Sep; 12(9): 508–30. doi: 10.1038/nrcardio.2015.82. Epub 2015 Jun 16. PMID: 26076950; PMCID: PMC4945698

Begg SJ, Vos T, Barker B, Stanley L and Lopez AD. 'Burden of disease and injury in Australia in the new millennium: measuring health loss from diseases, injuries and risk factors', *MJA*. 2008; 188: 36–40

https://www.healthdata.org/sites/default/files/files/country_profiles/GBD/ihme_gbd_country_report_united_kingdom.pdf

Exceptional survivors

Willcox BJ, He Q, Chen R, et al. 'Midlife Risk Factors and Healthy Survival in Men', *JAMA*. 2006; 296(19): 2343–2350. doi: 10.1001/jama.296.19.2343

Pignolo RJ. 'Exceptional Human Longevity', *Mayo Clin Proc*. 2019 Jan; 94(1): 110–124. doi: 10.1016/j.mayocp.2018.10.005. Epub 2018 Dec 10. PMID: 30545477

Gavrilov LA, Gavrilova NS. 'Predictors of Exceptional Longevity: Effects of Early-Life Childhood Conditions, Midlife Environment and Parental Characteristics', *Living 100 Monogr*. 2014; 2014: 1–18. PMID: 25664346; PMCID: PMC4318523

Willcox DC, Willcox BJ, Hsueh W, Suzuki M. 'Genetic determinants of exceptional human longevity: insights from the Okinawa Centenarian Study', *AGE*. 2006; 28: 313–332

Willcox BJ, Willcox DC, Ferrucci L. 'Secrets of Healthy Aging and Longevity From Exceptional Survivors Around the Globe: Lessons From Octogenarians to Supercentenarians', *The Journals of Gerontology: Series A*. November 2008; volume 63, issue 11, pp. 1181–1185. https://doi.org/10.1093/gerona/63.11.1181

Be critical of percentages – look for numbers

Noordzij M, van Diepen M, Caskey FC, Jager KJ. 'Relative risk versus absolute risk: one cannot be interpreted without the other', *Nephrology Dialysis Transplantation*. April 2017; volume 32, issue suppl_2, pp. ii13–ii18. https://doi.org/10.1093/ndt/gfw465

Schechtman E. 'Odds ratio, relative risk, absolute risk reduction, and the number needed to treat – which of these should we use?', *Value Health*. 2002 Sep–Oct; 5(5): 431–6. doi: 10.1046/J.1524-4733.2002.55150.x. PMID: 12201860

So what counts?

Ranganathan P, Pramesh CS, Aggarwal R. 'Common pitfalls in statistical analysis: Absolute risk reduction, relative risk reduction, and number needed to treat', *Perspect Clin Res*. 2016 Jan-Mar; 7(1): 51–3. doi: 10.4103/2229-3485.173773. PMID: 26952180; PMCID: PMC4763519

Inflammation may count

Reuben DB, Cheh AI, Harris TB, Ferrucci L, Rowe JW, Tracy RP, Seeman TE. 'Peripheral blood markers of inflammation predict mortality and functional decline in high-functioning community-dwelling older persons', *J Am Geriatr Soc*. 2002 Apr; 50(4): 638–44. doi: 10.1046/j.1532-5415.2002.50157.x. PMID: 11982663

Ko F, Yu Q, Xue QL, et al. 'Inflammation and mortality in a frail mouse model', *AGE*. 2012; 34: 705–715. https://doi.org/10.1007/s11357-011-9269-6

de Jager J, Dekker JM, Kooy A, Kostense PJ, Nijpels G, Heine RJ, Bouter LM, Stehouwer CD. 'Endothelial dysfunction and low-grade inflammation explain much of the excess cardiovascular mortality in individuals with type 2 diabetes: the Hoorn Study', *Arterioscler Thromb Vasc Biol*. 2006 May; 26(5): 1086–93. doi: 10.1161/01.ATV.0000215951.36219.a4. Epub 2006 Mar 2. PMID: 16514084

Bonaccio M, Di Castelnuovo A, Pounis G, De Curtis A, Costanzo S, Persichillo M, Cerletti C, Donati MB, de Gaetano G, Iacoviello L; Moli-sani Study Investigators. 'A score of low-grade inflammation and risk of mortality: prospective findings from the Moli-sani study', *Haematologica*. 2016 Nov; 101(11): 1434–1441. doi: 10.3324/haematol.2016.144055. Epub 2016 Oct 14. PMID: 27742767; PMCID: PMC5394885

Gialluisi A, Costanzo S, Castelnuovo AD, Bonaccio M, Bracone F, Magnacca S, De Curtis A, Cerletti C, Donati MB, de Gaetano G, Iacoviello L; Moli-sani Study Investigators. 'Combined influence of depression severity and low-grade inflammation on incident hospitalization and mortality risk in Italian adults', *J Affect Disord*. 2021 Jan 15; 279: 173–182. doi: 10.1016/j.jad.2020.10.004. Epub 2020 Oct 7. PMID: 33059220

Kälsch AI, Scharnagl H, Kleber ME, et al. 'Long- and short-term association of low-grade systemic inflammation with cardiovascular mortality in the LURIC study', *Clin Res Cardiol*. 2020; 109: 358–373. https://doi.org/10.1007/s00392-019-01516-9

How old are you really?

de Goeij MC, Halbesma N, Dekker FW, Wijsman CA, van Heemst D, Maier AB, Mooijaart SP, Slagboom PE, Westendorp RG, de Craen AJ. 'Renal function in familial longevity: the Leiden Longevity Study', *Exp Gerontol*. 2014 Mar; 51: 65–70. doi: 10.1016/j.exger.2013.12.012. Epub 2014 Jan 2. PMID: 24389060

Tarry-Adkins JL, Ozanne SE, Norden A, Cherif H, Hales CN. 'Lower antioxidant capacity and elevated p53 and p21 may be a link between gender disparity in renal telomere shortening, albuminuria, and longevity', *Am J Physiol Renal Physiol*. 2006 Feb; 290(2): F509–16. doi: 10.1152/ajprenal.00215.2005. Epub 2005 Sep 27. PMID: 16189290

Shlipak MG, Wassel Fyr CL, Chertow GM, Harris TB, Kritchevsky SB, Tylavsky FA, Satterfield S, Cummings SR, Newman AB, Fried LF. 'Cystatin C and mortality risk in the elderly: the health, aging, and body composition study', *J Am Soc Nephrol.* 2006 Jan; 17(1): 254–61. doi: 10.1681/ASN.2005050545. Epub 2005 Nov 2. PMID: 16267155

Mao Q, Zhao N, Wang Y, Li Y, Xiang C, Li L, Zheng W, Xu S, Zhao XH. 'Association of Cystatin C with Metabolic Syndrome and Its Prognostic Performance in Non-ST-Segment Elevation Acute Coronary Syndrome with Preserved Renal Function', *Biomed Res Int.* 2019 Jun 16; 2019: 8541402. doi: 10.1155/2019/8541402. PMID: 31317040; PMCID: PMC6601472

Pelaez A, Dinic M, Jean-Claude B, Roche F, Alamartine E, Cavalier E, Delanaye P, Maillard N, Mariat C. 'P0186 Serum cystatin C, inflammation and autonomic dysfunction: a hidden "ménage à trois"?', *Nephrology Dialysis Transplantation.* June 2020; volume 35, issue supplement_3. gfaa142.P0186. https://doi.org/10.1093/ndt/gfaa142.P0186

There's no such thing as normal

Nishida C, Ko GT, Kumanyika S. 'Body fat distribution and noncommunicable diseases in populations: overview of the 2008 WHO Expert Consultation on Waist Circumference and Waist-Hip Ratio' *Eur J Clin Nutr.* 2010 Jan; 64(1): 2–5. doi: 10.1038/ejcn.2009.139. Epub 2009 Nov 25. PMID: 19935820

Willadsen TG, Bebe A, Køster-Rasmussen R, Jarbøl DE, Guassora AD, Waldorff FB, Reventlow S, Olivarius Nde F. 'The role of diseases, risk factors and symptoms in the definition of multimorbidity – a systematic review' *Scand J Prim Health Care.* 2016 Jun; 34(2): 112–21. doi: 10.3109/02813432.2016.1153242. Epub 2016 Mar 8. PMID: 26954365; PMCID: PMC4977932

Turner EL, Dobson JE & Pocock SJ 'Categorisation of continuous risk factors in epidemiological publications: a survey of current practice' *Epidemiol Perspect Innov.* 2010; 7(9). https://doi.org/10.1186/1742-5573-7-9

Moynihan R, Doust J, Henry D. 'Preventing overdiagnosis: how to stop harming the healthy' *BMJ.* 2012 May 28; 344: e3502. doi: 10.1136/bmj.e3502. PMID: 22645185

Under pressure

MacMahon S, Neal B, Rodgers A. 'Hypertension – time to move on', *Lancet.* 2005 Mar 19–25; 365(9464): 1108–9. doi: 10.1016/S0140-6736(05)71148-X. PMID: 15781107

MacMahon S, Peto R, Cutler J, Collins R, Sorlie P, Neaton J, Abbott R, Godwin J, Dyer A, Stamler J. 'Blood pressure, stroke, and coronary heart disease. Part 1, Prolonged differences in blood pressure: prospective observational studies corrected for the regression dilution bias', *Lancet.* 1990 Mar 31; 335(8692): 765–74. doi: 10.1016/0140-6736(90)90878-9. PMID: 1969518

Collins R, Peto R, MacMahon S, Hebert P, Fiebach NH, Eberlein KA, Godwin J, Qizilbash N, Taylor JO, Hennekens CH. 'Blood pressure, stroke, and coronary heart disease. Part 2, Short-term reductions in blood pressure: overview of randomised drug trials in their epidemiological context', *Lancet.* 1990 Apr 7; 335(8693): 827–38. doi: 10.1016/0140-6736(90)90944-z. PMID: 1969567

Nissen SE, Tuzcu EM, Libby P, Thompson PD, Ghali M, Garza D, Berman L, Shi H, Buebendorf E, Topol EJ; CAMELOT Investigators. 'Effect of antihypertensive agents on cardiovascular events in patients with coronary disease and normal blood pressure: the CAMELOT study: a randomized controlled trial', *JAMA.* 2004 Nov 10; 292(18): 2217–25. doi: 10.1001/jama.292.18.2217. PMID: 15536108

Zhang D, Wang G, Joo H. 'A Systematic Review of Economic Evidence on Community Hypertension Interventions', *Am J Prev Med.* 2017 Dec; 53(6S2): S121–S130. doi: 10.1016/j.amepre.2017.05.008. PMID: 29153113; PMCID: PMC5819001

Unal B, Critchley JA, Fidan D, Capewell S. 'Life-years gained from modern cardiological treatments and population risk factor changes in England and Wales, 1981–2000', *Am J Public Health.* 2005 Jan; 95(1): 103–8. doi: 10.2105/AJPH.2003.029579. PMID: 15623868; PMCID: PMC1449860

Blacher J, Levy BI, Mourad JJ, Safar ME, Bakris G. 'From epidemiological transition to modern cardiovascular epidemiology: hypertension in the 21st century', *Lancet.* 2016 Jul 30; 388(10043): 530–2. doi: 10.1016/S0140-6736(16)00002-7. Epub 2016 Feb 6. PMID: 26856636

Berkelmans GFN, et al. 'Prediction of individual life-years gained without cardiovascular events from lipid, blood pressure, glucose, and aspirin treatment based on data of more than 500 000 patients with Type 2 diabetes mellitus', *European Heart Journal.* September 2019; volume 40, issue 34, 7, pp. 2899–2906. https://doi.org/10.1093/eurheartj/ehy839

Schorling E, Niebuhr D, Kroke A. 'Cost-effectiveness of salt reduction to prevent hypertension and CVD: A systematic review', *Public Health Nutrition*. 2017; 20(11): 1993–2003. doi: 10.1017/S1368980017000593

Lewington S, Clarke R, Qizilbash N, Peto R, Collins R; Prospective Studies Collaboration. 'Age-specific relevance of usual blood pressure to vascular mortality: a meta-analysis of individual data for one million adults in 61 prospective studies', *Lancet*. 2002 Dec 14; 360(9349): 1903–13. doi: 10.1016/s0140-6736(02)11911-8. Erratum in: *Lancet*. 2003 Mar 22; 361(9362): 1060. PMID: 12493255

Hird TR, Zomer E, Owen AJ, Magliano DJ, Liew D, Ademi Z. 'Productivity Burden of Hypertension in Australia', *Hypertension*. 2019 Apr; 73(4): 777–784. doi: 10.1161/HYPERTENSIONAHA.118.12606. PMID: 30798659

MacMahon S, Rodgers A. 'The epidemiological association between blood pressure and stroke: implications for primary and secondary prevention', *Hypertens Res*. 1994; 17: 23–32

Yusuf S, Sleight P, Pogue J, Bosch J, Davies R, Dagenais G. 'Effects of an angiotensin-converting-enzyme inhibitor, ramipril, on cardiovascular events in high-risk patients: the Heart Outcomes Prevention Evaluation Study Investigators', *N Engl J Med*. 2000; 342: 145–153. View record in Scopus | Cited By in Scopus (4859)

Blood Pressure Lowering Treatment Trialists' Collaboration. 'Effects of different blood-pressure-lowering regimens on major cardiovascular events: results of prospectively-designed overviews of randomised trials', *Lancet*. 2003; 362: 1527–1535

New Zealand Guidelines Group. 'Guidelines for the Detection and Management of Cardiovascular Disease', New Zealand Guidelines Group, Wellington. 2003. http://www.nzgg.org.nz (accessed Sept 14, 2004)

Collins R, Peto R, MacMahon S, Hebert P, Fiebach NH, Eberlein KA, Godwin J, Qizilbash N, Taylor JO, Hennekens CH. 'Blood pressure, stroke, and coronary heart disease. Part 2, Short-term reductions in blood pressure: overview of randomised drug trials in their epidemiological context', *Lancet*. 1990 Apr 7; 335(8693): 827–38. doi: 10.1016/0140-6736(90)90944-z. PMID: 1969567

Heart Outcomes Prevention Evaluation Study Investigators. 'Effects of an angiotensin-convertingenzyme inhibitor, ramipril, on cardiovascular events in high-risk patients', *N Engl J Med*. 2000; 342: 145–153

Fox KM. 'European Trial on Reduction of Cardiac Events With Perindopril in Stable Coronary Artery Disease Investigators. Efficacy of perindopril in reduction of cardiovascular events among patients with stable coronary artery disease: randomised, double-blind, placebo-controlled, multicentre trial (the EUROPA study)', *Lancet*. 2003; 362: 782–788

Pitt B, Byington RP, Furberg CD, et al; PREVENT Investigators. 'Effect of amlodipine on the progression of atherosclerosis and the occurrence of clinical events', *Circulation*. 2000; 102: 1503–1510

Perez MI, Musini VM, Wright JM. 'Effect of early treatment with anti-hypertensive drugs on short and long-term mortality in patients with an acute cardiovascular event', *Cochrane Database Syst Rev*. 2009 Oct 7; (4): CD006743. doi: 10.1002/14651858.CD006743.pub2. PMID: 19821384

Arguedas JA, Leiva V, Wright JM. 'Blood pressure targets in adults with hypertension', *Cochrane Database of Systematic Reviews*. 2020; issue 12. Art. No.: CD004349. doi: 10.1002/14651858.CD004349.pub3

Lv J, Perkovic V, Foote CV, Craig ME, Craig JC, Strippoli GF. 'Antihypertensive agents for preventing diabetic kidney disease', *Cochrane Database Syst Rev*. 2012 Dec 12; 12: CD004136. doi: 10.1002/14651858.CD004136.pub3. PMID: 23235603

Is your blood fat?
Kronmal RA, Cain KC, Ye Z, Omenn GS. 'Total serum cholesterol levels and mortality risk as a function of age. A report based on the Framingham data', *Arch Intern Med*. 1993 May 10; 153(9): 1065–73. PMID: 8481074

Grover SA, Paquet S, Levinton C, Coupal L, Zowall H. 'Estimating the benefits of modifying risk factors of cardiovascular disease: a comparison of primary vs secondary prevention', *Arch Intern Med*. 1998 Mar 23; 158(6): 655–62. doi: 10.1001/archinte.158.6.655. Erratum in: *Arch Intern Med*. 1998 Jun 8; 158(11): 1228. PMID: 9521231

Capewell S, Hayes DK, Ford ES, Critchley JA, Croft JB, Greenlund KJ, Labarthe DR. 'Life-Years Gained Among US Adults From Modern Treatments and Changes in the Prevalence of 6 Coronary Heart Disease Risk Factors Between 1980 and 2000', *Am J Epidemiol.* 2009; 170: 229–236

Browner WS, Westenhouse J, Tice JA. 'What if Americans ate less fat? A quantitative estimate of the effect on mortality', *JAMA.* 1991 Jun 26; 265(24): 3285–91. PMID: 1801770

Taylor WC, Pass TM, Shepard DS, Komaroff AL. 'Cholesterol reduction and life expectancy. A model incorporating multiple risk factors', *Ann Intern Med.* 1987 Apr; 106(4): 605–14. doi: 10.7326/0003-4819-106-4-605. Erratum in: *Ann Intern Med.* 1988 Feb; 108(2): 314. PMID: 3826960

Yudkin JS. 'Assessing coronary risk', *BMJ.* 1995 Jul 22; 311(6999): 260–1. doi: 10.1136/bmj.311.6999.260d. PMID: 7627065; PMCID: PMC2550313

Grover SA, Lowensteyn I, Esrey KL, Steinert Y, Joseph L, Abrahamowicz M. 'Do doctors accurately assess coronary risk in their patients? Preliminary results of the coronary health assessment study', *BMJ.* 1995 Apr 15; 310(6985): 975–8. doi: 10.1136/bmj.310.6985.975. PMID: 7728035; PMCID: PMC2549361

Hamilton VH, Racicot FE, Zowall H, Coupal L, Grover SA. 'The cost-effectiveness of HMG-CoA reductase inhibitors to prevent coronary heart disease. Estimating the benefits of increasing HDL-C', *JAMA.* 1995 Apr 5; 273(13): 1032–8. PMID: 7897787

Denke MA, Grundy SM. 'Efficacy of low-dose cholesterol-lowering drug therapy in men with moderate hypercholesterolemia', *Arch Intern Med.* 1995 Feb 27; 155(4): 393–9. PMID: 7848022

Grover SA, Gray-Donald K, Joseph L, Abrahamowicz M, Coupal L. 'Life expectancy following dietary modification or smoking cessation. Estimating the benefits of a prudent lifestyle', *Arch Intern Med.* 1994 Aug 8; 154(15): 1697–704. Erratum in: *Arch Intern Med.* 1995 Jan 9; 155(1): 61. PMID: 8042886

National Cholesterol Education Program (NCEP) Expert Panel on Detection, Evaluation, and Treatment of High Blood Cholesterol in Adults (Adult Treatment Panel III). 'Third Report of the National Cholesterol Education Program (NCEP) Expert Panel on Detection, Evaluation, and Treatment of High Blood Cholesterol in Adults (Adult Treatment Panel III) final report', *Circulation.* 2002 Dec 17; 106(25): 3143–421. PMID: 12485966

Grover SA, Abrahamowicz M, Joseph L, Brewer C, Coupal L, Suissa S. 'The benefits of treating hyperlipidemia to prevent coronary heart disease. Estimating changes in life expectancy and morbidity', *JAMA.* 1992 Feb 12; 267(6): 816–22. PMID: 1732653

Does size matter?
Allaire J, Vors C, Couture P, Lamarche B. 'LDL particle number and size and cardiovascular risk: anything new under the sun?', *Current Opinion in Lipidology.* June 2017; volume 28, issue 3, pp. 261–266. doi: 10.1097/MOL.0000000000000419

Pichler G, Amigo N, Tellez-Plaza M, Pardo-Cea MA, Dominguez-Lucas A, Marrachelli VG, Monleon D, Martin-Escudero JC, Ascaso JF, Chaves FJ, Carmena R, Redon J. 'LDL particle size and composition and incident cardiovascular disease in a South-European population: The Hortega-Liposcale Follow-up Study', *Int J Cardiol.* 2018 Aug 1; 264: 172–178. doi: 10.1016/j.ijcard.2018.03.128. Epub 2018 Mar 29. PMID: 29628276

HDL – not simply good
Nicholls SJ, Nelson AJ. 'HDL and cardiovascular disease', *Pathology.* 2019 Feb; 51(2): 142–147. doi: 10.1016/j.pathol.2018.10.017. Epub 2019 Jan 3. PMID: 30612759

Kosmas CE, Martinez I, Sourlas A, Bouza KV, Campos FN, Torres V, Montan PD, Guzman E. 'High-density lipoprotein (HDL) functionality and its relevance to atherosclerotic cardiovascular disease', *Drugs Context.* 2018 Mar 28; 7: 212525. doi: 10.7573/dic.212525. PMID: 29623098; PMCID: PMC5877920

Allard-Ratick MP, Kindya BR, Khambhati J, et al. 'HDL: Fact, fiction, or function? HDL cholesterol and cardiovascular risk', *European Journal of Preventive Cardiology.* May 2019. doi: 10.1177/2047487319848214

Ruiz-Ramie JJ, Barber JL, Sarzynski MA. 'Effects of exercise on HDL functionality', *Curr Opin Lipidol.* 2019 Feb; 30(1): 16–23. doi: 10.1097/MOL.0000000000000568. PMID: 30480581; PMCID: PMC6492243

Triglycerides

Pradhan A, Bhandari M, Vishwakarma P, Sethi R. 'Triglycerides and Cardiovascular Outcomes – Can We REDUCE-IT?', *Int J Angiol*. 2020 Mar; 29(1): 2–11. doi: 10.1055/s-0040-1701639. Epub 2020 Feb 25. PMID: 32132810; PMCID: PMC7054063

Sandesara PB, Virani SS, Fazio S, Shapiro MD. 'The Forgotten Lipids: Triglycerides, Remnant Cholesterol, and Atherosclerotic Cardiovascular Disease Risk', *Endocrine Reviews*. April 2019; volume 40, issue 2, pp. 537–557. https://doi.org/10.1210/er.2018-00184

Halcox JP, Banegas JR, Roy C, et al. 'Prevalence and treatment of atherogenic dyslipidemia in the primary prevention of cardiovascular disease in Europe: EURIKA, a cross-sectional observational study', *BMC Cardiovasc Disord*. 2017; 17: 160. https://doi.org/10.1186/s12872-017-0591-5

Sniderman AD, Couture P, Martin SS, DeGraaf J, Lawler PR, Cromwell WC, Wilkins JT, Thanassoulis G. 'Hypertriglyceridemia and cardiovascular risk: a cautionary note about metabolic confounding', *J Lipid Res*. 2018 Jul; 59(7): 1266–1275. doi: 10.1194/jlr.R082271. Epub 2018 May 16. PMID: 29769239; PMCID: PMC6027915

Fish oil and survival

Siscovick DS, Barringer TA, Fretts AM, Wu JH, Lichtenstein AH, Costello RB, Kris-Etherton PM, Jacobson TA, Engler MB, Alger HM, Appel LJ, Mozaffarian D; American Heart Association Nutrition Committee of the Council on Lifestyle and Cardiometabolic Health; Council on Epidemiology and Prevention; Council on Cardiovascular Disease in the Young; Council on Cardiovascular and Stroke Nursing; and Council on Clinical Cardiology. 'Omega-3 Polyunsaturated Fatty Acid (Fish Oil) Supplementation and the Prevention of Clinical Cardiovascular Disease: A Science Advisory From the American Heart Association', *Circulation*. 2017 Apr 11; 135(15): e867–e884. doi: 10.1161/CIR.0000000000000482. Epub 2017 Mar 13. PMID: 28289069; PMCID: PMC6903779

https://www.abc.net.au/radionational/programs/healthreport/omega-3-supplements-dont-protect-against-heart-attack-or-stroke/10050886

Abdelhamid AS, Brown TJ, Brainard JS, Biswas P, Thorpe GC, Moore HJ, Deane KH, AlAbdulghafoor FK, Summerbell CD, Worthington HV, Song F, Hooper L. 'Omega-3 fatty acids for the primary and secondary prevention of cardiovascular disease', *Cochrane Database Syst Rev*. 2018 Jul 18; 7(7): CD003177. doi: 10.1002/14651858.CD003177.pub3. Update in: *Cochrane Database Syst Rev*. 2018 Nov 30; 11: CD003177. PMID: 30019766; PMCID: PMC6513557

https://www.abc.net.au/radionational/programs/healthreport/fish-oil-supplements-for-heart-health/12888668

Nicholls SJ, Lincoff AM, Garcia M, et al. 'Effect of High-Dose Omega-3 Fatty Acids vs Corn Oil on Major Adverse Cardiovascular Events in Patients at High Cardiovascular Risk: The STRENGTH Randomized Clinical Trial', *JAMA*. 2020; 324(22): 2268–2280. doi: 10.1001/jama.2020.22258

The polypill

Fiuza-Luces C, Garatachea N, Berger NA, Lucia A. 'Exercise is the real polypill', *Physiology (Bethesda)*. 2013 Sep; 28(5): 330–58. doi: 10.1152/physiol.00019.2013. PMID: 23997192

Lonn E, Bosch J, Teo KK, Pais P, Xavier D, Yusuf S. 'The polypill in the prevention of cardiovascular diseases: key concepts, current status, challenges, and future directions', *Circulation*. 2010 Nov 16; 122(20): 2078–88. doi: 10.1161/CIRCULATIONAHA.109.873232. PMID: 21098469

Wang TJ, Muñoz D, Blot WJ. 'Polypill for Cardiovascular Disease Prevention in an Underserved Population. Reply', *N Engl J Med*. 2020 Jan 2; 382(1): 95. doi: 10.1056/NEJMc1914047. PMID: 31875511; PMCID: PMC7061282

Wald NJ, Wald DS. 'The polypill concept', *Heart*. 2010 Jan; 96(1): 1–4. doi: 10.1136/hrt.2009.186429. PMID: 20019207

Wald DS, Morris JK, Wald NJ. 'Randomized Polypill crossover trial in people aged 50 and over', *PLoS One*. 2012; 7(7): e41297. doi: 10.1371/journal.pone.0041297. Epub 2012 Jul 18. PMID: 22815989; PMCID: PMC3399742

Wald NJ, Law MR. 'A strategy to reduce cardiovascular disease by more than 80%', *BMJ*. 2003 Sep 13; 327(7415): 586. Erratum for: *BMJ*. 326: 1419. PMCID: PMC194119

Living longer with more sex

Ebrahim S, May M, Ben Shlomo Y, McCarron P, Frankel S, Yarnell J, Davey Smith G. 'Sexual intercourse and risk of ischaemic stroke and coronary heart disease: the Caerphilly study', *J Epidemiol Community Health.* 2002 Feb; 56(2): 99–102. doi: 10.1136/jech.56.2.99. PMID: 11812807; PMCID: PMC1732071

Palmore EB. PhD, 'Predictors of the Longevity Difference: A 25-Year Follow-Up', *The Gerontologist,* December 1982; volume 22, issue 6, pp. 513–518. https://doi.org/10.1093/geront/22.6.513

Cheitlin MD. 'Sexual activity and cardiac risk', *Am J Cardiol.* 2005 Dec 26; 96(12B): 24M–28M. doi: 10.1016/j.amjcard.2005.07.007. Epub 2005 Nov 15. PMID: 16387562

Living longer with less salt

Refer to Our Salt Addiction references.

Life and your abdomen

Chang SH, Pollack LM, Colditz GA. 'Life Years Lost Associated with Obesity-Related Diseases for U.S. Non-Smoking Adults', *PLoS One.* 2013 Jun 18; 8(6): e66550. doi: 10.1371/journal.pone.0066550. PMID: 23823705; PMCID: PMC3688902

Chang SH, Yu YC, Carlsson NP, Liu X, Colditz GA. 'Racial disparity in life expectancies and life years lost associated with multiple obesity-related chronic conditions', *Obesity (Silver Spring).* 2017 May; 25(5): 950–957. doi: 10.1002/oby.21822. Epub 2017 Mar 22. PMID: 28329429; PMCID: PMC5404943

Grover SA, Kaouache M, Rempel P, Joseph L, Dawes M, Lau DC, Lowensteyn I. 'Years of life lost and healthy life-years lost from diabetes and cardiovascular disease in overweight and obese people: a modelling study', *Lancet Diabetes Endocrinol.* 2015 Feb; 3(2): 114–22. doi: 10.1016/S2213-8587(14)70229-3. Epub 2014 Dec 5. PMID: 25483220

Lung T, Jan S, Tan EJ, Killedar A, Hayes A. 'Impact of overweight, obesity and severe obesity on life expectancy of Australian adults', *Int J Obes (Lond).* 2019 Apr; 43(4): 782–789. doi: 10.1038/s41366-018-0210-2. Epub 2018 Oct 3. PMID: 30283076

Walter S, Kunst A, Mackenbach J, Hofman A, Tiemeier H. 'Mortality and disability: the effect of overweight and obesity', *Int J Obes (Lond).* 2009 Dec; 33(12): 1410–8. doi: 10.1038/ijo.2009.176. PMID: 19786964

Hruby A, Hu FB. 'The Epidemiology of Obesity: A Big Picture', *Pharmacoeconomics.* 2015 Jul; 33(7): 673–89. doi: 10.1007/s40273-014-0243-x. PMID: 25471927; PMCID: PMC4859313

Madala MC, Franklin BA, Chen AY, Berman AD, Roe MT, Peterson ED, Ohman EM, Smith SC Jr, Gibler WB, McCullough PA; CRUSADE Investigators. 'Obesity and age of first non-ST-segment elevation myocardial infarction', *J Am Coll Cardiol.* 2008 Sep 16; 52(12): 979–85. doi: 10.1016/j.jacc.2008.04.067. PMID: 18786477

Suwaidi JA, Wright RS, Grill JP, Hensrud DD, Murphy JG, Squires RW, Kopecky SL. 'Obesity is associated with premature occurrence of acute myocardial infarction', *Clin Cardiol.* 2001 Aug; 24(8): 542–7. doi: 10.1002/clc.4960240804. PMID: 11501605; PMCID: PMC6655201

Keller K, Münzel T, Ostad MA. 'Sex-specific differences in mortality and the obesity paradox of patients with myocardial infarction ages >70 y', *Nutrition.* 2018 Feb; 46: 124–130. doi: 10.1016/j.nut.2017.09.004. Epub 2017 Sep 22. PMID: 29108730

Murphy NF, MacIntyre K, Stewart S, Hart CL, Hole D, McMurray JJ. 'Long-term cardiovascular consequences of obesity: 20-year follow-up of more than 15 000 middle-aged men and women (the Renfrew-Paisley study)', *Eur Heart J.* 2006 Jan; 27(1): 96–106. doi: 10.1093/eurheartj/ehi506. Epub 2005 Sep 23. PMID: 16183687

Stevens J, Katz E, Huxley R. 'Associations between gender, age and waist circumference', *Eur J Clin Nutr.* 2010; 64: 6–15. https://doi.org/10.1038/ejcn.2009.101

McCarthy H, Jarrett K, Crawley H. 'The development of waist circumference percentiles in British children aged 5.0–16.9 y', *Eur J Clin Nutr.* 2001; 55: 902–907. https://doi.org/10.1038/sj.ejcn.1601240

Sui X, LaMonte MJ, Laditka JN, Hardin JW, Chase N, Hooker SP, Blair SN. 'Cardiorespiratory fitness and adiposity as mortality predictors in older adults', *JAMA.* 2007 Dec 5; 298(21): 2507–16. doi: 10.1001/jama.298.21.2507. PMID: 18056904; PMCID: PMC2692959

Power M, Schulkin J. 'Sex differences in fat storage, fat metabolism, and the health risks from obesity: Possible evolutionary origins', *British Journal of Nutrition.* 2008; 99(5): 931–940. doi: 10.1017/

S0007114507853347

Lear SA, Humphries KH, Kohli S, Birmingham CL. 'The use of BMI and waist circumference as surrogates of body fat differs by ethnicity', *Obesity (Silver Spring)*. 2007 Nov; 15(11): 2817–24. doi: 10.1038/oby.2007.334. PMID: 18070773

Freiberg MS, Pencina MJ, D'Agostino RB, Lanier K, Wilson PW, Vasan RS. 'BMI vs. waist circumference for identifying vascular risk', *Obesity (Silver Spring)*. 2008 Feb; 16(2): 463–9. doi: 10.1038/oby.2007.75. PMID: 18239660

Ashwell M, Gunn P, Gibson S. 'Waist-to-height ratio is a better screening tool than waist circumference and BMI for adult cardiometabolic risk factors: systematic review and meta-analysis', *Obes Rev*. 2012 Mar; 13(3): 275–86. doi: 10.1111/j.1467-789X.2011.00952.x. Epub 2011 Nov 23. PMID: 22106927

Adab P, Pallan M, Whincup PH. 'Is BMI the best measure of obesity?', *BMJ*. 2018 Mar 29; 360: k1274. doi: 10.1136/bmj.k1274. Erratum in: *BMJ*. 2018 May 23; 361: k2293. PMID: 29599212

Nuttall FQ. 'Body Mass Index: Obesity, BMI, and Health: A Critical Review', *Nutr Today*. 2015 May; 50(3): 117–128. doi: 10.1097/NT.0000000000000092. Epub 2015 Apr 7. PMID: 27340299; PMCID: PMC4890841

Peeters A, Magliano DJ, Backholer K, et al. 'Changes in the rates of weight and waist circumference gain in Australian adults over time: a longitudinal cohort study', *BMJ Open*. 2014; 4: e003667. doi: 10.1136/bmjopen-2013-003667

Ross R, Neeland IJ, Yamashita S, et al. 'Waist circumference as a vital sign in clinical practice: a Consensus Statement from the IAS and ICCR Working Group on Visceral Obesity', *Nat Rev Endocrinol*. 2020; 16: 177–189. https://doi.org/10.1038/s41574-019-0310-7

Lopez A, Adair T. 'Slower increase in life expectancy in Australia than in other high income countries: the contributions of age and cause of death', *Medical Journal of Australia*. 2019; 210. doi: 10.5694/mja2.50144

Hayes AJ, Lung TW, Bauman A, Howard K. 'Modelling obesity trends in Australia: unravelling the past and predicting the future', *Int J Obes (Lond)*. 2017; 41: 178–185

Global BMI Mortality Collaboration; Di Angelantonio E, Bhupathiraju SN, Wormser D, et al. 'Body-mass index and all-cause mortality: individual-participant-data meta-analysis of 239 prospective studies in four continents', *Lancet*. 2016; 388: 776–786

The metabolic syndrome

Alberti KG, Eckel RH, Grundy SM, et al. 'Harmonizing the metabolic syndrome: a joint interim statement of the International Diabetes Federation Task Force on Epidemiology and Prevention; National Heart, Lung, and Blood Institute; American Heart Association; World Heart Federation; International Atherosclerosis Society; and International Association for the Study of Obesity', *Circulation*. 2009; 120: 1640–5

Zimmet P, Alberti KG, Kaufman F, Tajima N, Silink M, Arslanian S, Wong G, Bennett P, Shaw J, Caprio S; IDF Consensus Group. 'The metabolic syndrome in children and adolescents – an IDF consensus report', *Pediatr Diabetes*. 2007 Oct; 8(5): 299–306. doi: 10.1111/j.1399-5448.2007.00271.x. PMID: 17850473

Alberti KG, Zimmet P, Shaw J. 'Metabolic syndrome – a new world-wide definition. A Consensus Statement from the International Diabetes Federation', *Diabet Med*. 2006 May; 23(5): 469–80. doi: 10.1111/j.1464-5491.2006.01858.x. PMID: 16681555

Assmann G, Guerra R, Fox G, Cullen P, Schulte H, Willett D, Grundy SM. 'Harmonizing the definition of the metabolic syndrome: comparison of the criteria of the Adult Treatment Panel III and the International Diabetes Federation in United States American and European populations', *Am J Cardiol*. 2007 Feb 15; 99(4): 541–8. doi: 10.1016/j.amjcard.2006.08.045. Epub 2007 Jan 2. PMID: 17293200

Laying waste to your waist (this is the weight loss bit)

Elfhag K, Rössner S. 'Who succeeds in maintaining weight loss? A conceptual review of factors associated with weight loss maintenance and weight regain', *Obes Rev*. 2005 Feb; 6(1): 67–85. doi: 10.1111/j.1467-789X.2005.00170.x. PMID: 15655039

Wing RR, Phelan S. 'Long-term weight loss maintenance', *The American Journal of Clinical Nutrition*. July 2005; volume 82, issue 1, pp. 222S–225S. https://doi.org/10.1093/ajcn/82.1.222S

Fuglestad PT, Jeffery RW, Sherwood NE. 'Lifestyle patterns associated with diet, physical activity, body mass index and amount of recent weight loss in a sample of successful weight losers', *Int J Behav Nutr Phys Act*. 2012 Jun 26; 9: 79. doi: 10.1186/1479-5868-9-79. PMID: 22734914; PMCID: PMC3494571

Exercise, HIIT and longevity
You E, Ellis KA, Cox K, Lautenschlager NT. 'Targeted physical activity for older adults with mild cognitive impairment and subjective cognitive decline', *Med J Aust*. 2019 May; 210(9): 394–395. e1. doi: 10.5694/mja2.50153. Epub 2019 Apr 25. PMID: 31020997

Gremeaux V, Gayda M, Lepers R, Sosner P, Juneau M, Nigam A. 'Exercise and longevity', *Maturitas*. 2012 Dec; 73(4): 312–7. doi: 10.1016/j.maturitas.2012.09.012. Epub 2012 Oct 11. PMID: 23063021

Kujala UM. 'Is physical activity a cause of longevity? It is not as straightforward as some would believe. A critical analysis', *British Journal of Sports Medicine*. 2018; 52: 914–918

Wewege M, van den Berg R, Ward RE, Keech A. 'The effects of high-intensity interval training vs. moderate-intensity continuous training on body composition in overweight and obese adults: a systematic review and meta-analysis', *Obes Rev*. 2017 Jun; 18(6): 635–646. doi: 10.1111/obr.12532. Epub 2017 Apr 11. PMID: 28401638

Lee I, Hsieh C, Paffenbarger RS. 'Exercise Intensity and Longevity in Men: The Harvard Alumni Health Study', *JAMA*. 1995; 273(15): 1179–1184. doi: 10.1001/jama.1995.03520390039030

Lee IM, Paffenbarger RS, Hennekens CH. 'Physical activity, physical fitness and longevity', *Aging Clin Exp Res*. 1997; 9: 2–11. https://doi.org/10.1007/BF03340123

Poirier P. 'Exercise, heart rate variability, and longevity: the cocoon mystery?', *Circulation*. 2014 May 27; 129(21): 2085–7. doi: 10.1161/CIRCULATIONAHA.114.009778. Epub 2014 May 5. PMID: 24799512

Levine HJ. 'Rest heart rate and life expectancy', *J Am Coll Cardiol*. 1997; 30: 1104–1106

Dekker JM, Crow RS, Folsom AR, Hannan PJ, Liao D, Swenne CA, Schouten EG. 'Low heart rate variability in a 2-minute rhythm strip predicts risk of coronary heart disease and mortality from several causes: the ARIC Study–Atherosclerosis Risk in Communities', *Circulation*. 2000; 102: 1239–1244

Capewell S, Hayes DK, Ford ES, Critchley JA, Croft JB, Greenlund KJ, Labarthe DR. 'Life-Years Gained Among US Adults From Modern Treatments and Changes in the Prevalence of 6 Coronary Heart Disease Risk Factors Between 1980 and 2000', *American Journal of Epidemiology*. 15 July 2009; volume 170, issue 2, pp. 229–236. https://doi.org/10.1093/aje/kwp150

Janssen I, Carson V, Lee IM, Katzmarzyk PT, Blair SN. 'Years of life gained due to leisure-time physical activity in the U.S.', *Am J Prev Med*. 2013 Jan; 44(1): 23–9. doi: 10.1016/j.amepre.2012.09.056. PMID: 23253646; PMCID: PMC3798023

Manuel DG, Perez R, Sanmartin C, Taljaard M, Hennessy D, Wilson K, Tanuseputro P, Manson H, Bennett C, Tuna M, Fisher S, Rosella LC. 'Measuring Burden of Unhealthy Behaviours Using a Multivariable Predictive Approach: Life Expectancy Lost in Canada Attributable to Smoking, Alcohol, Physical Inactivity, and Diet', *PLoS Med*. 2016 Aug 16; 13(8): e1002082. doi: 10.1371/journal.pmed.1002082. PMID: 27529741; PMCID: PMC4986987

Venturelli M, Schena F, Richardson RS. 'The role of exercise capacity in the health and longevity of centenarians', *Maturitas*. 2012 Oct; 73(2): 115–20. doi: 10.1016/j.maturitas.2012.07.009. Epub 2012 Aug 9. PMID: 22883374; PMCID: PMC3618983

Minois N. 'Longevity and aging: beneficial effects of exposure to mild stress', *Biogerontology*. 2000; 1(1): 15–29. doi: 10.1023/a:1010085823990. PMID: 11707916

Vina J, Sanchis-Gomar F, Martinez-Bello V, Gomez-Cabrera MC. 'Exercise acts as a drug; the pharmacological benefits of exercise', *Br J Pharmacol*. 2012 Sep; 167(1): 1–12. doi: 10.1111/j.1476-5381.2012.01970.x. PMID: 22486393; PMCID: PMC3448908

van Saase JL, Noteboom WM, Vandenbroucke JP. 'Longevity of men capable of prolonged vigorous physical exercise: a 32 year follow up of 2259 participants in the Dutch eleven cities ice skating tour', *BMJ*. 1990 Dec 22–29; 301(6766): 1409–11. doi: 10.1136/bmj.301.6766.1409. PMID: 2279154; PMCID: PMC1679864

Cadilhac DA, Cumming TB, Sheppard L, et al. 'The economic benefits of reducing physical inactivity:

an Australian example', *Int J Behav Nutr Phys Act*. 2011; 8: 99. https://doi.org/10.1186/1479-5868-8-99

Grace F, Herbert P, Elliott AD, Richards J, Beaumont A, Sculthorpe NF. 'High intensity interval training (HIIT) improves resting blood pressure, metabolic (MET) capacity and heart rate reserve without compromising cardiac function in sedentary aging men', *Exp Gerontol*. 2018 Aug; 109: 75–81. doi: 10.1016/j.exger.2017.05.010. Epub 2017 May 13. PMID: 28511954

Su L, Fu J, Sun S, Zhao G, Cheng W, Dou C, Quan M. 'Effects of HIIT and MICT on cardiovascular risk factors in adults with overweight and/or obesity: A meta-analysis', *PLoS One*. 2019 Jan 28; 14(1): e0210644. doi: 10.1371/journal.pone.0210644. PMID: 30689632; PMCID: PMC6349321

https://www.thelancet.com/series/physical-activity-2016

http://new.globalphysicalactivityobservatory.com/

Wu S, Cohen D, Shi Y, Pearson M, Sturm R. 'Economic analysis of physical activity interventions', *Am J Prev Med*. 2011 Feb; 40(2): 149–58. doi: 10.1016/j.amepre.2010.10.029. PMID: 21238863; PMCID: PMC3085087

Jetté M, Sidney K, Blümchen G. 'Metabolic equivalents (METS) in exercise testing, exercise prescription, and evaluation of functional capacity', *Clin Cardiol*. 1990 Aug; 13(8): 555–65. doi: 10.1002/clc.4960130809. PMID: 2204507

Mendes MA, da Silva I, Ramires V, Reichert F, Martins R, Ferreira R, Tomasi E. 'Metabolic equivalent of task (METs) thresholds as an indicator of physical activity intensity', *PLoS One*. 2018 Jul 19; 13(7): e0200701. doi: 10.1371/journal.pone.0200701. PMID: 30024953; PMCID: PMC6053180

Strasser B, Pesta D. 'Resistance training for diabetes prevention and therapy: experimental findings and molecular mechanisms', *Biomed Res Int*. 2013; 2013: 805217. doi: 10.1155/2013/805217. Epub 2013 Dec 22. PMID: 24455726; PMCID: PMC3881442

Pan B, Ge L, Xun YQ, Chen YJ, Gao CY, Han X, Zuo LQ, Shan HQ, Yang KH, Ding GW, Tian JH. 'Exercise training modalities in patients with type 2 diabetes mellitus: a systematic review and network meta-analysis', *Int J Behav Nutr Phys Act*. 2018 Jul 25; 15(1): 72. doi: 10.1186/s12966-018-0703-3. PMID: 30045740; PMCID: PMC6060544

Di Meo S, Iossa S, Venditti P. 'Improvement of obesity-linked skeletal muscle insulin resistance by strength and endurance training', *J Endocrinol*. 2017 Sep; 234(3): R159–R181. doi: 10.1530/JOE-17-0186. PMID: 28778962

A warning about getting ripped

Raevuori A, Hoek HW, Susser E, Kaprio J, Rissanen A, Keski-Rahkonen A. 'Epidemiology of Anorexia Nervosa in Men: A Nationwide Study of Finnish Twins', *PLoS ONE*. 2009; 4(2): e4402. https://doi.org/10.1371/journal.pone.0004402

https://www.nationaleatingdisorders.org/learn/general-information/research-on-males

Lavender JM, Brown TA, Murray SB. 'Men, Muscles, and Eating Disorders: an Overview of Traditional and Muscularity-Oriented Disordered Eating', *Curr Psychiatry Rep*. 2017 Jun; 19(6): 32. doi: 10.1007/s11920-017-0787-5. PMID: 28470486; PMCID: PMC5731454

Calzo JP, Horton NJ, Sonneville KR, Swanson SA, Crosby RD, Micali N, Eddy KT, Field AE. 'Male eating disorder symptom patterns and health correlates from 13 to 26 years of age', *J Am Acad Child Adolesc Psychiatry*. 2016; 55: 693–700

Compte EJ, Sepulveda AR, Torrente F. 'A two-stage epidemiological study of eating disorders and muscle dysmorphia in male university students in Buenos Aires', *Int J Eat Disord*. 2015; 48: 1092–101

Griffiths S, Murray SB, Touyz SW. 'Disordered eating and the muscular ideal', *J Eat Disord*. 2013; 1: 15

Tod D, Edwards C, Cranswick I. 'Muscle dysmorphia: current insights' *Psychol Res Behav Manag*. 2016 Aug 3; 9: 179–88. doi: 10.2147/PRBM.S97404. PMID: 27536165; PMCID: PMC4977020

Karpik A, Machniak M, Chwałczynska A. 'Evaluation of protein content in the diet of amateur male bodybuilder' *Am J Mens Health*. 2020 Nov–Dec; 14(6): 1557988320970267. doi: 10.1177/1557988320970267. PMID: 33256520; PMCID: PMC7711235

Badenes-Ribera L, Rubio-Aparicio M, Sánchez-Meca J, Fabris MA, Longobardi C. 'The association between muscle dysmorphia and eating disorder symptomatology: a systematic review and meta-analysis' *J Behav Addict*. 2019 Sep 1; 8(3): 351–371. doi: 10.1556/2006.8.2019.44. Epub 2019 Sep 11. PMID: 31505966; PMCID: PMC7044626

Nagata JM, Ganson KT, Griffiths S, Mitchison D, Garber AK, Vittinghoff E, Bibbins-Domingo K,

Murray SB. 'Prevalence and correlates of muscle-enhancing behaviors among adolescents and young adults in the United States' *Int J Adolesc Med Health*. 2020 Jun 5. doi: 10.1515/ijamh-2020-0001

Can my mum blame the menopause?
Asghari M, Mirghafourvand M, Mohammad-Alizadeh-Charandabi S, Malakouti J, Nedjat S. 'Effect of aerobic exercise and nutrition educationon quality of life and early menopause symptoms: A randomized controlled trial', *Women Health*. 2017 Feb; 57(2): 173–188. doi: 10.1080/03630242.2016.1157128. Epub 2016 Feb 24. PMID: 26909662

Witkowski S, Serviente C. 'Endothelial dysfunction and menopause: is exercise an effective countermeasure?', *Climacteric*. 2018 Jun; 21(3): 267–275. doi: 10.1080/13697137.2018.1441822. Epub 2018 Mar 15. PMID: 29542349

Gliemann L, Hellsten Y. 'The exercise timing hypothesis: can exercise training compensate for the reduction in blood vessel function after menopause if timed right?', *J Physiol*. 2019 Oct; 597(19): 4915–4925. doi: 10.1113/JP277056. Epub 2019 Jun 30. PMID: 31077368

Sydora BC, MSc, PhD1; Turner C, BSc1; Malley A, BSc1; Davenport M, PhD2; Yuksel N, BScPharm, PharmD, FCSHP, NCMP3; Shandro T, MD4,5; Ross S, PhD1. 'Can walking exercise programs improve health for women in menopause transition and postmenopausal? Findings from a scoping review', *Menopause*. August 2020, volume 27, issue 8, pp. 952–963. doi: 10.1097/GME.0000000000001554

Orri JC, Hughes EM, Mistry DG, Scala AH. 'Is Vigorous Exercise Training Superior to Moderate for CVD Risk after Menopause?', *Sports Med Int Open*. 2017 Sep 6; 1(5): E166–E171. doi: 10.1055/s-0043-118094. PMID: 30539103; PMCID: PMC6226081

What you need to know about smoking (vaping comes later)
Rosenberg MA, Feuer EJ, Yu B, Sun J, Henley SJ, Shanks TG, Anderson CM, McMahon PM, Thun MJ, Burns DM. 'Chapter 3: Cohort life tables by smoking status, removing lung cancer as a cause of death', *Risk Anal*. 2012 Jul; 32 Suppl 1(Suppl 1): S25–38. doi: 10.1111/j.1539-6924.2011.01662.x. PMID: 22882890; PMCID: PMC3594098

Owen AJ, Maulida SB, Zomer E, et al. 'Productivity burden of smoking in Australia: a life table modelling study', *Tobacco Control*. 2019; 28: 297–304

Brønnum-Hansen H, Juel K. 'Abstention from smoking extends life and compresses morbidity: a population based study of health expectancy among smokers and never smokers in Denmark', *Tobacco Control*. 2001; 10: 273–278

Buchwald J, Chenoweth MJ, Palviainen T, et al. 'Genome-wide association meta-analysis of nicotine metabolism and cigarette consumption measures in smokers of European descent', *Mol Psychiatry*. 2020. https://doi.org/10.1038/s41380-020-0702-z

Not just lack of will
Lariscy JT. 'Smoking-attributable mortality by cause of death in the United States: An indirect approach', *SSM Popul Health*. 2019 Jan 11; 7: 100349. doi: 10.1016/j.ssmph.2019.100349. PMID: 30723766; PMCID: PMC6351587

Hughes JR. 'Comorbidity and smoking', *Nicotine Tob Res*. 1999; 1 Suppl 2: S149–52; discussion S165–6. doi: 10.1080/14622299050011981. PMID: 11768173

Kalman D, Morissette SB, George TP. 'Co-morbidity of smoking in patients with psychiatric and substance use disorders', *Am J Addict*. 2005 Mar–Apr; 14(2): 106–23. doi: 10.1080/10550490590924728. PMID: 16019961; PMCID: PMC1199553

Huisman M, Kunst AE, Mackenbach JP. 'Inequalities in the prevalence of smoking in the European Union: comparing education and income', *Prev Med*. 2005 Jun; 40(6): 756–64. doi: 10.1016/j.ypmed.2004.09.022. PMID: 15850876

Stopping smoking before it starts and beware vaping
Charlesworth A, Glantz SA. 'Smoking in the movies increases adolescent smoking: a review', *Pediatrics*. 2005 Dec; 116(6): 1516–28. doi: 10.1542/peds.2005-0141. PMID: 16322180

Chapman S, Wakefield M. 'Smoking cessation strategies', *BMJ (Clinical research edition)*. 2012; 344; e1732. doi: 10.1136/bmj.e1732

Thomas DP, Briggs VL, Couzos S, Panaretto KS, van der Sterren AE, Stevens M, Borland R. 'Use of nicotine replacement therapy and stop-smoking medicines in a national sample of Aboriginal and Torres Strait Islander smokers and ex-smokers', *Medical Journal of Australia*. 2015; 202: S78–S84. https://doi.org/10.5694/mja15.00205

Hammond D, Reid JL, Rynard VL, Fong GT, Cummings KM, McNeill A, et al. 'Prevalence of vaping and smoking among adolescents in Canada, England, and the United States: repeat national cross sectional surveys', *BMJ*. 2019; 365: l2219 doi: 10.1136/bmj.l2219

Hammond D, Reid JL, Cole AG, Leatherdale ST. 'Electronic cigarette use and smoking initiation among youth: a longitudinal cohort study', *CMAJ*. 2017; 189: E1328–36. doi: 10.1503/cmaj.161002. PMID: 29084759

Leventhal AM, Stone MD, Andrabi N, et al. 'Association of e-cigarette vaping and progression to heavier patterns of cigarette smoking', *JAMA*. 2016; 316: 1918–20. doi: 10.1001/jama.2016.14649. PMID: 27825000

East K, Hitchman SC, Bakolis I, et al. 'The association between smoking and electronic cigarette use in a cohort of young people', *J Adolesc Health*. 2018; 62: 539–47. doi: 10.1016/j.jadohealth.2017.11.301. PMID: 29499983

Levy DT, Warner KE, Cummings KM, et al. 'Examining the relationship of vaping to smoking initiation among US youth and young adults: a reality check', *Tob Control*. 2018; published online 20 Nov. doi: 10.1136/tobaccocontrol-2018-054446. PMID: 30459182CrossRefPubMedGoogle Scholar

Smoking versus weight gain – which matters most?

Filozof C, Fernández Pinilla MC, Fernández-Cruz A. 'Smoking cessation and weight gain' *Obes Rev*. 2004 May; 5(2): 95–103. doi: 10.1111/j.1467-789X.2004.00131.x. PMID: 15086863

Kawachi I, Troisi RJ, Rotnitzky AG, Coakley EH, Colditz GA. 'Can physical activity minimize weight gain in women after smoking cessation?' *American Journal of Public Health*. 1996; 86, 999–1004. https://doi.org/10.2105/AJPH.86.7.999

Your life and other people's smoke

Leone A, Giannini D, Bellotto C, Balbarini A. 'Passive smoking and coronary heart disease' *Curr Vasc Pharmacol*. 2004 Apr; 2(2): 175–82. doi: 10.2174/1570161043476366. PMID: 15320518

Centers for Disease Control and Prevention (CDC). 'Smoking-attributable mortality, years of potential life lost, and productivity losses – United States, 2000–2004' *Morb Mortal Wkly Rep (MMWR)*. 2008 Nov 14; 57(45): 1226–8. PMID: 19008791

What you need to know about alcohol

Stockwell T, Zhao J, Panwar S, Roemer A, Naimi T, Chikritzhs T. 'Do "Moderate" Drinkers Have Reduced Mortality Risk? A Systematic Review and Meta-Analysis of Alcohol Consumption and All-Cause Mortality', *Journal of Studies on Alcohol and Drugs*. 2016; 77: 2, 185–198

Bruce ML, Leaf PJ, Rozal GPM, et al. 'Psychiatric status and 9-year mortality in the New Haven Epidemiologic Catchment Area study', *American Journal of Psychiatry*. 1994; 151: 716–721

Naimi TS, Stockwell T, Zhao J, Xuan Z, Dangardt F, Saitz R, Liang W, Chikritzhs T. 'Selection biases in observational studies affect associations between "moderate" alcohol consumption and mortality', *Addiction*. 2017; 112: 207–214. doi: 10.1111/add.13451

Rehm J, Patra J, Popova S. 'Alcohol-attributable mortality and potential years of life lost in Canada 2001: implications for prevention and policy', *Addiction*. 2006 Mar; 101(3): 373–84. doi: 10.1111/j.1360-0443.2005.01338.x. PMID: 16499510

Sjögren H, Eriksson A, Broström G, Ahlm K. 'Quantification of alcohol-related mortality in Sweden', *Alcohol Alcohol*. 2000 Nov–Dec; 35(6): 601–11. doi: 10.1093/alcalc/35.6.601. PMID: 11093968

Anstey KJ, Windsor TD, Rodgers B, Jorm AF, Christensen H. 'Lower cognitive test scores observed in alcohol abstainers are associated with demographic, personality, and biological factors: the PATH Through Life Project', *Addiction*. 2005; 100: 1291–1301

Anstey KJ, Jorm AF, Reglade-Meslin C, Maller JJ, Kumar R, von Sanden C, Windsor TD, Rodgers B, Wen W, Sachdev P. 'Weekly alcohol consumption, brain atrophy and white matter hyperintensities in a community based sample aged 60–64', *Psychosomatic Medicine*. 2006; 68: 778–785

Sachdev PS, Chen X, Wen W, Anstey KJ. 'Light to moderate alcohol use is associated with increased cortical gray matter in middle-aged men: a voxel-based morphometric study', *Psychiatry Research*. 2008; 163(1): 61–9

What is it about turning 40?
Doyle G. *Untamed*. 2020. The Dial Press

What do the stats in Australia say?
Australian Gender Equality Council – Resources section. https://www.agec.org.au/resources/
Australian Gender Equality Council. 'Australia's gender equality scorecard'. November 2019.
https://www.agec.org.au/wp-content/uploads/2020/02/2018-19-Gender-Equality-Scorecard.pdf
Australian Human Rights Commission. 'A Conversation in Gender Equality'. March 2017.
https://www.agec.org.au/wp-content/uploads/2018/09/AHRC-A-Conversation-on-Gender-Equality-2017.pdf
The Australian Women's Working Futures Project, The University of Sydney. 'Women and the Future of Work Report 1'. 2018
https://www.agec.org.au/wp-content/uploads/2018/09/Women-and-the-Future-of-Work-Report-2017.pdf
https://www.agec.org.au/wp-content/uploads/2018/09/Time-to-Talk-What-Has-to-Change-for-Women-at-Work-2018.pdf
Parker K, Patten E. *The Sandwich Generation*. 2013. Pew Research Center
'Unpacking the mental load: How to know if you're doing too much – and how to stop'
https://assets.jeanhailes.org.au/JHMagazine/JeanHailes_Magazine_2019_Vol2.pdf?_ga=2.49545382.1661518074.1602115758-1729957488.1602115758
Kulkarni J. 'Gender Differences in Mental Health', The Alfred and Monash University.
https://psychscenehub.com/video/gender-differences-mental-health-professor-jayashri-kulkarni/
Melbourne Institute – Applied Economic & Social Research, The University of Melbourne. 'The Household, Income and Labour Dynamics in Australia Survey: Selected Findings from Waves 1 to 16'. 2018.

So what about divorce?
Australian Institute of Family Studies. 'Couple relationships Australian Families Then & Now'. July 2020.
https://aifs.gov.au/sites/default/files/publication-documents/2007_aftn_couples.pdf
Australian Institute of Family Studies. 'Divorce rates in Australia'. https://aifs.gov.au/facts-and-figures/divorce-rates-australia

Looking after kids
Australian Institute of Family Studies. 'Life During Covid-19: Families in Australia Survey Report no:1 Early Findings'. July 2020.
https://aifs.gov.au/sites/default/files/publication-documents/covid-19-survey-report_1_early_findings_0.pdf
https://melbourneinstitute.unimelb.edu.au/__data/assets/pdf_file/0005/2839919/2018-HILDA-SR-for-web.pdf

Let's talk about sex
The Australian Study of Health and Relationships (ASHR). 'Sex in Australia 2'. https://www.ashr.edu.au/wp-content/uploads/2015/06/sex_in_australia_2_summary_data.pdf
Thomas HN, Hamm M, Hess R, Thurston RC. 'Changes in sexual function among midlife women: "I'm older... and I'm wiser"', *Menopause*. 2018 Mar; 25(3): 286–292. doi: 10.1097/GME.0000000000000988. PMID: 29088016; PMCID: PMC5821528
Meston CM, Hamilton LD, Harte CB. 'Sexual motivation in women as a function of age', *J Sex Med*. 2009 Dec; 6(12): 3305–19. doi: 10.1111/j.1743-6109.2009.01489.x. Epub 2009 Sep 14. Erratum in: *J Sex Med*. 2010 Nov; 7(11): 3803. PMID: 19751384; PMCID: PMC2978963

Maybe mid-life doesn't have to be a crisis at all
Gilbert E. *Eat Pray Love*. 2006. Penguin
Magon N, Chauhan M, Malik S, Shah D. 'Sexuality in midlife: Where the passion goes?', *J Midlife Health*. 2012 Jul; 3(2): 61–5. doi: 10.4103/0976-7800.104452. PMID: 23372319; PMCID:

PMC3555026

Bain & Company. 'Better Together: Increasing Male Engagement in Gender Equality Efforts in Australia'. 2019. https://www.wgea.gov.au/sites/default/files/documents/CEW-BAIN_REPORT_Better_Together_19-03-2019.pdf

Fair Work Ombudsman. 'Paid parental leave'. https://www.fairwork.gov.au/leave/maternity-and-parental-leave/paid-parental-leave

Baxter J. 'Fathers and Work: A statistical overview', Australian Institute of Family Studies. 2019. https://aifs.gov.au/aifs-conference/fathers-and-work

Crabb A. *The Wife Drought – Why Women Need Wives and Men Need Lives*. 2015. Penguin

· https://www.womenonboards.net/en-au/resources/boardroom-diversity-index

https://www.wgea.gov.au/publications/gender-equitable-parental-leave

Endometriosis and its curious genetic links

AIHW. 'Endometriosis in Australia: prevalence and hospitalisations'. Published August 2019

Adewuyi EO, Mehta D, Sapkota Y; International Endogene Consortium; 23andMe Research Team: Auta A, Yoshihara K, Nyegaard M, Griffiths LR, Montgomery GW, Chasman DI, Nyholt DR. 'Genetic analysis of endometriosis and depression identifies shared loci and implicates causal links with gastric mucosa abnormality', *Hum Genet.* 2021 Mar; 140(3): 529–552. doi: 10.1007/s00439-020-02223-6. Epub 2020 Sep 21. PMID: 32959083

Adewuyi EO, Sapkota Y; International Endogene Consortium (IEC); 23andMe Research Team; International Headache Genetics Consortium (IHGC); Auta A, Yoshihara K, Nyegaard M, Griffiths LR, Montgomery GW, Chasman DI, Nyholt DR. 'Shared Molecular Genetic Mechanisms Underlie Endometriosis and Migraine Comorbidity', *Genes (Basel).* 2020 Feb 29; 11(3): 268. doi: 10.3390/genes11030268. PMID: 32121467; PMCID: PMC7140889

When do my eggs clap out? And when do his sperm?

Igarashi H, Takahashi T, Nagase S. 'Oocyte aging underlies female reproductive aging: biological mechanisms and therapeutic strategies', *Reprod Med Biol.* 2015 May 9; 14(4): 159–169. doi: 10.1007/s12522-015-0209-5. PMID: 29259413; PMCID: PMC5715832

Joseph JF, Parr MK. 'Synthetic androgens as designer supplements', *Curr Neuropharmacol.* 2015 Jan; 13(1): 89–100. doi: 10.2174/1570159X13666141210224756. PMID: 26074745; PMCID: PMC4462045

El Osta R, Almont T, Diligent C, Hubert N, Eschwège P, Hubert J. 'Anabolic steroids abuse and male infertility', *Basic Clin Androl.* 2016 Feb 6; 26: 2. doi: 10.1186/s12610-016-0029-4. PMID: 26855782; PMCID: PMC4744441

Harris ID, Fronczak C, Roth L, Meacham RB. 'Fertility and the aging male', *Rev Urol.* 2011; 13(4): e184–90. PMID: 22232567; PMCID: PMC3253726

Sandin S et al. 'Autism risk associated with parental age and with increasing difference in age between the parents' *Molecular Psychiatry.* 2016 May; 21(5): 693–700

Gaskins AJ, Rich-Edwards JW, Missmer SA, Rosner B, Chavarro JE. 'Association of Fecundity With Changes in Adult Female Weight', *Obstet Gynecol.* 2015 Oct; 126(4): 850–858. doi: 10.1097/AOG.0000000000001030. PMID: 26348178; PMCID: PMC4580510

Boutari C, Pappas PD, Mintziori G, Nigdelis MP, Athanasiadis L, Goulis DG, Mantzoros CS. 'The effect of underweight on female and male reproduction', *Metabolism.* 2020 Jun; 107: 154229. doi: 10.1016/j.metabol.2020.154229. Epub 2020 Apr 11. PMID: 32289345

Guo D, Xu M, Zhou Q, Wu C, Ju R, Dai J. 'Is low body mass index a risk factor for semen quality? A PRISMA-compliant meta-analysis', *Medicine (Baltimore).* 2019 Aug; 98(32): e16677. doi: 10.1097/MD.0000000000016677. PMID: 31393367; PMCID: PMC6709190

The flip side … when you still have all your eggs

Remsberg KE, Demerath EW, Schubert CM, Chumlea WC, Sun SS, Siervogel RM. 'Early menarche and the development of cardiovascular disease risk factors in adolescent girls: the Fels Longitudinal Study', *J Clin Endocrinol Metab.* 2005 May; 90(5): 2718–24. doi: 10.1210/jc.2004-1991. Epub 2005 Feb 22. PMID: 15728207

Jorm AF, Christensen H, Rodgers B, Jacomb PA, Easteal S. 'Association of adverse childhood experiences, age of menarche and adult reproductive behavior: Does the androgen receptor gene play a role?', *American Journal of Medical Genetics (Neuropsychiatric Genetics)*. 2004; 125B

Low L-F, Anstey KJ, Jorm AF, Rodgers B, Christensen H. 'Reproductive period and cognitive function in a representative sample of naturally postmenopausal women aged 60–64', *Climacteric*. 2005; 8: 380–389

Chisholm JS, Quinlivan JA, Petersen RW, Coall DA. 'Early stress predicts age at menarche and first birth, adult attachment, and expected lifespan', *Hum Nat*. 2005 Sep; 16(3): 233–65. doi: 10.1007/s12110-005-1009-0. PMID: 26189749

Kelsey JL, Gammon MD, John EM. 'Reproductive factors and breast cancer', *Epidemiol Rev*. 1993; 15(1): 36–47. doi: 10.1093/oxfordjournals.epirev.a036115. PMID: 8405211

Thomas F, Renaud F, Benefice E, de Meeus T, Guegan J-F. 'International Variability of Ages at Menarche and Menopause: Patterns and Main Determinants', *Human Biology*. 2001; volume 73, number 2, pp. 271–290

Adair LS, Gordon-Larsen P. 'Maturational timing and overweight prevalence in US adolescent girls', *Am J Public Health*. 2001 Apr; 91(4): 642–4. doi: 10.2105/ajph.91.4.642. PMID: 11291382; PMCID: PMC1446647

Giles LC, Glonek GF, Moore VM, Davies MJ, Luszcz MA. 'Lower age at menarche affects survival in older Australian women: results from the Australian Longitudinal Study of Ageing', *BMC Public Health*. 2010 Jun 15; 10: 341. doi: 10.1186/1471-2458-10-341. PMID: 20546623; PMCID: PMC2908577

Frontini MG, Srinivasan SR, Berenson GS. 'Longitudinal changes in risk variables underlying metabolic Syndrome X from childhood to young adulthood in female subjects with a history of early menarche: the Bogalusa Heart Study', *Int J Obes Relat Metab Disord*. 2003 Nov; 27(11): 1398–404. doi: 10.1038/sj.ijo.0802422. PMID: 14574352

Marshall LM, Spiegelman D, Goldman MB, Manson JE, Colditz GA, Barbieri RL, Stampfer MJ, Hunter DJ. 'A prospective study of reproductive factors and oral contraceptive use in relation to the risk of uterine leiomyomata', *Fertil Steril*. 1998 Sep; 70(3): 432–9. doi: 10.1016/s0015-0282(98)00208-8. PMID: 9757871

Li CI, Malone KE, Daling JR, Potter JD, Bernstein L, Marchbanks PA, Strom BL, Simon MS, Press MF, Ursin G, Burkman RT, Folger SG, Norman S, McDonald JA, Spirtas R. 'Timing of menarche and first full-term birth in relation to breast cancer risk', *Am J Epidemiol*. 2008 Jan 15; 167(2): 230–9. doi: 10.1093/aje/kwm271. Epub 2007 Oct 26. PMID: 17965112; PMCID: PMC3804121

https://www.ncbi.nlm.nih.gov/pmc/articles/PMC2994234

Part 4: The wellbeing thing

Wellness and resilience: two annoying words

Rosenman S, Rodgers B. 'Childhood adversity and adult personality', *Aust & NZ J Psychiatry*. 2006; 40: 482–490

van der Wal SJ, Gorter R, Reijnen A, et al. 'Cohort profile: the Prospective Research In Stress Related Military Operations (PRISMO) study in the Dutch Armed Forces', *BMJ Open*. 2019; 9: e026670. doi: 10.1136/ bmjopen-2018-026670

Baker DG, Nash WP, Litz BT, et al. 'Predictors of risk and resilience for post-traumatic stress disorder among ground combat Marines: methods of the Marine Resiliency Study', *Prev Chronic Dis*. 2012; 9: e97

Naifeh JA, Herberman Mash HB, Stein MB, Fullerton CS, Kessler RC, Ursano RJ. 'The Army Study to Assess Risk and Resilience in Servicemembers (Army STARRS): progress toward understanding suicide among soldiers', *Molecular Psychiatry*. 2019; 24: 34–48. https://doi.org/10.1038/s41380-018-0197-z

Sudom KA, Lee JE, Zamorski MA. 'A longitudinal pilot study of resilience in Canadian military personnel', *Stress Health*. 2014 Dec; 30(5): 377–85. doi: 10.1002/smi.2614. PMID: 25476962

Rocklein Kemplin K, Paun O, Godbee DC, Brandon JW. 'Resilience and Suicide in Special Operations Forces: State of the Science via Integrative Review', *J Spec Oper Med*. 2019 Summer; 19(2): 57–66. PMID: 31201752

Rocklein-Kemplin K, Paun O, Sons N, Brandon JW. 'The Myth of Hyperresilience Evolutionary Concept Analysis of Resilience in Special Operations Forces', *J Spec Oper Med*. 2018 Spring; 18(1): 54–60. PMID: 29533434

Stein MB, Campbell-Sills L, Ursano RJ, Rosellini AJ, Colpe LJ, He F, Heeringa SG, Nock MK, Sampson NA, Schoenbaum M, Sun X, Jain S, Kessler RC; Army STARRS Collaborators. 'Childhood Maltreatment and Lifetime Suicidal Behaviors Among New Soldiers in the US Army: Results From the Army Study to Assess Risk and Resilience in Servicemembers (Army STARRS)', *J Clin Psychiatry.* 2018 Mar/Apr; 79(2): 16m10900. doi: 10.4088/JCP.16m10900. PMID: 28541647; PMCID: PMC6460907

Campbell-Sills L, Kessler RC, Ursano RJ, Sun X, Taylor CT, Heeringa SG, Nock MK, Sampson NA, Jain S, Stein MB. 'Predictive validity and correlates of self-assessed resilience among U.S. Army soldiers', *Depress Anxiety.* 2018 Feb; 35(2): 122–131. doi: 10.1002/da.22694. Epub 2017 Nov 2. PMID: 29095544; PMCID: PMC6013057

Pyne JM, Constans JI, Nanney JT, Wiederhold MD, Gibson DP, Kimbrell T, Kramer TL, Pitcock JA, Han X, Williams DK, Chartrand D, Gevirtz RN, Spira J, Wiederhold BK, McCraty R, McCune TR. 'Heart Rate Variability and Cognitive Bias Feedback Interventions to Prevent Post-deployment PTSD: Results from a Randomized Controlled Trial', *Mil Med.* 2019 Jan 1; 184(1–2): e124–e132. doi: 10.1093/milmed/usy171. PMID: 30020511; PMCID: PMC6751385

Mjelde FV, Smith K, Lunde P, Espevik R. 'Military teams – A demand for resilience', *Work.* 2016 May 27; 54(2): 283–94. doi: 10.3233/WOR-162298. PMID: 27259180

van der Wal SJ, Vermetten E, Elbert G. 'Long-term development of post-traumatic stress symptoms and associated risk factors in military service members deployed to Afghanistan: Results from the PRISMO 10-year follow-up', *Eur Psychiatry.* 2020 Dec 21; 64(1): e10. doi: 10.1192/j.eurpsy.2020.113. PMID: 33342444

Bonanno GA, Mancini AD, Horton JL, Powell TM, Leardmann CA, Boyko EJ, Wells TS, Hooper TI, Gackstetter GD and Smith TC, for the Millennium Cohort Study Team. 'Trajectories of trauma symptoms and resilience in deployed US military service members: prospective cohort study', *The British Journal of Psychiatry.* 2012; 200: 317–323. doi: 10.1192/bjp.bp.111.096552

Smith BN, Vaughn RA, Vogt D, King DW, King LA, Shipherd JC. 'Main and interactive effects of social support in predicting mental health symptoms in men and women following military stressor exposure', *Anxiety Stress Coping.* 2013; 26(1): 52–69. doi: 10.1080/10615806.2011.634001. Epub 2011 Nov 21. PMID: 22098413

Hossack MR, MD, USAF, MC; Reid MW, PhD; Aden JK, PhD; Gibbons T, PhD, GS-14, DAF MT, ASCP, MS CLS; Noe JC, MT (ASCP), PhD; Willis AM, MD, PhD, MC, FS, USAF. 'Adverse Childhood Experience, Genes, and PTSD Risk in Soldiers: A Methylation Study', *Military Medicine.* March–April 2020, volume 185, issue 3–4, pp. 377–384. https://doi.org/10.1093/milmed/usz292

Stevanović A, Frančišković T, Vermetten E. 'Relationship of early-life trauma, war-related trauma, personality traits, and PTSD symptom severity: a retrospective study on female civilian victims of war', *Eur J Psychotraumatol.* 2016 Apr 6; 7: 30964. doi: 10.3402/ejpt.v7.30964. PMID: 27056034; PMCID: PMC4824847

Kimhi S, Marciano H, Eshel Y, Adini B. 'Resilience and demographic characteristics predicting distress during the COVID-19 crisis', *Soc Sci Med.* 2020 Nov; 265: 113389. doi: 10.1016/j.socscimed.2020.113389. Epub 2020 Sep 25. PMID: 33039732; PMCID: PMC7518838

Work–life balance: yet more annoying words

Fleetwood S. 'Why work–life balance now?' *The International Journal of Human Resource Management.* 2007; 18(3) 387–400. doi: 10.1080/09585190601167441

Byrne U. 'Work-life balance: Why are we talking about it at all?' *Business Information Review.* 2005; 22(1): 53–59. doi:10.1177/0266382105052268

So should we be talking about burnout?

Broom DH, DíSouza RM, Strazdins L, Butterworth P, Parslow R, Rodgers B. (2006) 'The lesser evil: bad jobs or unemployment? A survey of mid-aged Australians', *Social Science and Medicine.* 2006; 63: 575–586

D'Souza RM, Strazdins L, Clements MS, Broom DH, Parslow R, Rodgers B. 'The health effects of jobs: status, working conditions or both?', *Australian and New Zealand Journal of Public Health.* 2005; 29: 222–228

Parslow RA, Jorm AF, Christensen H, Rodgers B, Strazdins L, D'Souza RM. 'The associations between work stress and mental health: A comparison of organizationally employed and self-employed workers', *Work and Stress.* 2004; 18: 3, 231–244

Wilson SH, Walker GM. 'Unemployment and health: a review', *Public Health*. 1993 May; 107(3): 153–62. doi: 10.1016/s0033-3506(05)80436-6. PMID: 8511234 https://www.mindgarden.com/312-mbi-general-survey

Maslach C, 'Job Burnout: New Directions in Research and Intervention', *Current Directions in Psychological Science*. First published October 1, 2003. Research article. https://doi.org/10.1111/1467-8721.01258

Maslach C, Leiter MP. 'Understanding the burnout experience: recent research and its implications for psychiatry', *World Psychiatry*. 2016 Jun; 15(2): 103–11. doi: 10.1002/wps.20311. PMID: 27265691; PMCID: PMC4911781

Gómez-Gascón T, Martín-Fernández J, Gálvez-Herrer M, et al. 'Effectiveness of an intervention for prevention and treatment of burnout in primary health care professionals', *BMC Fam Pract*. 2013; 14: 173. https://doi.org/10.1186/1471-2296-14-173

Korczak D, Wastian M, Schneider M. 'Therapy of the burnout syndrome', *GMS Health Technol Assess*. 2012; 8: Doc05. doi: 10.3205/hta000103. Epub 2012 Jun 14. PMID: 22984372; PMCID: PMC3434360

Kakiashvili T, Leszek J, Rutkowski K. 'The medical perspective on burnout', *IJOMEH*. 2013; 26: 401–412. https://doi.org/10.2478/s13382-013-0093-3

It's usually better to think about strengths

Wessells MG. 'Strengths-based community action as a source of resilience for children affected by armed conflict', *Glob Ment Health (Camb)*. 2016 Jan 21; 3: e1. doi: 10.1017/gmh.2015.23. PMID: 28596870; PMCID: PMC5314737

Ibrahim N, Michail M, Callaghan P. 'The strengths based approach as a service delivery model for severe mental illness: a meta-analysis of clinical trials', *BMC Psychiatry*. 2014 Aug 29; 14: 243. doi: 10.1186/s12888-014-0243-6. PMID: 25189400; PMCID: PMC415452

Tse S, Tsoi EW, Hamilton B, O'Hagan M, Shepherd G, Slade M, Whitley R, Petrakis M. 'Uses of strength-based interventions for people with serious mental illness: A critical review', *Int J Soc Psychiatry*. 2016 May; 62(3): 281–91. doi: 10.1177/0020764015623970. Epub 2016 Feb 1. PMID: 26831826

Mautone JA, Pendergast LL, Cassano M, Blum NJ, Power TJ. 'Behavioral Health Screening: Validation of a Strength-Based Approach', *J Dev Behav Pediatr*. 2020 Oct–Nov; 41(8): 587–595. doi: 10.1097/DBP.0000000000000832. PMID: 32576785

Yu DS, Li PW, Zhang F, Cheng ST, Ng TK, Judge KS. 'The effects of a dyadic strength-based empowerment program on the health outcomes of people with mild cognitive impairment and their family caregivers: a randomized controlled trial', *Clin Interv Aging*. 2019 Oct 4; 14: 1705–1717. doi: 10.2147/CIA.S213006. PMID: 31686796; PMCID: PMC6783396

Frankowski BL, Leader IC, Duncan PM. 'Strength-based interviewing', *Adolesc Med State Art Rev*. 2009 Apr; 20(1): 22–40, vii–viii. PMID: 19492689

Rogoff B, Coppens AD, Alcalá L, Aceves-Azuara I, Ruvalcaba O, López A, Dayton A. 'Noticing Learners' Strengths Through Cultural Research', *Perspect Psychol Sci*. 2017 Sep; 12(5): 876–888. doi: 10.1177/1745691617718355. PMID: 28972848

Sederer LI. 'The Social Determinants of Mental Health', *Psychiatr Serv*. 2016 Feb; 67(2): 234–5. doi: 10.1176/appi.ps.201500232. Epub 2015 Nov 2. PMID: 26522677

Distress and depression: two sides of the same coin?

Russ TC, Stamatakis E, Hamer M, Starr JM, Kivimäki M, Batty GD. 'Association between psychological distress and mortality: individual participant pooled analysis of 10 prospective cohort studies', *BMJ*. 2012 Jul 31; 345: e4933. doi: 10.1136/bmj.e4933. PMID: 22849956; PMCID: PMC3409083

Hamer M, Kivimaki M, Stamatakis E, Batty GD. 'Psychological distress as a risk factor for death from cerebrovascular disease', *CMAJ*. 2012 Sep 18; 184(13): 1461–6. doi: 10.1503/cmaj.111719. Epub 2012 Jun 18. PMID: 22711734; PMCID: PMC3447014

Butterworth P, Rodgers B, Windsor TD. 'Financial hardship, socio-economic position and depression: Results from the PATH Through Life Survey', *Social Science and Medicine*. July 2009; 69(2): 229–237

Chipman P, Jorm AF, Prior M, Sanson A, Smart D, Tan X, Easteal S. 'No interaction between the serotonin transporter polymorphism (5_HTTLPR) and childhood adversity or recent stressful life events on symptoms of anxiety, depression: Results from two community surveys',

American Journal of Medical Genetics Part B (Neuropsychiatric Genetics). 2007; 144B: 561–565

Jorm AF, Windsor TD, Dear KBG, Anstey KJ, Christensen H, Rodgers B. 'Age group differences in psychological distress: the role of psychosocial risk factors that very with age', *Psychological Medicine.* 2005; 35: 1253–1263

Batterham PJ, Christensen H, Mackinnon AJ. 'Modifiable risk factors predicting major depressive disorder at four year follow-up: a decision tree approach', *BMC Psychiatry.* 2009; 9: 75. https://doi.org/10.1186/1471-244X-9-75

Coleman JRI, Gaspar HA, Bryois J; Bipolar Disorder Working Group of the Psychiatric Genomics Consortium; Major Depressive Disorder Working Group of the Psychiatric Genomics Consortium; Breen G. 'The Genetics of the Mood Disorder Spectrum: Genome-wide Association Analyses of More Than 185,000 Cases and 439,000 Controls', *Biol Psychiatry.* 2020 Jul 15; 88(2): 169–184. doi: 10.1016/j.biopsych.2019.10.015. Epub 2019 Nov 1. PMID: 31926635

https://nswmentalhealthcommission.com.au/indicator-2-psychological-distress

McLachlan KJJ, Gale CR. 'The effects of psychological distress and its interaction with socioeconomic position on risk of developing four chronic diseases', *J Psychosom Res.* 2018 Jun; 109: 79–85. doi: 10.1016/j.jpsychores.2018.04.004. Epub 2018 Apr 14. PMID: 29680578; PMCID: PMC5959313

Hankins, M. 'The reliability of the twelve-item general health questionnaire (GHQ-12) under realistic assumptions', *BMC Public Health.* 2008; 8: 355. https://doi.org/10.1186/1471-2458-8-355

Anjara SG, Bonetto C, Van Bortel T, et al. 'Using the GHQ-12 to screen for mental health problems among primary care patients: psychometrics and practical considerations', *Int J Ment Health Syst.* 2020; 14: 62. https://doi.org/10.1186/s13033-020-00397-0

Andrews G, Slade T. 'Interpreting scores on the Kessler Psychological Distress Scale (K10)', *Aust NZ J Public Health.* 2001 Dec; 25(6): 494–7. doi: 10.1111/j.1467-842x.2001.tb00310.x. PMID: 11824981

https://patient.info/doctor/patient-health-questionnaire-phq-9

Spitzer RL, Kroenke K, Williams JB, et al. 'A brief measure for assessing generalized anxiety disorder: the GAD-7', *Arch Intern Med.* 2006 May 22; 166(10): 1092–7

Green JG, McLaughlin KA, Berglund PA, Gruber MJ, Sampson NA, Zaslavsky AM, et al. 'Childhood adversities and adult psychiatric disorders in the national comorbidity survey replication I: associations with first onset of DSM-IV disorders', *Arch Gen Psychiatry.* 2010; 67: 113–123 [PubMed: 20124111]

Nanni V, Uher R, Danese A. 'Childhood maltreatment predicts unfavorable course of illness and treatment outcome in depression: a meta-analysis', *Am J Psychiatry.* 2012; 169: 141–151 [PubMed: 22420036] 5

Kessler RC. 'The effects of stressful life events on depression', *Annu Rev Psychol.* 1997; 48: 191–214 [PubMed: 9046559]

McLaughlin KA, Conron KJ, Koenen KC, Gilman SE. 'Childhood adversity, adult stressful life events, and risk of past-year psychiatric disorder: a test of the stress sensitization hypothesis in a population-based sample of adults', *Psychol Med.* 2010; 40: 1647–1658 [PubMed: 20018126]

Aiming for wellbeing

Sachdev PS, Parslow RA, Lux O, Salonikas C, Wen W, Naidoo D, Christensen H, Jorm AF. 'Relationship of homocysteine, folic acid and vitamin B12 with depression in a middle-aged community sample', *Psychological Medicine.* 2005; 35: 529–538

Reynolds EH. 'Folic acid, ageing, depression, and dementia', *BMJ.* 2002 Jun 22; 324(7352): 1512–5. doi: 10.1136/bmj.324.7352.1512. PMID: 12077044; PMCID: PMC1123448

McManus S, Bebbington P, Jenkins R, Brugha T. 'Mental Health and Wellbeing in England: Adult Psychiatric Morbidity Survey 2014: a Survey Carried Out for NHS Digital by NatCen Social Research and the Department of Health Sciences, University of Leicester', *NHS Digital.* 2016

Bender A, Hagan KE, Kingston N. 'The association of folate and depression: A meta-analysis', *J Psychiatr Res.* 2017 Dec; 95: 9–18. doi: 10.1016/j.jpsychires.2017.07.019. Epub 2017 Jul 22. PMID: 28759846

Khosravi M, Sotoudeh G, Amini M, et al. 'The relationship between dietary patterns and depression mediated by serum levels of Folate and vitamin B12', *BMC Psychiatry.* 2020; 20: 63. https://doi.org/10.1186/s12888-020-2455-2

Cockayne NL, Duffy SL, Bonomally R, et al. 'The Beyond Ageing Project Phase 2 – a double-blind, selective prevention, randomised, placebo-controlled trial of omega-3 fatty acids and sertraline in an older age cohort at risk for depression: study protocol for a randomized controlled trial', *Trials*. 2015; 16: 247. https://doi.org/10.1186/s13063-015-0762-6

Sachdev PS, Parslow RA, Lux O, Salonikas C, Wen W, Naidoo D, Christensen H, Jorm AF. 'Relationship of homocysteine, folic acid and vitamin B12 with depression in a middle-aged community sample', *Psychological Medicine*. 2005; 35: 529–538

Sleep-iety/How much sleep should you be getting?

Refinetti R. 'Chronotype Variability and Patterns of Light Exposure of a Large Cohort of United States Residents', *Yale J Biol Med*. 2019 Jun 27; 92(2): 179–186. PMID: 31249478; PMCID: PMC6585522

Facer-Childs ER, Boiling S, Balanos GM. 'The effects of time of day and chronotype on cognitive and physical performance in healthy volunteers', *Sports Med Open*. 2018 Oct 24; 4(1): 47. doi: 10.1186/s40798-018-0162-z. PMID: 30357501; PMCID: PMC6200828

Mazri FH, Manaf ZA, Shahar S, Mat Ludin AF. 'The Association between Chronotype and Dietary Pattern among Adults: A Scoping Review', *Int J Environ Res Public Health*. 2019 Dec 20; 17(1): 68. doi: 10.3390/ijerph17010068. PMID: 31861810; PMCID: PMC6981497

Kalmbach DA, Schneider LD, Cheung J, Bertrand SJ, Kariharan T, Pack AI, Gehrman PR. 'Genetic Basis of Chronotype in Humans: Insights From Three Landmark GWAS', *Sleep*. 2017 Feb 1; 40(2): zsw048. doi: 10.1093/sleep/zsw048. PMID: 28364486; PMCID: PMC6084759

Mongrain V, Carrier J, Dumont M. 'Chronotype and sex effects on sleep architecture and quantitative sleep EEG in healthy young adults', *Sleep*. 2005 Jul; 28(7): 819–27. doi: 10.1093/sleep/28.7.819. PMID: 16124660

Age matters too

Chaput JP, Dutil C, Sampasa-Kanyinga H. 'Sleeping hours: what is the ideal number and how does age impact this?', *Nat Sci Sleep*. 2018 Nov 27; 10: 421–430. doi: 10.2147/NSS.S163071. PMID: 30568521; PMCID: PMC6267703

Okely AD, et al. 'A collaborative approach to adopting/adapting guidelines – The Australian 24-Hour Movement Guidelines for the early years (Birth to 5 years): an integration of physical activity, sedentary behavior, and sleep', *BMC Public Health*. 2017 Nov 20; 17(Suppl 5): 869. doi: 10.1186/s12889-017-4867-6. PMID: 29219094; PMCID: PMC5773882

Sleep deprivation

Chen JC, Espeland MA, Brunner RL, Lovato LC, Wallace RB, Leng X, Phillips LS, Robinson JG, Kotchen JM, Johnson KC, Manson JE, Stefanick ML, Sarto GE, Mysiw WJ. 'Sleep duration, cognitive decline, and dementia risk in older women', *Alzheimers Dement*. 2016 Jan; 12(1): 21–33. doi: 10.1016/j.jalz.2015.03.004. Epub 2015 Jun 15. PMID: 26086180; PMCID: PMC4679723

de Almondes KM, Costa MV, Malloy-Diniz LF, Diniz BS. 'Insomnia and risk of dementia in older adults: Systematic review and meta-analysis', *J Psychiatr Res*. 2016 Jun; 77: 109–15. doi: 10.1016/j.jpsychires.2016.02.021. Epub 2016 Mar 8. PMID: 27017287

Sprecher KE, Bendlin BB, Racine AM, Okonkwo OC, Christian BT, Koscik RL, Sager MA, Asthana S, Johnson SC, Benca RM. 'Amyloid burden is associated with self-reported sleep in nondemented late middle-aged adults', *Neurobiol Aging*. 2015 Sep; 36(9): 2568–76. doi: 10.1016/j.neurobiolaging.2015.05.004. Epub 2015 May 14. PMID: 26059712; PMCID: PMC4523445

Ju YS, Ooms SJ, Sutphen C, Macauley SL, Zangrilli MA, Jerome G, Fagan AM, Mignot E, Zempel JM, Claassen JAHR, Holtzman DM. 'Slow wave sleep disruption increases cerebrospinal fluid amyloid-β levels', *Brain*. 2017 Aug 1; 140(8): 2104–2111. doi: 10.1093/brain/awx148. PMID: 28899014; PMCID: PMC5790144

Lucey BP, McCullough A, Landsness EC, Toedebusch CD, McLeland JS, Zaza AM, Fagan AM, McCue L, Xiong C, Morris JC, Benzinger TLS, Holtzman DM. 'Reduced non-rapid eye movement sleep is associated with tau pathology in early Alzheimer's disease', *Sci Transl Med*. 2019 Jan 9; 11(474): eaau6550. doi: 10.1126/scitranslmed.aau6550. Erratum in: *Sci Transl Med*. 2020 Jan 8; 12(525): PMID: 30626715; PMCID: PMC6342564

Worley SL. 'The Extraordinary Importance of Sleep: The Detrimental Effects of Inadequate Sleep on Health and Public Safety Drive an Explosion of Sleep Research', *P T*. 2018 Dec; 43(12): 758–763. PMID: 30559589; PMCID: PMC6281147

https://www.abc.net.au/radionational/programs/healthreport/cognitive-behavioural-therapy-for-insomnia-sleep/11427238

Goldstein-Piekarski AN, Greer SM, Saletin JM, Harvey AG, Williams LM, Walker MP. 'Sex, Sleep Deprivation, and the Anxious Brain', *J Cogn Neurosci*. 2018 Apr; 30(4): 565–578. doi: 10.1162/jocn_a_01225. Epub 2017 Dec 15. PMID: 29244642; PMCID: PMC6143348

Oh CM, Kim HY, Na HK, Cho KH, Chu MK. 'The Effect of Anxiety and Depression on Sleep Quality of Individuals With High Risk for Insomnia: A Population-Based Study', *Front Neurol*. 2019 Aug 13; 10: 849. doi: 10.3389/fneur.2019.00849. PMID: 31456736; PMCID: PMC6700255

Asnis GM, Thomas M, Henderson MA. 'Pharmacotherapy Treatment Options for Insomnia: A Primer for Clinicians', *Int J Mol Sci*. 2015 Dec 30; 17(1): 50. doi: 10.3390/ijms17010050. PMID: 26729104; PMCID: PMC4730295

Therapy: now probably counts more than then

Eysenck HJ. 'The effects of psychotherapy: an evaluation', *J Consult Psychol*. 1952 Oct; 16(5): 319–24. doi: 10.1037/h0063633. PMID: 13000035

Strupp HH. 'Implications of the empirically supported treatment movement for psychoanalysis', *Psychoanal. Dialogues*. 2001; 11: 605–619. doi: 10.1080/10481881109348631

https://theconversation.com/counselling-doesnt-work-in-the-long-term-86446

Bower P, Knowles S, Coventry PA, Rowland N. 'Counselling for mental health and psychosocial problems in primary care', *Cochrane Database Syst Rev*. 2011 Sep 7; 2011(9): CD001025. doi: 10.1002/14651858.CD001025.pub3. PMID: 21901675; PMCID: PMC7050339

MacPherson H, Richmond S, Bland M, Brealey S, Gabe R, et al. 'Acupuncture and Counselling for Depression in Primary Care: A Randomised Controlled Trial', *PLoS Med*. 2013; 10(9): e1001518. doi:10.1371/journal.pmed.1001518

Mindfulness – does it work?

Hofmann SG, Gómez AF. 'Mindfulness-Based Interventions for Anxiety and Depression', *Psychiatr Clin North Am*. 2017 Dec; 40(4): 739–749. doi: 10.1016/j.psc.2017.08.008. Epub 2017 Sep 18. PMID: 29080597; PMCID: PMC5679245

Gu J, Strauss C, Bond R, Cavanagh K. 'How do mindfulness-based cognitive therapy and mindfulness-based stress reduction improve mental health and wellbeing? A systematic review', *Clin Psychol Rev*. 2015; 37: 1–12. doi: 10.1016/j.cpr. 2015.01.006 [PubMed: 25689576]

Hofmann SG, Asmundson GJG. 'Acceptance and mindfulness-based therapy: New wave or old hat?', *Clin Psychol Rev*. 2008; 28(1): 1–16. doi: 10.1016/j.cpr.2007.09.003 [PubMed: 17904260]

Khoury B, Lecomte T, Fortin G, et al. 'Mindfulness-based therapy: A comprehensive meta-analysis', *Clin Psychol Rev*. 2013; 33(6): 763–771. doi: 10.1016/j.cpr.2013.05.005 [PubMed: 23796855]

Strauss C, Cavanagh K, Oliver A, Pettman D, Laks J. 'Mindfulness-based interventions for people diagnosed with a current episode of an anxiety or depressive disorder: A meta-analysis of randomised controlled trials', *PLoS ONE*. 2014; 9(4): e96110. doi: 10.1371/journal.pone.0096110 [PubMed: 24763812]

Fjorback LO, Arendt M, Ornbol E, Fink P, Walach H. 'Mindfulness-based stress reduction and mindfulness-based cognitive therapy: a systematic review of randomized controlled trials', *Acta Psychiatr Scand*. 2011; 124(2): 102–119. doi: 10.1111/j.1600-0447.2011.01704.x [PubMed: 21534932]

Schell LK, Monsef I, Wöckel A, Skoetz N. 'Mindfulness-based stress reduction for women diagnosed with breast cancer', *Cochrane Database of Systematic Reviews*. 2019; issue 3. Art. No.: CD011518. doi: 10.1002/14651858.CD011518.pub2

So what about yoga?

https://www.cochrane.org/news/cochrane-library-special-collection-yoga-improving-health-and-well-being

Yang ZY, Zhong HB, Mao C, Yuan JQ, Huang Y, Wu XY, Gao YM, Tang JL. 'Yoga for asthma', *Cochrane Database of Systematic Reviews*. 2016; issue 4. Art. No.: CD010346. doi: 10.1002/14651858.CD010346.pub2

Broderick J, Vancampfort D. 'Yoga as part of a package of care versus non-standard care for schizophrenia', *Cochrane Database of Systematic Reviews*. 2019; issue 4. Art. No.: CD012807. doi: 10.1002/14651858.CD012807.pub2

Marc I, Toureche N, Ernst E, Hodnett ED, Blanchet C, Dodin S, Njoya MM. 'Mind-body interventions during pregnancy for preventing or treating women's anxiety', *Cochrane Database of Systematic Reviews.* 2011; issue 7. Art. No.: CD007559. doi: 10.1002/14651858. CD007559.pub2

Howe TE, Rochester L, Neil F, Skelton DA, Ballinger C. 'Exercise for improving balance in older people', *Cochrane Database of Systematic Reviews.* 2011; issue 11. Art. No.: CD004963. doi: 10.1002/14651858.CD004963.pub3

Mishra SI, Scherer RW, Geigle PM, Berlanstein DR, Topaloglu O, Gotay CC, Snyder C. 'Exercise interventions on health-related quality of life for cancer survivors', *Cochrane Database of Systematic Reviews.* 2012; issue 8. Art. No.: CD007566. doi: 10.1002/14651858.CD007566.pub2

Mooventhan A, Nivethitha L. 'Evidence based effects of yoga in neurological disorders', *J Clin Neurosci.* 2017 Sep; 43: 61–67. doi: 10.1016/j.jocn.2017.05.012. Epub 2017 Jun 7. PMID: 28599839

Danhauer SC, Addington EL, Sohl SJ, Chaoul A, Cohen L. 'Review of yoga therapy during cancer treatment', *Support Care Cancer.* 2017 Apr; 25(4): 1357–1372. doi: 10.1007/s00520-016-3556-9. Epub 2017 Jan 7. PMID: 28064385; PMCID: PMC5777241

Cramer H, Lauche R, Klose P, Lange S, Langhorst J, Dobos GJ. 'Yoga for improving health-related quality of life, mental health and cancer-related symptoms in women diagnosed with breast cancer', *Cochrane Database Syst Rev.* 2017 Jan 3; 1(1): CD010802. doi: 10.1002/14651858. CD010802.pub2. PMID: 28045199; PMCID: PMC6465041

Meister K, Becker S. 'Yoga bei psychischen Störungen [Yoga for mental disorders]', *Nervenarzt.* 2018 Sep; 89(9): 994–998. German. doi: 10.1007/s00115-018-0537-x. PMID: 29858642

Gong H, Ni C, Shen X, Wu T, Jiang C. 'Yoga for prenatal depression: a systematic review and meta-analysis', *BMC Psychiatry.* 2015 Feb 5; 15: 14. doi: 10.1186/s12888-015-0393-1. PMID: 25652267; PMCID: PMC4323231

Lin PJ, Kleckner IR, Loh KP, Inglis JE, Peppone LJ, Janelsins MC, Kamen CS, Heckler CE, Culakova E, Pigeon WR, Reddy PS, Messino MJ, Gaur R, Mustian KM. 'Influence of Yoga on Cancer-Related Fatigue and on Mediational Relationships Between Changes in Sleep and Cancer-Related Fatigue: A Nationwide, Multicenter Randomized Controlled Trial of Yoga in Cancer Survivors', *Integr Cancer Ther.* 2019 Jan–Dec; 18: 1534735419855134. doi: 10.1177/1534735419855134. PMID: 31165647; PMCID: PMC6552348

And pilates?

Yamato TP, Maher CG, Saragiotto BT, Hancock MJ, Ostelo RW, Cabral CM, Menezes Costa LC, Costa LO. 'Pilates for low back pain', *Cochrane Database Syst Rev.* 2015 Jul 2; (7): CD010265. doi: 10.1002/14651858.CD010265.pub2. PMID: 26133923

Fernández-Rodríguez R, Álvarez-Bueno C, Ferri-Morales A, Torres-Costoso AI, Cavero-Redondo I, Martínez-Vizcaíno V. 'Pilates Method Improves Cardiorespiratory Fitness: A Systematic Review and Meta-Analysis', *J Clin Med.* 2019 Oct 23; 8(11): 1761. doi: 10.3390/jcm8111761. PMID: 31652806; PMCID: PMC6912807

Dias NT, Ferreira LR, Fernandes MG, Resende APM, Pereira-Baldon VS. 'A Pilates exercise program with pelvic floor muscle contraction: Is it effective for pregnant women? A randomized controlled trial', *Neurourol Urodyn.* 2018 Jan; 37(1): 379–384. doi: 10.1002/nau.23308. Epub 2017 May 23. PMID: 28543751

Chmielewska D, Stania M, Kucab-Klich K, Błaszczak E, Kwaśna K, Smykla A, Hudziak D, Dolibog P. 'Electromyographic characteristics of pelvic floor muscles in women with stress urinary incontinence following sEMG-assisted biofeedback training and Pilates exercises', *PLoS One.* 2019 Dec 2; 14(12): e0225647. doi: 10.1371/journal.pone.0225647. PMID: 31790463; PMCID: PMC6886793

Roller M, Kachingwe A, Beling J, Ickes DM, Cabot A, Shrier G. 'Pilates Reformer exercises for fall risk reduction in older adults: A randomized controlled trial', *J Bodyw Mov Ther.* 2018 Oct; 22(4): 983–998. doi: 10.1016/j.jbmt.2017.09.004. Epub 2017 Sep 9. PMID: 30368346

Part 5: Dominated by devices

Dodgen-Magee D. *Deviced! Balancing Life and Technology in a Digital World.* Rowman & Littlefield 2018

Karacic S, Oreskovic S. 'Internet Addiction Through the Phase of Adolescence: A Questionnaire Study', *JMIR Ment Health.* 2017 Apr 3; 4(2): e11. doi: 10.2196/mental.5537. PMID: 28373154; PMCID: PMC5394260

DR NORMAN SWAN

Balhara YPS, Verma K, Bhargava R. 'Screen time and screen addiction: Beyond gaming, social media and pornography – A case report', *Asian J Psychiatr.* 2018 Jun; 35: 77–78. doi: 10.1016/j.ajp.2018.05.020. Epub 2018 May 26. PMID: 29803121

Alhassan AA, Alqadhib EM, Taha NW, Alahmari RA, Salam M, Almutairi AF. 'The relationship between addiction to smartphone usage and depression among adults: a cross sectional study', *BMC Psychiatry.* 2018 May 25; 18(1): 148. doi: 10.1186/s12888-018-1745-4. PMID: 29801442; PMCID: PMC5970452

Cash H, Rae CD, Steel AH, Winkler A. 'Internet Addiction: A Brief Summary of Research and Practice', *Curr Psychiatry Rev.* 2012; 8(4): 292–298. doi: 10.2174/157340012803520513

Madhav KC, Sherchand SP, Sherchan S. 'Association between screen time and depression among US adults', *Prev Med Rep.* 2017 Aug 16; 8: 67–71. doi: 10.1016/j.pmedr.2017.08.005. PMID: 28879072; PMCID: PMC5574844

Hunt MG, Marx R, Lipson C, Young J. 'No More FOMO: Limiting Social Media Decreases Loneliness and Depression', *Journal of Social and Clinical Psychology.* Volume 37, no. 10. Published online: 5 Dec 2018. https://doi.org/10.1521/jscp.2018.37.10.751

https://www.pewresearch.org/fact-tank/2019/07/25/americans-going-online-almost-constantly/

Vizcaino M, Buman M, DesRoches C, et al. 'Reliability of a new measure to assess modern screen time in adults', *BMC Public Health.* 2019; 19: 1386. https://doi.org/10.1186/s12889-019-7745-6

Part 6: The sex thing

Sex-iety

Mason-Jones AJ, Sinclair D, Mathews C, Kagee A, Hillman A, Lombard C. 'School-based interventions for preventing HIV, sexually transmitted infections, and pregnancy in adolescents', *Cochrane Database Syst Rev.* 2016 Nov 8; 11(11): CD006417. doi: 10.1002/14651858.CD006417.pub3. PMID: 27824221; PMCID: PMC5461872

Wright PJ, Bridges AJ, Sun C, Ezzell MB, Johnson JA. 'Personal Pornography Viewing and Sexual Satisfaction: A Quadratic Analysis', *J Sex Marital Ther.* 2018 Apr 3; 44(3): 308–315. doi: 10.1080/0092623X.2017.1377131. Epub 2017 Oct 9. PMID: 28885897

Dwulit AD, Rzymski P. 'The Potential Associations of Pornography Use with Sexual Dysfunctions: An Integrative Literature Review of Observational Studies', *J Clin Med.* 2019 Jun 26; 8(7): 914. doi: 10.3390/jcm8070914. PMID: 31247949; PMCID: PMC6679165

Milas G, Wright P, Štulhofer A. 'Longitudinal Assessment of the Association Between Pornography Use and Sexual Satisfaction in Adolescence', *J Sex Res.* 2020 Jan; 57(1): 16–28. doi: 10.1080/00224499.2019.1607817. Epub 2019 May 1. PMID: 31042055

Willoughby BJ, Leonhardt ND. 'Behind Closed Doors: Individual and Joint Pornography Use Among Romantic Couples', *J Sex Res.* 2020 Jan; 57(1): 77–91. doi: 10.1080/00224499.2018.1541440. Epub 2018 Nov 28. PMID: 30485135

Landripet I, Štulhofer A. 'Is Pornography Use Associated with Sexual Difficulties and Dysfunctions among Younger Heterosexual Men?', *J Sex Med.* 2015 May; 12(5): 1136–9. doi: 10.1111/jsm.12853. Epub 2015 Mar 26. PMID: 25816904

McNabney SM, Hevesi K, Rowland DL. 'Effects of Pornography Use and Demographic Parameters on Sexual Response during Masturbation and Partnered Sex in Women', *Int J Environ Res Public Health.* 2020 Apr 30; 17(9): 3130. doi: 10.3390/ijerph17093130. PMID: 32365874; PMCID: PMC7246896

Poulsen FO, Busby DM, Galovan AM. 'Pornography use: who uses it and how it is associated with couple outcomes', *J Sex Res.* 2013; 50(1): 72–83. doi: 10.1080/00224499.2011.648027. Epub 2012 Mar 26. PMID: 22449010.

Sniewski L, Farvid P, Carter P. 'The assessment and treatment of adult heterosexual men with self-perceived problematic pornography use: A review', *Addict Behav.* 2018 Feb; 77: 217–224. doi: 10.1016/j.addbeh.2017.10.010. Epub 2017 Oct 16. PMID: 29069616

Sklenarik S, Potenza MN, Gola M, Kor A, Kraus SW, Astur RS. 'Approach bias for erotic stimuli in heterosexual male college students who use pornography', *J Behav Addict.* 2019 Jun 1; 8(2): 234–241. doi: 10.1556/2006.8.2019.31. PMID: 31257916; PMCID: PMC7044553

Gola M, Wordecha M, Sescousse G, Lew-Starowicz M, Kossowski B, Wypych M, Makeig S, Potenza MN, Marchewka A. 'Can Pornography be Addictive? An fMRI Study of Men Seeking Treatment for

Problematic Pornography Use', *Neuropsychopharmacology*. 2017 Sep; 42(10): 2021–2031. doi: 10.1038/npp.2017.78. Epub 2017 Apr 14. PMID: 28409565; PMCID: PMC5561346

Séguin LJ, Rodrigue C, Lavigne J. 'Consuming Ecstasy: Representations of Male and Female Orgasm in Mainstream Pornography', *J Sex Res*. 2018 Mar–Apr; 55(3): 348–356. doi: 10.1080/00224499.2017.1332152. Epub 2017 Jun 20. PMID: 28632461

Peter J, Valkenburg PM. 'Adolescents and Pornography: A Review of 20 Years of Research', *J Sex Res*. 2016 May–Jun; 53(4–5): 509–31. doi: 10.1080/00224499.2016.1143441. Epub 2016 Mar 30. PMID: 27105446

Mattebo M, Tydén T, Häggström-Nordin E, Nilsson KW, Larsson M. 'Pornography consumption among adolescent girls in Sweden', *Eur J Contracept Reprod Health Care*. 2016 Aug; 21(4): 295–302. doi: 10.1080/13625187.2016.1186268. Epub 2016 May 24. PMID: 27218610

Johnson JA, Ezzell MB, Bridges AJ, Sun CF. 'Pornography and Heterosexual Women's Intimate Experiences with a Partner', *J Womens Health (Larchmt)*. 2019 Sep; 28(9): 1254–1265. doi: 10.1089/jwh.2018.7006. Epub 2019 Apr 18. PMID: 30998084

Sun C, Bridges A, Johnson JA, Ezzell MB. 'Pornography and the Male Sexual Script: An Analysis of Consumption and Sexual Relations', *Arch Sex Behav*. 2016 May; 45(4): 983–94. doi: 10.1007/s10508-014-0391-2. Epub 2014 Dec 3. Erratum in: *Arch Sex Behav*. 2016 May; 45(4): 995. PMID: 25466233

Identity and sex: is this right? … Is that wrong?

Mooney-Somers J, Deacon R, Anderst A, Philios L, Keeffe S, Price K, Parkhill N, Akbany A, Rybak L. 'Women in contact with the Sydney LGBTIQ communities: Report of the SWASH Lesbian, Bisexual and Queer Women's Health Survey 2016, 2018, 2020'. 2020

Deacon RM, Mooney-Somers J. 'Smoking prevalence among lesbian, bisexual and queer women in Sydney remains high: Analysis of trends and correlates', *Drug and Alcohol Review*. July 2017; 36: 546–554. doi: 10.1111/dar.12477

Douglas C, Deacon R, Mooney-Somers J. 'Pap smear rates among Australian community-attached lesbian and bisexual women: some good news but disparities persist', *Sexual Health*. 2015; 12: 249–256. http://dx.doi.org/10.1071/SH14210

Hill AO, Bourne A, McNair R, Carman M, Lyons A. 'Private Lives 3: The health and wellbeing of LGBTIQ people in Australia', *ARCSHS Monograph Series No. 122*. Melbourne, Australia: Australian Research Centre in Sex, Health and Society, La Trobe University. 2020

National LGBTI Health Alliance. 'Snapshot of mental health and suicide prevention statistics for LGBTI people'. February 2020

Darlington Statement: https://darlington.org.au/statement/

TransHub: https://www.transhub.org.au/101/trans-lgbt

Bourne A, Hammond G, Hickson F, Reid D, Schmidt AJ, Weatherburn P; EMIS Network. 'What constitutes the best sex life for gay and bisexual men? Implications for HIV prevention', *BMC Public Health*. 2013 Nov 20; 13: 1083. doi: 10.1186/1471-2458-13-1083. PMID: 24256555; PMCID: PMC4225579

https://www.ashr.edu.au/wp-content/uploads/2015/06/sex_in_australia_2_summary_data.pdf

Philpot S, Prestage G, Holt M, et al. 'Gay and Bisexual Men's Perceptions of Pre-exposure Prophylaxis (PrEP) in a Context of High Accessibility: An Australian Qualitative Study', *AIDS Behav*. 2020; 24: 2369–2380. https://doi.org/10.1007/s10461-020-02796-3

https://www.mentalhealth.org.uk/statistics/mental-health-statistics-lgbtiq-people

Staying safe and fertile

https://www.tht.org.uk/news/rise-stis-underlines-need-urgent-action

Make pleasure a principle

Beasley C. 'The challenge of pleasure: Re-imagining sexuality and sexual health', *Health Sociology Review*. 2008; 17(2): 151–163. doi: 10.5172/hesr.451.17.2.151

Hirst J. '"It's got to be about enjoying yourself": young people, sexual pleasure, and sex and relationships education', *Sex Education*. 2013; 13(4): 423–436. doi: 10.1080/14681811.2012.747433

Philpott A, Knerr W, Boydell V. 'Pleasure and prevention: When good sex is safer sex', *Reproductive Health Matters*. 2006: 14(28): 23–31

Ingham R. '"We didn't cover that at school": Education against pleasure or education for pleasure?', *Sex Education*. 2005; 5(4): 375–88

Carmody M. 'Ethical erotics: Reconceptualising anti-rape education', *Sexualities*. 2005; 8(4): 465–80

Staying safe and fertile

https://www.cdc.gov/std/chlamydia/stdfact-chlamydia-detailed.htm

https://www.aihw.gov.au/reports/men-women/male-health/contents/how-healthy/sexual-health

Is it love? Is intimacy love? And the limerence thing

Goldenberg T, Stephenson R, Bauermeister J. 'Cognitive and Emotional Factors Associated with Sexual Risk-Taking Behaviors Among Young Men Who Have Sex with Men', *Arch Sex Behav*. 2019 May; 48(4): 1127–1136. doi: 10.1007/s10508-018-1310-8. Epub 2019 Jan 3. PMID: 30607713; PMCID: PMC6872980

Weinrich JD. 'The periodic table model of the gender transpositions: Part II. Limerent and lusty sexual attractions and the nature of bisexuality', *J Sex Res*. 1988 Jan; 24(1): 113–29. doi: 10.1080/00224498809551402. PMID: 22375639

Bauermeister JA. 'Sexual Partner Typologies Among Single Young Men Who Have Sex with Men', *AIDS Behav*. 2015 Jun; 19(6): 1116–28. doi: 10.1007/s10461-014-0932-7. PMID: 25358726; PMCID: PMC4417101

Are we on the same page? Negotiating the path from 'dating' to monogamy

Philpot SP, Duncan D, Ellard J, Bavinton BR, Grierson J, Prestage G. 'Negotiating gay men's relationships: how are monogamy and non-monogamy experienced and practised over time?', *Culture, Health & Sexuality*. 2018: 20(8): 915–928. doi: 10.1080/13691058.2017.1392614

Bavinton BR, Duncan D, Grierson J, et al. 'The Meaning of "Regular Partner" in HIV Research Among Gay and Bisexual Men: Implications of an Australian Cross-Sectional Survey', *AIDS Behav*. 2016; 20: 1777–1784. https://doi.org/10.1007/s10461-016-1354-5

Worth H, Reid A, McMillan K. 'Somewhere over the rainbow: love, trust and monogamy in gay relationships', *Journal of Sociology*. 2002; 38(3): 237–253. doi: 10.1177/144078302128756642

Duncan D, Prestage G, Grierson J. 'Trust, Commitment, Love and Sex: HIV, Monogamy, and Gay Men', *Journal of Sex & Marital Therapy*. 2014; 41. doi: 10.1080/0092623X.2014.915902.

Duncombe J, Harrison K, Allan G, Marsden D. 'The State of Affairs: Explorations in Infidelity and Commitment Psychology Press', 8 Apr 2014

Joye Swan D, Thompson SC. 'Monogamy, the Protective Fallacy: Sexual versus Emotional Exclusivity and the Implication for Sexual Health Risk', *The Journal of Sex Research*. 2016; 53(1): 64–73. doi: 10.1080/00224499.2014.1003771

Insta sex: beware the algorithm

Baker N, Ferszt G, Breines JG. 'A Qualitative Study Exploring Female College Students' Instagram Use and Body Image', *Cyberpsychol Behav Soc Netw*. 2019 Apr; 22(4) :277–282. doi: 10.1089/cyber.2018.0420. Epub 2019 Mar 11. PMID: 30855190

Turner PG, Lefevre CE. 'Instagram use is linked to increased symptoms of orthorexia nervosa', *Eat Weight Disord*. 2017 Jun; 22(2): 277–284. doi: 10.1007/s40519-017-0364-2. Epub 2017 Mar 1. PMID: 28251592; PMCID: PMC5440477

Gültzow T, Guidry JPD, Schneider F, Hoving C. 'Male Body Image Portrayals on Instagram', *Cyberpsychol Behav Soc Netw*. 2020 May; 23(5): 281–289. doi: 10.1089/cyber.2019.0368. Epub 2020 Apr 15. PMID: 32286866

Griffiths S, Murray SB, Krug I, McLean SA. 'The Contribution of Social Media to Body Dissatisfaction, Eating Disorder Symptoms, and Anabolic Steroid Use Among Sexual Minority Men', *Cyberpsychol Behav Soc Netw*. 2018 Mar; 21(3): 149–156. doi: 10.1089/cyber.2017.0375. Epub 2018 Jan 24. PMID: 29363993; PMCID: PMC5865626

Tiggemann M, Hayden S, Brown Z, Veldhuis J. 'The effect of Instagram "likes" on women's social comparison and body dissatisfaction', *Body Image*. 2018 Sep; 26: 90–97. doi: 10.1016/j.bodyim.2018.07.002. Epub 2018 Jul 21. PMID: 30036748

Prichard I, Kavanagh E, Mulgrew KE, Lim MSC, Tiggemann M. 'The effect of Instagram #fitspiration images on young women's mood, body image, and exercise behaviour', *Body Image*. 2020 Jun; 33: 1–6. doi: 10.1016/j.bodyim.2020.02.002. Epub 2020 Feb 13. PMID: 32062021

Is porn addiction a thing?
Willis M, Canan SN, Jozkowski KN, Bridges AJ. 'Sexual Consent Communication in Best-Selling Pornography Films: A Content Analysis', *The Journal of Sex Research*. 2020; 57(1): 52–63. doi: 10.1080/00224499.2019.1655522

Rissel C, Richters J, de Visser RO, McKee A, Yeung A, Caruana T. 'A Profile of Pornography Users in Australia: Findings From the Second Australian Study of Health and Relationships', *J Sex Res*. 2017 Feb; 54(2): 227–240. doi: 10.1080/00224499.2016.1191597. Epub 2016 Jul 15. PMID: 27419739

Lim MSC, Agius PA, Carrotte ER, Vella AM, Hellard ME. 'Young Australians' use of pornography and associations with sexual risk behaviours', *Aust NZ J Public Health*. 2017; online. doi: 10.1111/1753-6405.12678

Is sex addiction a thing?
Reid RC, Kafka MP. 'Controversies about hypersexual disorder and the DSM-5', *Current Sexual Health Reports*. 2014; 6: 259–64

Asiff M, Sidi H, Masiran R, Kumar J, Das S, Hatta NH, Alfonso C. 'Hypersexuality as a Neuropsychiatric Disorder: The Neurobiology and Treatment Options', *Curr Drug Targets*. 2018; 19(12): 1391–1401. doi: 10.2174/1389450118666170321144931. PMID: 28325146

Walton MT, Cantor JM, Bhullar N, Lykins AD. 'Hypersexuality: A Critical Review and Introduction to the "Sexhavior Cycle"', *Arch Sex Behav*. 2017 Nov; 46(8): 2231–2251. doi: 10.1007/s10508-017-0991-8. Epub 2017 Jul 7. PMID: 28687897

For men – cis and trans
O'Connell HE, Haller B, Hoe V. 'Moving from critical clitoridectomy', *Aust NZ J Obstet Gynaecol*. 2020; 60: 637–639. https://doi.org/10.1111/ajo.13243

Hoag N, Keast JR, O'Connell HE. 'The "G-Spot" Is Not a Structure Evident on Macroscopic Anatomic Dissection of the Vaginal Wall', *J Sex Med*. 2017 Dec; 14(12): 1524–1532. doi: 10.1016/j.jsxm.2017.10.071. PMID: 29198508

Pan S, Leung C, Shah J, Kilchevsky A. 'Clinical anatomy of the G-spot', *Clin Anat*. 2015 Apr; 28(3): 363–7. doi: 10.1002/ca.22523. Epub 2015 Mar 4. PMID: 25740385

O'Connell HE, Eizenberg N, Rahman M, Cleeve J. 'The anatomy of the distal vagina: Towards unity', *J Sex Med*. 2008; 5: 1883–1891

O'Connell HE, Sanjeevan KV, Hutson JM. 'Anatomy of the clitoris', *J Urol*. 2005 Oct; 174(4 Pt 1): 1189–95. doi: 10.1097/01.ju.0000173639.38898.cd. PMID: 16145367

O'Connell HE, DeLancey JO. 'Clitoral anatomy in nulliparous, healthy, premenopausal volunteers using unenhanced magnetic resonance imaging', *J Urol*. 2005 Jun; 173(6): 2060–3. doi: 10.1097/01.ju.0000158446.21396.c0. PMID: 15879834; PMCID: PMC1283096

Wallen K, Lloyd EA. 'Female sexual arousal: genital anatomy and orgasm in intercourse', *Horm Behav*. 2011 May; 59(5): 780–92. doi: 10.1016/j.yhbeh.2010.12.004. Epub 2010 Dec 30. PMID: 21195073; PMCID: PMC3894744

Shirazi T, Renfro KJ, Lloyd E, Wallen K. 'Women's Experience of Orgasm During Intercourse: Question Semantics Affect Women's Reports and Men's Estimates of Orgasm Occurrence', *Arch Sex Behav*. 2018 Apr; 47(3): 605–613. doi: 10.1007/s10508-017-1102-6. Epub 2017 Oct 27. Erratum in: *Arch Sex Behav*. 2017 Nov 10. PMID: 29079939

Shaeer O, Skakke D, Giraldi A, Shaeer E, Shaeer K. 'Female Orgasm and Overall Sexual Function and Habits: A Descriptive Study of a Cohort of U.S. Women', *J Sex Med*. 2020 Jun; 17(6): 1133–1143. doi: 10.1016/j.jsxm.2020.01.029. Epub 2020 Mar 20. PMID: 32201145

Siegler AJ, Boos E, Rosenberg ES, Cecil MP, Sullivan PS. 'Validation of an Event-Level, Male Sexual Pleasure Scale (EMSEXpleasure) Among Condom-Using Men in the U.S.', *Arch Sex Behav*. 2018 Aug; 47(6): 1745–1754. doi: 10.1007/s10508-017-1103-5. Epub 2018 Feb 1. PMID: 29392486; PMCID: PMC6035083

Valenti LM, Suchil C, Beltran G, Rogers RC, Massey EA, Astorino TA. 'Effect of Sexual Intercourse on Lower Extremity Muscle Force in Strength-Trained Men', *J Sex Med*. 2018 Jun; 15(6): 888–893. doi: 10.1016/j.jsxm.2018.04.636. Epub 2018 May 9. PMID: 29753800

Nelson KM, Leickly E, Yang JP, Pereira A, Simoni JM. 'The influence of sexually explicit online media on sex: do men who have sex with men believe they "do what they see"?', *AIDS Care*. 2014; 26(7): 931–4. doi: 10.1080/09540121.2013.871219. Epub 2014 Jan 2. PMID: 24382316; PMCID:

PMC3989406

Brennan J. 'Size Matters: Penis Size and Sexual Position in Gay Porn Profiles', *J Homosex*. 2018; 65(7): 912–933. doi: 10.1080/00918369.2017.1364568. Epub 2017 Sep 5. PMID: 28820665

Chou NH, Huang YJ, Jiann BP. 'The Impact of Illicit Use of Amphetamine on Male Sexual Functions', *J Sex Med*. 2015 Aug; 12(8): 1694–702. doi: 10.1111/jsm.12926. Epub 2015 Jul 6. PMID: 26147855

Harte CB, Meston CM. 'Recreational use of erectile dysfunction medications and its adverse effects on erectile function in young healthy men: the mediating role of confidence in erectile ability', *J Sex Med*. 2012 Jul; 9(7): 1852–9. doi: 10.1111/j.1743-6109.2012.02755.x. Epub 2012 May 8. PMID: 22568639

Hammoud MA, Jin F, Lea T, Maher L, Grierson J, Prestage G. 'Off-Label Use of Phosphodiesterase Type 5 Inhibitor Erectile Dysfunction Medication to Enhance Sex Among Gay and Bisexual Men in Australia: Results From the FLUX Study', *J Sex Med*. 2017 Jun; 14(6): 774–784. doi: 10.1016/j.jsxm.2017.04.670. PMID: 28583339

For women – cis and trans

Tuiten A, van Rooij K, Bloemers J, et al. 'Efficacy and Safety of On-Demand Use of 2 Treatments Designed for Different Etiologies of Female Sexual Interest/Arousal Disorder: 3 Randomized Clinical Trials', *J Sex Med*. 2018; 15: 201–216

Gelman F, Atrio J. 'Flibanserin for hypoactive sexual desire disorder: place in therapy', *Ther Adv Chronic Dis*. 2017; 8(1): 16–25. doi: 10.1177/ 2040622316679933

Zheng J, Islam RM, Skiba MA, Bell RJ, Davis SR. 'Associations between androgens and sexual function in premenopausal women: a cross-sectional study', *Lancet Diabetes Endocrinol*. 2020 Aug; 8(8): 693–702. doi: 10.1016/S2213-8587(20)30239-4. PMID: 32707117

Islam RM, Bell RJ, Green S, Page MJ, Davis SR. 'Safety and efficacy of testosterone for women: a systematic review and meta-analysis of randomised controlled trial data', *Lancet Diabetes Endocrinol*. 2019 Oct; 7(10): 754–766. doi: 10.1016/S2213-8587(19)30189-5. Epub 2019 Jul 25. PMID: 31353194

Fooladi E, Bell RJ, Jane F, Robinson PJ, Kulkarni J, Davis SR. 'Testosterone improves antidepressant-emergent loss of libido in women: findings from a randomized, double-blind, placebo-controlled trial', *J Sex Med*. 2014 Mar; 11(3): 831–9. doi: 10.1111/jsm.12426. Epub 2014 Jan 16. PMID: 24433574

Davis S, Papalia MA, Norman RJ, O'Neill S, Redelman M, Williamson M, Stuckey BG, Wlodarczyk J, Gard'ner K, Humberstone A. 'Safety and efficacy of a testosterone metered-dose transdermal spray for treating decreased sexual satisfaction in premenopausal women: a randomized trial', *Ann Intern Med*. 2008 Apr 15; 148(8): 569–77. doi: 10.7326/0003-4819-148-8-200804150-00001. PMID: 18413618

Reed BG, Nemer LB, Carr BR. 'Has testosterone passed the test in premenopausal women with low libido? A systematic review', *International Journal of Women's Health*. 2016; 8: 599–607

Leddy LS, Yang CC, Stuckey BG, Sudworth M, Haughie S, Sultana S, Maravilla KR. 'Influence of sildenafil on genital engorgement in women with female sexual arousal disorder', *J Sex Med*. 2012 Oct; 9(10): 2693–7. doi: 10.1111/j.1743-6109.2012.02796.x. Epub 2012 May 23. PMID: 22620487

Joffe HV, Chang C, Sewell C, Easley O, Nguyen C, Dunn S, Lehrfeld K, Lee L, Kim MJ, Slagle AF, Beitz J. 'FDA Approval of Flibanserin – Treating Hypoactive Sexual Desire Disorder', *N Engl J Med*. 2016 Jan 14; 374(2): 101–4. doi: 10.1056/NEJMp1513686. Epub 2015 Dec 9. PMID: 26649985

Tuiten A, Michiels F, Böcker KB, Höhle D, van Honk J, de Lange RP, van Rooij K, Kessels R, Bloemers J, Gerritsen J, Janssen P, de Leede L, Meyer JJ, Everaerd W, Frijlink HW, Koppeschaar HP, Olivier B, Pfaus JG. 'Genotype scores predict drug efficacy in subtypes of female sexual interest/arousal disorder: A double-blind, randomized, placebo-controlled cross-over trial', *Women's Health (Lond)*. 2018 Jan–Dec; 14: 1745506518788970. doi: 10.1177/1745506518788970. PMID: 30016917; PMCID: PMC6052493

Croft HA. 'Understanding the Role of Serotonin in Female Hypoactive Sexual Desire Disorder and Treatment Options', *J Sex Med*. 2017; 14: 1575–1584

Kleinplatz PJ, Charest M, Paradis N, et al. 'Treatment of Low Sexual Desire or Frequency Using a Sexual Enhancement Group Couples Therapy Approach', *J Sex Med*. 2020; 17: 1288–1296

Hogue JV, Rosen NO, Bockaj A, Impett EA, Muise A. 'Sexual communal motivation in couples coping with low sexual interest/arousal: Associations with sexual well-being and sexual goals', *PLoS One*. 2019 Jul 17; 14(7): e0219768. doi: 10.1371/journal.pone.0219768. PMID: 31314799; PMCID: PMC6636740

Field N, Mercer CH, Sonnenberg P, Tanton C, Clifton S, Mitchell KR, Erens B, Macdowall W, Wu F, Datta J, Jones KG, Stevens A, Prah P, Copas AJ, Phelps A, Wellings K, Johnson AM. 'Associations between health and sexual lifestyles in Britain: findings from the third National Survey of Sexual Attitudes and Lifestyles (Natsal-3)', *Lancet*. 2013 Nov 30; 382(9907): 1830–44. doi: 10.1016/S0140-6736(13)62222-9. Epub 2013 Nov 26. PMID: 24286788; PMCID: PMC3898988

Kong L, Li T, Li L. 'The impact of sexual intercourse during pregnancy on obstetric and neonatal outcomes: a cohort study in China', *J Obstet Gynaecol*. 2019 May; 39(4): 455–460. doi: 10.1080/01443615.2018.1533930. Epub 2019 Feb 16. PMID: 30773958

Hannaford PC, Selvaraj S, Elliott AM, Angus V, Iversen L, Lee AJ. 'Cancer risk among users of oral contraceptives: cohort data from the Royal College of Practitioner's oral contraception study', *BMJ*. Cited 12 Sept 2007; online. doi: 10.1136/bmj.39289.649410.55

Hannaford PC, Iverson L, Macfarlane TV, Elliott AM, Angus V, Lee AJ. 'Mortality among contraceptive pill users: cohort evidence from Royal College of General Practitioners' Oral Contraception Study', *BMJ*. 2010; 340: c927

Hall KS, Kusunoki Y, Gatny H, Barber J. 'Stress symptoms and frequency of sexual intercourse among young women', *J Sex Med*. 2014 Aug; 11(8): 1982–90. doi: 10.1111/jsm.12607. Epub 2014 Jun 3. PMID: 24894425; PMCID: PMC4115031

DiCenso A, Guyatt G, Willan A, Griffith L. 'Interventions to reduce unintended pregnancies among adolescents: systematic review of randomised controlled trials', *BMJ*. 2002 Jun 15; 324(7351): 1426. doi: 10.1136/bmj.324.7351.1426. PMID: 12065267; PMCID: PMC115855

Reissing ED, Andruff HL, Wentland JJ. 'Looking back: the experience of first sexual intercourse and current sexual adjustment in young heterosexual adults', *J Sex Res*. 2012; 49(1): 27–35. doi: 10.1080/00224499.2010.538951. Epub 2011 May 24. PMID: 21161815

Kalaaji A, Dreyer S, Maric I, Schnegg J, Jönsson V. 'Female Cosmetic Genital Surgery: Patient Characteristics, Motivation, and Satisfaction', *Aesthet Surg J*. 2019 Nov 13; 39(12): 1455–1466. doi: 10.1093/asj/sjy309. PMID: 30423019

Kalaaji A, Dreyer S, Brinkmann J, Maric I, Nordahl C, Olafsen K. 'Quality of Life After Breast Enlargement With Implants Versus Augmentation Mastopexy: A Comparative Study', *Aesthet Surg J*. 2018 Nov 12; 38(12): 1304–1315. doi: 10.1093/asj/sjy047. PMID: 29481590

Clerico C, Lari A, Mojallal A, Boucher F. 'Anatomy and Aesthetics of the Labia Minora: The Ideal Vulva?', *Aesthetic Plast Surg*. 2017 Jun; 41(3): 714–719. doi: 10.1007/s00266-017-0831-1. Epub 2017 Mar 10. Erratum in: *Aesthetic Plast Surg*. 2017 Jun; 41(3): 720. PMID: 28314908

Hunter JG. 'Labia Minora, Labia Majora, and Clitoral Hood Alteration: Experience-Based Recommendations', *Aesthet Surg J*. 2016 Jan; 36(1): 71–9. doi: 10.1093/asj/sjv092. Epub 2015 Oct 24. PMID: 26499942

Hamori CA. 'Postoperative clitoral hood deformity after labiaplasty', *Aesthet Surg J*. 2013 Sep 1; 33(7): 1030–6. doi: 10.1177/1090820X13502202. Epub 2013 Sep 4. PMID: 24005612

Learner HI, Rundell C, Liao LM, Creighton SM. '"Botched labiaplasty": a content analysis of online advertising for revision labiaplasty', *J Obstet Gynaecol*. 2020 Oct; 40(7): 1000–1005. doi: 10.1080/01443615.2019.1679732. Epub 2019 Dec 12. PMID: 31826680

Zwier S. '"What Motivates Her": Motivations for Considering Labial Reduction Surgery as Recounted on Women's Online Communities and Surgeons' Websites', *Sex Med*. 2014 Apr; 2(1): 16–23. doi: 10.1002/sm2.20. PMID: 25356297; PMCID: PMC4184612

Sharp G, Tiggemann M, Mattiske J. 'A Retrospective Study of the Psychological Outcomes of Labiaplasty', *Aesthet Surg J*. 2017 Mar 1; 37(3): 324–331. doi: 10.1093/asj/sjw190. PMID: 28207030

Sex and being trans

Callander D, Wiggins J, Rosenberg S, Cornelisse VJ, Duck-Chong E, Holt M, Pony M, Vlahakis E, MacGibbon J, Cook T. 'The 2018 Australian Trans and Gender Diverse Sexual Health Survey: Report of Findings'. 2019. The Kirby Institute, UNSW Sydney: Sydney, NSW

Bungener SL, Steensma TD, Cohen-Kettenis PT, de Vries ALC. 'Sexual and Romantic Experiences of Transgender Youth Before Gender-Affirmative Treatment', *Pediatrics*. 2017 Mar; 139(3):

e20162283. doi: 10.1542/peds.2016-2283. PMID: 28242863

Bungener SL, de Vries ALC, Popma A, Steensma TD. 'Sexual Experiences of Young Transgender Persons During and After Gender-Affirmative Treatment', *Pediatrics*. 2020 Dec; 146(6): e20191411. doi: 10.1542/peds.2019-1411. PMID: 33257402

Ristori J, Cocchetti C, Castellini G, Pierdominici M, Cipriani A, Testi D, Gavazzi G, Mazzoli F, Mosconi M, Meriggiola MC, Cassioli E, Vignozzi L, Ricca V, Maggi M, Fisher AD. 'Hormonal Treatment Effect on Sexual Distress in Transgender Persons: 2-Year Follow-Up Data', *J Sex Med*. 2020 Jan; 17(1): 142–151. doi: 10.1016/j.jsxm.2019.10.008. Epub 2019 Nov 15. PMID: 31735612

Holmberg M, Arver S, Dhejne C. 'Supporting sexuality and improving sexual function in transgender persons', *Nat Rev Urol*. 2019 Feb; 16(2): 121–139. doi: 10.1038/s41585-018-0108-8. PMID: 30375495

Kerckhof ME, Kreukels BPC, Nieder TO, Becker-Hébly I, van de Grift TC, Staphorsius AS, Köhler A, Heylens G, Elaut E. 'Prevalence of Sexual Dysfunctions in Transgender Persons: Results from the ENIGI Follow-Up Study', *J Sex Med*. 2019 Dec; 16(12): 2018–2029. doi: 10.1016/j.jsxm.2019.09.003. Epub 2019 Oct 24. Erratum in: *J Sex Med*. 2020 Apr; 17(4): 830. PMID: 31668732

Defreyne J, Kreukels B, T'Sjoen G, Staphorsius A, Den Heijer M, Heylens G, Elaut E. 'No correlation between serum testosterone levels and state-level anger intensity in transgender people: Results from the European Network for the Investigation of Gender Incongruence', *Horm Behav*. 2019 Apr; 110: 29–39. doi: 10.1016/j.yhbeh.2019.02.016. Epub 2019 Mar 2. PMID: 30822410

Motta G, Crespi C, Mineccia V, Brustio PR, Manieri C, Lanfranco F. 'Does Testosterone Treatment Increase Anger Expression in a Population of Transgender Men?', *J Sex Med*. 2018 Jan; 15(1): 94–101. doi: 10.1016/j.jsxm.2017.11.004. Epub 2017 Nov 27. PMID: 29175227

Nikkelen SWC, Kreukels BPC. 'Sexual Experiences in Transgender People: The Role of Desire for Gender-Confirming Interventions, Psychological Well-Being, and Body Satisfaction', *J Sex Marital Ther*. 2018 May 19; 44(4): 370–381. doi: 10.1080/0092623X.2017.1405303. Epub 2018 Jan 31. PMID: 29144853

Bartolucci C, Gómez-Gil E, Salamero M, Esteva I, Guillamón A, Zubiaurre L, Molero F, Montejo AL. 'Sexual quality of life in gender-dysphoric adults before genital sex reassignment surgery', *J Sex Med*. 2015 Jan; 12(1): 180–8. doi: 10.1111/jsm.12758. Epub 2014 Nov 17. PMID: 25401972

Part 7: What about the kids?

Child development and tennis

Peters I et al. 'Social determinants of psychological wellness for children and adolescents in rural NSW', *BMC Public Health*. 2019; 19: 1616. https://doi.org/10.1186/s12889-019-7961-0

https://massaimh.org/wp-content/uploads/2020/02/Brazelton%E2%80%99s-Neurodevelopmental-and-Relational-Touchpoints-and-Infant-Mental-Health-Horsteing.pdf

Brazelton TB, Nugent K. *Neonatal Behavioral Assessment Scale*. 3rd edition. 1995; London, Mac Keith Press

Brazelton TB, Greenspan S. *The Irreducible Needs of Children: What Every Child Must Have to Grow, Learn, and Flourish*. 2000; Cambridge, MA, Da Capo Press

Are we wrecking our kids by letting them use screens?

Wrobel A. 'Young children's use of digital technologies: Risks and opportunities for early childhood development [CoLab Evidence Report]'. 2019. Retrieved from https://colab.telethonkids.org.au/resources/

McClure ER, Chentsova-Dutton YE, Barr RF, Holochwost SJ, Gerrod Parrott W. '"Facetime doesn't count": Video chat as an exception to media restrictions for infants and toddlers', *International Journal of Child-Computer Interaction*. 2015; volume 6, pp. 1–6. ISSN 2212-8689. https://doi.org/10.1016/j.ijcci.2016.02.002

Content is queen

International Literacy Association. 'Digital resources in early childhood literacy development [Position statement and research brief]'. Newark DE: Author. 2019

Screen guidelines for toddlers
Lerner C, Barr R. 'Screen Sense: Setting the Record Straight – Research-Based Guidelines for Screen Use for Children under 3 Years Old', *Zero to Three*. Mar 2015; volume 35, no. 4, pp. 1–10
https://www.esafety.gov.au/parents/big-issues/time-online

Adolescents
Karacic S, Oreskovic S. 'Internet addiction through the phase of adolescence: a questionnaire study' *JMIR Ment Health*. 2017 Apr–Jun; 4(2)
Shakir T et al. 'Social media and its impact on adolescents' *Pediatrics*. 2018 Jan; 141(1)

For parents of adolescents: delay is better
Dewaele A, Van Houtte M, Symons K, Buysse A. 'Exploring First Sexual Intercourse, Sexual Orientation, and Sexual Health in Men', *J Homosex*. 2017; 64(13): 1832–1849. doi: 10.1080/00918369.2016.1267467. Epub 2016 Dec 2. PMID: 27911671
Nogueira Avelar E, Silva R, Wijtzes A, van de Bongardt D, van de Looij-Jansen P, Bannink R, Raat H. 'Early Sexual Intercourse: Prospective Associations with Adolescents Physical Activity and Screen Time', *PLoS One*. 2016 Aug 11; 11(8): e0158648. doi: 10.1371/journal.pone.0158648. PMID: 27513323; PMCID: PMC4981454
Collins RL, Strasburger VC, Brown JD, Donnerstein E, Lenhart A, Ward LM. 'Sexual Media and Childhood Well-being and Health', *Pediatrics*. 2017 Nov; 140(Suppl 2): S162–S166. doi: 10.1542/peds.2016-1758X. PMID: 29093054
Collins RL, Elliott MN, Berry SH, Kanouse DE, Kunkel D, Hunter SB, Miu A. 'Watching sex on television predicts adolescent initiation of sexual behavior', *Pediatrics*. 2004 Sep; 114(3): e280–9. doi: 10.1542/peds.2003-1065-L. PMID: 15342887
Chandra A, Martino SC, Collins RL, Elliott MN, Berry SH, Kanouse DE, Miu A. 'Does watching sex on television predict teen pregnancy? Findings from a national longitudinal survey of youth', *Pediatrics*. 2008 Nov; 122(5): 1047–54. doi: 10.1542/peds.2007-3066. PMID: 18977986
Lin WH, Liu CH, Yi CC. 'Exposure to sexually explicit media in early adolescence is related to risky sexual behavior in emerging adulthood', *PLoS One*. 2020 Apr 10; 15(4): e0230242. doi: 10.1371/journal.pone.0230242. PMID: 32275669; PMCID: PMC7147756
Vasilenko SA, Kugler KC, Rice CE. 'Timing of First Sexual Intercourse and Young Adult Health Outcomes', *J Adolesc Health*. 2016 Sep; 59(3): 291–297. doi: 10.1016/j.jadohealth.2016.04.019. Epub 2016 Jun 3. PMID: 27265422; PMCID: PMC5002249

How do I prevent my child getting into drugs?
Teesson M, et al; the Health4Life Team. 'Study protocol of the Health4Life Initiative: A cluster randomised controlled trial of an eHealth school-based program targeting multiple lifestyle risk behaviours among young Australians', *BMJ Open*. 2020; 10(7)
Toumbourou JW, Hall J, Varcoe J, Leung R. 'Review of key risk and protective factors for child development and wellbeing (antenatal to age 25)', Australian Research Alliance for Children and Young People. 2014
Baker S. 'Brain development in early childhood [CoLab Evidence Report]'. 2017. Retrieved from https://colab.telethonkids.org.au/resources/
Hunter Institute of Mental Health. 'Issues paper: the importance of the early childhood years'. 2016. Retrieved from https://himh.org.au/
Afuseh E, Pike CA, Oruche UM. 'Individualized approach to primary prevention of substance use disorder: age-related risks', *Subst Abuse Treat Prev Policy*. 2020; 15: 58. https://doi.org/10.1186/s13011-020-00300-7
Mewton L, Visontay R, Chapman C, Newton N, Slade T, Kay-Lambkin F, Teesson M. 'Universal primary prevention of alcohol and drug use and related harms: An overview of reviews', Report prepared for the Australian National Advisory Council on Alcohol and Other Drugs. 2017. ISBN: 978-0-6488048-1-9
Poole JC, Kim HS, Dobson KS, Hodgins DC. 'Adverse Childhood Experiences and Disordered Gambling: Assessing the Mediating Role of Emotion Dysregulation', *J Gambl Stud*. 2017 Dec; 33(4): 1187–1200. doi: 10.1007/s10899-017-9680-8. PMID: 28258336.
Teesson M, Newton N, Slade T, Chapman C, Birrell L, Mewton L, Mather M, Hides L, McBride N,

Allsop S, Andrews G. 'Combined prevention for substance use, depression and anxiety in adolescence: A cluster randomised controlled trial of an online universal intervention', *Lancet Digital Health*. 2020; 2(2): 74–84
https://www.drinkaware.co.uk/research/research-and-evaluation-reports/consumption-underage-drinking-in-the-uk

Acknowledgements

This book didn't emerge from a flash of inspiration in the shower. It's the result of decades of broadcast journalism in health. I don't think I've ever publicly thanked the interviewing committee at the ABC who gave me my first job there. They allowed me to forge a new career outside medicine. They were: Robyn Williams. Malcolm Long, Kirsten Garrett and John Challis. Kirsten told me later when the recommendation went up the line for approval, the response was why would a doctor want to join the ABC? Is he yet another Commie, was the poorly hidden subtext. That's a question best left unanswered till the KGB's files on the ABC are eventually opened. I don't have a media degree so I learned broadcasting and journalism as an apprentice watching and being taught by Robyn, Tim Bowden (who also showed me the dark art of filling in ABC expense forms), the late Tony Barrell (one of the most creative people I've ever worked with and who, decades before Twitter, had worked out that brevity was the future), Tom Molomby and many many others.

The highly talented Eliza Harvey was my researcher but that doesn't go close to describing her contribution, which included – to put it mildly – assertive instructions and feedback to keep me on message and on track. Eliza extended the path forged by her mother, one of my closest friends and confidantes, Geraldine Doogue.

The book also wouldn't have happened without my agent, Gaby Naher of Left Bank Literary, who guided, encouraged and made it happen. Candice Bruce, a terrific writer and close friend, recommended Gaby as the best. She was right. Louise Adler was also significant in getting me off my bottom. I'm also grateful to Michael O'Connor at Williams and Connolly in Washington DC.

Thanks to the unparalleled team at Hachette who helped realise the idea and facilitated its execution: Vanessa Radnidge, Karen Ward, Susin Chow, Emma Rusher, Rosina Di Marzo and Eve Le Gall. Professional and tireless doesn't come close.

I've already credited the highly energetic Jack Mortlock, who came up with the idea when he was at Tonic, of a series of Q&A sessions which had the same title.

The whole thing about the Greek Paradox goes back many years to my early time in journalism when I met John Powles at Monash University. John was a leading thinker in social medicine and one of the pioneers of what was then called the 'new' public health, investigating the non-health – upstream – causes of health and illness. He moved on to the University of Cambridge and, sadly, died a few years ago. He loved paradoxes and exposed this one before anyone else.

Many people gave me advice and criticism and made a difference. However, they bear no responsibility for what I eventually wrote. They are, in no particular order:

Maree Teesson, Ian Hickie, Nick Kates (who's been one of my closest friends since adolescence), Catherine Itsiopoulos, Tania Thodis, Steve Philpot, Liz Scott, Catherine Boland, James Bolster, Julie Mooney-Somers, Emily Banks, Bill

Bowtell, Paul Zimmet, Dallas English, Candice Bruce, David Cameron-Smith, Adrian Bauman and Teddy Cook.

Georgia Swan read an early draft and gave her usual fearless and funny feedback. Ghada Ali, a very talented young producer at *The Drum*, did so too. I needed a reality check from the audience I was primarily targeting – and got it. Betsy Woodruff-Swan, my daughter-in-law and a formidable journalist, read it with a North American eye for the US version.

I couldn't have done this book without the patience of the people I worked with closely during the first year of COVID, which is when I wrote this: James Bullen, Tegan Taylor, Will Ockenden, Jonathan Webb, Tanya Nolan, Joel Werner and the terrific producers at *7.30*, particularly Amy Donaldson, Callum Denness, Alex McDonald, Raveen Hunjan, Clay Hichens and Executive Producer, Justin Stevens.

Katie Hamann put up with me during a tough year and also read the draft, which is always a risky thing, but Katie's skills as a producer and editor supervened.

My children are my nourishment: Jonathan, Anna and Georgia. I love them more than they'll ever know.

Index